Koro

Arabinda Narayan Chowdhury

Koro

Clinical and Historical Developments of the Culturally Defined Genital Retraction Disorder

palgrave
macmillan

Arabinda Narayan Chowdhury
Bradgate Mental Health Unit
Glenfield Hospital
Leicester, UK

Department of Psychiatry
Institute of Postgraduate Medical
Education & Research
Kolkata, India

ISBN 978-3-030-87961-7 ISBN 978-3-030-87962-4 (eBook)
https://doi.org/10.1007/978-3-030-87962-4

This Palgrave Macmillan imprint is published by the registered company Springer Nature Switzerland AG
The registered company address is: Gewerbestrasse 11, 6330 Cham, Switzerland

To
My wife Dr. Shyamali Chowdhury
My daughter Dr. Monali Chowdhury
For their generous allowance of time and deep inspiration for my research.

Kettering: March 2021

Foreword

Since George Cheyne's book *The English Malady* in 1734, medical psychologists have periodically wondered as to whether certain types of mental derangements might be attributed to distinct cultural or geographical areas. Cheyne himself suggested that the frequency of melancholia and suicide in England could be related to the national temperament, diet (alcohol and beef), and the weather (nasty).

Our modern discipline of cultural psychiatry developed out of the hospital-based medicine of the nineteenth century, from studies of institutionalized insane Europeans, but also from accounts of peculiar mental reactions in the colonized world coming from travelers, missionaries, and imperial officials. Some of the classic patterns were described to Europeans in the Victorian period—latah, koro, amok, susto, piblokto, artic hysteria, spirit possession states. Some, like amok, passed into the English vernacular. Many became memorable through their association with exotic or bizarre sexual patterns: all my fellow medical students were superficially familiar with the subject of Professor Chowdhury's monograph, the genital retrac*tion syndrome* or Koro, known to us facetiously then as the "disappearing penis syndrome." Hilarity, yes. Understanding, no.

Into the consolidation of psychiatric nosologies in the nineteenth century, these "exotic"curiosities for European asylum medicine could not be fitted easily. Emil Kraepelin, a German physician who had placed the severe psychiatric disorders (the psychoses) into two great classes—schizophrenia and manic-depression—made a journey to Java to ascertain the universality of mental illness. He found he could include such local categories as amok, koro, and latah into his Western hospital-derived schema. There the matter rested until 1951 when a Hong Kong, British trained psychiatrist, P. M. Yap proposed bundling up all the exotic non-Western patterns into the category of "culture-bound syndromes," the concept of culture now having a greater salience than race or climate thanks to the growth of social anthropology. These syndromes, specific to a particular culture area, remained marginal to the first great international studies of mental illness conducted by the World Health Organization such as the InternatIoal Pilot Study of Schizophrenia. In the 1950s. They were referenced occasionally by social anthropologists and were listed in the margins of psychiatric textbooks. Whether these patterns were distinct diseases or merely local variants of schizophrenia or manic-depression was occasionally discussed briefly.

The development of medical sociology and medical anthropology from the 1970s onward led to a general social scientific emphasis on the cultural and historical factors in these patterns, as important influences if not actual causes. Could the culture-bound syndromes be specified by culture alone or specified by both culture and biology? The anthropologists interested obviously favored the former; the cross-cultural psychiatrists involved preferred the latter, retaining some notion of biological causality. I remember that when teaching in China in 1985 we received news of the great Hainan Island Koro Epidemic which affected over three hundred people. The Chinese doctors I was teaching immediately assumed that the illness was microbiological or nutritional, my Western colleagues however noting that the course of infection closely followed the trajectory of a series of government investigations into corruption in local districts which passed around the island. An investigation into kuru in New Guinea went the other way. Kuru was a wasting illness which was assumed to be hysterical, but was later attributed to a slow virus and so disappeared from the list of culture-bound syndromes. The very category has become redundant. Some of the classic patterns have been identified as merely exaggerations of cultural preoccupations (latah), or local treatments for spirit possession (zar, tarantism), as historical legacies of violent restitution (amok) or the consequences of European imperialism (piblokto). Were they so unique? My UCL colleague Sushrut Jadhav in his ethnographic study of the experience of depression in the White London population found that anxieties about sexual performance and indeed about the retraction of the penis into the abdomen were not uncommon.

What were once, for Europeans, bizarre cultural morbidities, are now to be considered with the range of evidence characteristic of Chowdhury's excellent compendium. His synopsis of knowledge is indeed magnificent and stands besides Ron Simons' exemplary text on latah for sheer detail and analysis. It is unlikely to be bettered.

Roland Littlewood
Professor of Anthropology
and Psychiatry
University College London
London, UK

Preface

This book is a documentation of Koro as reflected in the Koro publications (mainly in English language journals) from 1895 to 2020. Year-wise documentation of reports shows the development history of Koro as a clinical concept of a culture-bound syndrome. It also depicts the diversity of its clinical presentation over the years.

The book is divided into five main parts. The *current status* of Koro is discussed in Introduction (Chapters 1 and 2). The *Historical Perspective* is discussed next with three chapters (Chapters 3, 4, and 5). The next part is the *Literature review* and is described under four chapters (Chapters 6, 7, 8, and 9). The last two chapters are devoted to risk assessment (Chapter 10) and the research methodology of Koro (Chapter 11).

The first chapter—Introduction, covers Koro's current concept and global epidemiology. The penis-image perception is clinically relevant and has a close phenomenological link with Koro perception, so a brief discussion on perceptual deviations in penis image is included in Chapter 2.

Chapter 3 covers the historical perspective of Koro's Chinese cultural linkage. It also highlighted the animal symbolism in Koro's concept and etymological link, viz., Fox and Tortoise connections in Chapter 4.

Chapter 5 describes chronologically the *development of the cultural concept* behind Koro and how gradually the cultural tag is lost after 126 years of existence.

The next section is the main body of a *critical review of published literature* on Koro (mainly in English language journals). There is an arbitrary division in presenting the Koro reports, viz. from the Western medical press and India separately. Western publications are divided into three separate chapters: Chapter 6 from 1895 up to the Singapore Koro epidemic of 1970. Chapter 7 contains the publications during the last three decades of the twentieth century, viz., from 1971 to 2000, and Chapter 8 includes the publications during the first two decades of the twenty-first century, viz., from 2001 to 2020.

In the literature review sections, some Koro cases and some epidemic demography are discussed in detail with clinical analysis. Readers can understand the varied clinical spectrum of Koro and identify what is missing in the report (marked as "Observation"). Some Koro-related issues are also discussed, like coital death, depersonalization, and the debate over culture-bound syndromes, and mass psychogenic illnesses in Africa. All these might help map an exact frame of Koro in terms of the recent development in this area. Some contemporary newspaper coverage of epidemics is included, which depicts the mass and professional response of the incidents in real time. Each entry in the chapter is separately numbered, which shows the trend of number of publications in the designated periods.

Chapter 9: India is now a Koro-prone country and experiencing at least six large epidemics. So the publications are kept separately to view the details of the epidemics and the trend of *Indian Koro research.*

Chapter 10 highlighted the *public health risk of Koro,* both epidemic and sporadic forms.

Chapter 11 provided a general guideline as the *standards for research methodology* in Koro research with a suggested conceptual model of Koro as a disease category.

It is hoped that this documentation, being distilled from this review of the last 126 years Koro reportings, will help the reader to have a concise insight about Koro illness, including its clinical features, diverse associations, cultural root and progress, the public health risk aspect and guidance for further research.

Leicester, UK

Arabinda Narayan Chowdhury

Acknowledgments

I joined my rural teaching posting as Lecturer in the Department of Psychiatry, North Bengal Medical College, Darjeeling district, West Bengal, India, in April 1982. From July, a massive Koro epidemic started in the four districts of the region. This firsthand experience with Koro offered a great opportunity, and I, with my colleagues, began to collect data on Koro illness. Gradually, we developed more insight into this psychiatric epidemic of Koro in the region. Since then, I have kept my attention to this disorder and, over the years, met many new clinical presentations and challenges relating to Koro. India is becoming a Koro-prone country, and we have had at least six large-scale Koro epidemics since 1982. My long research experience with this disorder prompted me to write this book by compiling all published research (mainly in English language journals). The researchers and psychiatrists may have a coherent insight into this peculiar psychopathology, from historical roots to the current global scenario. They may exercise perfect research methodology or explore new avenues to enrich our understanding of Koro. Despite over four hundred publications on Koro, there is no composite book available on this issue. This critical evaluation of published research helps understand Koro's varied clinical aspects and provides more insight into Koro's diagnostic precision.

I am very grateful to all the Koro patients of the region. My sincere thanks to colleagues of North Bengal Medical College, Siliguri, Jalpaiguri, and Koch Bihar District Hospitals, many local village leaders, NGO members, folk healers, and general practitioners. They helped me over the years in my research. I had the privilege to meet many great personalities in this journey who supported me and gave valuable ideas and suggestions to carry out my Koro research. The list is long, but I must mention some of them as a mark of my respect, gratitude, and sincere thanks for their help and guidance.

Late Prof. Deepali Dutta of Gauhati University, Assam, shared her Koro research experience (1983). Late Prof. Srilekha Biswas was my head at North Bengal Medical College. She helped me in all the ways possible to carry out the Koro field research in North Bengal's districts and helped me organize two symposiums.

Prof. Anthony J. Marsella of Hawaii University, whom I met in the WHO workshop on Biological Psychiatry at Lucknow, spend hours suggesting how to do research data processing (1984). I am privileged to get suggestions and reprints from several Koro researchers: Dr. A. L. Gwee and Dr. P. W. Ngui (Singapore), Dr. H. Rin (Taiwan), Dr. Beng Yeong Ng and Dr. E. E. Heok Kua (Singapore), Dr. J. W. Edwards (USA), Dr. S. Moketi (Indonesia), Dr. J. P. Hes (Israel), Dr. W. M. Luiceer (Tanzania), Dr. J. Westermeyer (USA), Dr. M. L. Ng (Hong Kong), Dr. M. H. Connors and Dr. D. Mitchell (Australia).

Late Prof. D. N. Nandi, my teacher, commented on a few of my Koro papers. Late Prof. Ajita Chakraborty, my teacher, discussed several psycho-social issues relating to the Koro epidemic in Northeast India and gave her own Koro research file for my use (1987). Late Prof. N. C. Chowdhury, Head, Department of Sociology and Social Anthropology, North Bengal University, my Anthropology teacher, helped me design many research instruments and actively taught me anthropological research methods (1984–1992).

Prof. Subir Kumar Dutta and Prof. Monoj Kumar Bhattacharya, both were Ex-Dean, Faculty of Medicine, University of Calcutta, were always supportive and inspired me in all my research activities (1987–2005).

Prof. Arther Kleinman, I met him at the Central Institute of Psychiatry, Ranchi, and he commented on my Koro presentation there (1985). Professor M. G. Weiss, Head of Epidemiology at Swiss Tropical Institute, Basel, helped me with different suggestions, provided important reprints, attended the Social Psychiatry symposium at North Bengal Medical College, and visited a few of my Koro patients at Mal Bazar, Jalpaiguri. He also invited me to present my Koro research at the Swiss Tropical Institute at Basel (1985–2006).

Dr. Alain Bottero of Salpetriere Hospital, Paris, attended the Koro Symposium at North Bengal Medical College and visited one Tea Garden to interview some local healers who treated many Koro patients during the epidemic (1986). Professor Felice Leih-Mak, Head of Psychiatry Department, Hong Kong University, commented on my Koro research when I met her at her department in Hong Kong (1992).

Prof. Roland Littlewood, Professor of Psychiatry and Anthropology, University College of London, commented on my Koro research when I met him in London in 1995. Prof. L. J. Kirmayer, Head of Psychiatry, McGill University, Canada, commented on my Koro research (1996). Professor Parameshvara Deva, Head of Psychiatry Department of Malay University, visited my Institute at Kolkata. I presented my Koro research at his faculty in Kuala Lumpur at his invitation in 1996. Professor A. N. Singh, Professor of Psychiatry and Pharmacology, Toxicology and Neurosciences, Queen's University, Ontario, Canada, always supported my research activities (1997–2005).

Late Prof. Wen-Shing Tseng, Head Department of Psychiatry, University of the Hawaii School of Medicine, Honolulu, and President and founder of World Association of Cultural Psychiatry, since 2005, supported me in my research and encouraged me to present my Koro research at the International WACP conferences.

Smt. Leena Chakraborty, IAS, Secretary of Health, Government of West Bengal, entrusted me to study a mini Koro epidemic in certain villages of South 24 Parganas district, West Bengal, in 1993.

Last but not least, over the years, I received support and suggestions from my students and later my colleagues Dr. Piyal Sen (UK), Dr. Samrat Sengupta (UK), Drs. Krishna Das Sen, Gautam K Bandyopadhyay, Nirmal Bera, Himadri Mukherjee, Dhrubojyoti Bagchi, Saikat

Basu, Sayanti Ghosh, Arabinda Brahma, Sohini Banerjee, and Sri Mrinal K Biswas at the Institute of Psychiatry, Kolkata for their help in different steps of my Koro research.

I am thankful to my colleagues in India Dr. D.Chakraborty, Prof. P. B. Behere, Prof. P. D. Das, Prof. H. R.Phookan, and in the UK, Dr. Rajesh Jacob, Dr. Mohan Chawla, Dr. Shusrut Jadav, Dr. Satya Dev Nagri, Dr. Anand Madasamy, Dr. Aravind Lowe, Dr. Barid Bhattacharya, Dr. Shiva Margani, and Dr. Nilanjana Ray, for their help at different stages of my research.

I am deeply obliged and thankful to Prof. Roland Littlewood for writing a foreword and to Prof. Kamaldeep Bhui to introduce the book and Prof. Kua Ee Heok for his comment on the book.

I am expressing my sincere thanks and gratitude to Dr. Fabida Aria, Consultant Psychiatrist and Associate Medical Director, Leicestershire Partnership NHS Trust and Royal College of Psychiatry regional advisor for Leicestershire, Northamptonshire, and Rutland, for her continued help and encouragement and critical review of some chapters, despite her heavy and busy professional engagements.

I am thankful to McLaven Tanya, Deputy Librarian, Bradgate Hospital Library, University Hospital Leicester, who always has a smiling face in my repeated literature searching on Koro publications. My special thanks go to Dr. R.Haeussier of Winchester University for his help in German and Dutch translation of some of the earlier Koro papers.

I would like to express my sincere thanks to all the anonymous peer reviewers for their constructive criticisms and supportive comments that help me to reorganize the book in its present form.

March 2021

Arabinda Narayan Chowdhury
Kettering, Northamptonshire, UK

Introduction

This remarkable ethnographic and scientific treatise on Koro is the product of a lifetime of scholarship by Professor Arabinda Chowdhury. In this well-researched and illustrated volume, Professor Chowdhury describes what has been called a culture-bound syndrome of Koro, as an important and valid lay and health concept in many countries and cultures. He describes the clinical features in China and India, exploring physiological processes that account for it, and even shows a case study published in the Lancet in the 1800s. Through a detailed dissection of the clinical presentations, he relates the descriptions to origins in cultural belief systems and expectations and folklore, and traces the linguistic and ethnographic origins of local concepts of Koro. Although in most textbooks Koro is described briefly, and simplistically, from the perspective of an exotic syndrome, Professor Chowdhury explores clinical descriptions in the context of culturally rich thick descriptions to understand the origins of distress and help seeking, and thus therapeutics. Students of cultural psychiatry, cultural psychology, anthropology, and psychosexual medicine will find the book a fascinatingly detailed encyclopedia of global knowledge on Koro that cannot be found elsewhere.

Prof. Kamaldeep Bhui, CBE, M.D., FRC. Psych. FRCP(E), FRSA, PFHEA
Professor of Psychiatry, University of Oxford
Hon. Consultant Psychiatrist East London NHS Foundation Trust
Editor in Chief, British Journal of Psychiatry

Comment

This is a scholarly book and very well-researched by the author. It traces the history and geography of koro. It should be read by not just medical historians but also health professionals, traditional medicine physicians, anthropologists, sociologists, policymakers, and researchers in transcultural medicine.

Although koro first appeared in a Dutch medical journal in 1895, it was well described in ancient Chinese medical texts over two thousand years ago. The literature search by the author shows that there are published papers now in every continent on the planet.

In the geopolitics of the twenty-first century, there is no hint that Asians want to believe that koro is just an Asian phenomenon. However, for the APA to categorize it as an OCD-spectrum disorder shows a lack of understanding of historical and cultural perspectives.

I am certain this book will be in the libraries of all medical schools around the world—providing a balanced view of socio-cultural phenomenon in mental health.

Professor Kua Ee Heok, MBBS,
M.D., FRCPsych
Department of Psychological
Medicine, Yong Loo Lin School
of Medicine
National University of Singapore
Singapore, Singapore

Tan Geok Yin
Professor of Psychiatry and
Neuroscience
Department of Psychological
Medicine, Yong Loo Lin School
of Medicine
National University of Singapore
Singapore, Singapore

Contents

Abbreviations

AJP	*American Journal of Psychiatry*
BID	Two Times Daily
BJP	*British Journal of Psychiatry*
CBS	Culture-Bound Syndrome
CBT	*Cognitive Behavior Therapy*
CNS	Central Nervous System
DSM	Diagnostic and Statistical Manual of Mental Disorders, published by the American Psychiatric Association (APA). Current edition is 5
ECT	Electro-Convulsive Therapy
EEG	Electroencephalogram
EMI	Explanatory Model of Illness
I.M.	Intra-Muscular
I.V.	Intra-Venous
ICD	International Classification of Diseases, published by WHO. Current edition is 11
MDP	Manic-Depressive Psychosis
MMSE	Mimi Mental State Examination, a scale to assess cognitive impairment
MRI	*Magnetic Resonance Imaging*. A medical imaging technique used in radiology to form pictures of brain and other body parts

Nocte	At night
TID	Three Times Daily
TPRR	*Transcultural Psychiatric Research Review*
YBOCS	Yale-Brown Obsessive-Compulsive Scale. A rating scale for the assessment of the severity and type of symptoms in patients with Obsessive-Compulsive Disorder

Medications Mentioned

Anti-Anxiety	Clonazepam; Perphenazine; Alprazolam; Chlordiazepoxide; Lorazepam; Diazepam; Propranolol
Anti-Depressant	Imipramine; Trimipramine; Amitriptyline; Doxepin; Fluoxetine; Fluvoxamine; Dothiepin; Sertraline; Paroxetine; Citalopram; Escitalopram; Trazadone; Venlafaxin; Amoxapine; Desipramine
Anti-epileptic	Carbamazepine, Clonazepam
Antihistamine	Cyproheptadine; Promethazine
Anti-Psychotic	Trifluoperazine; Largactil; Risperidone; Haloperidol; Haloperidol decanoate IM injection; Olanzapine; Amisulpride; Clozapine; Depot flupenthixol; Zuclopentixol decanoate; Thioridazine; Quetiapine; Perphenazine; Paliperidone
Mood Stabilizer	Lithium; Sodium valproate
Sedative	Nitrazepam; Bromazepam

List of Figures

List of Tables

Part I

Introduction: Current Status

1

Koro: Definition, Etymology, and Clinical Features

Definition

Koro is a culturally related psychogenic syndrome, clinically characterized by acute panic reaction concerning the perception of genital hyperinvolution and fear of impending death. In the male, shrinking or retraction of penis and or testes into the abdomen, and in female, shrinkage of vulval labia into the abdomen and or nipple or breast into the chest cavity are the cardinal features.

Clinical Features

The symptom manifestations have four distinct features: (i) *Cognitive* (*Perceptual)*: perception of shrinkage and/or retraction of the penis/testes (or nipple and or labia) due to an intra-abdominal (or intra-thoracic) pull; (ii) *Psychological:* fear of impending death (or sexual disability) out of this penile (or breast and or labial) involution or dissolution, (iii) *Emotional:* there are accompanying symptoms of an intense panic

A. N. Chowdhury, *Koro*,
https://doi.org/10.1007/978-3-030-87962-4_1

reaction with feelings of collapse, palpitations, sweating, nausea, breathlessness, visual blurring, body-spasms, pain, and paresthesia, and (iv) *Behavioral:* patients' (or others') idiosyncratic remedial measures or maneuvers to prevent the apparent disappearance of the penis or vulva into the abdominal cavity or the breast into the chest. This last component may be prone to penile or nipple injury or other health hazards as a complication.

Historical Background

Koro is a Malay term, and in Chinese, it is called **Shook yang or Suo-yang**. Historically, Koro is known as a localized culture-bound syndrome, predominantly found in southern China's Chinese inhabitants. It is also found in the countries of Southeast Asia to which the south Chinese people have migrated, viz. Malaysia, Indonesia (Borneo), Thailand, and Singapore. The clinical concept and the term "Koro" were first introduced to the Western medical press as a disease indigenous to southern Sulawesi people by a Dutch physician Dr. J. C. Blonk, in 1895 from Nederlandsch-Indie.

The earliest modern Chinese reference is that of Pao Sian-Ow, a traditional Chinese physician, who in his treatise "New Collection of Remedies of Value," published in 1834 (Fig. 1.1) stated that "during intercourse, the man may be seized suddenly with acute abdominal pain. The limbs become cold and the complexion dusky, the penis retracts into the abdomen. If treatment is not instituted at once and effective, the case will die. The disease is due to the invasion of cold vapors, and the treatment is to employ the 'heaty' drugs" (Gwee, 1963, 1968).

The disorder has a centuries-old tradition in Chinese medicine, philosophy, and culture. It has many references in ancient Chinese classical medical texts (recorded from 403–221 BC with new additions and revisions throughout different dynasties). Both the terms Koro and Suo or Shook yang have a close folk-etymological connection with the tortoise in the Indonesian and the Chinese cultures, respectively. Ng and Kua (1996) stated that Koro or Suo-Yang's earliest historical record is found in the Yellow Emperor's "Classic of Internal Medicine" in a dialogue

APPENDIX I

NEW COLLECTION OF REMEDIES OF VALUE BY PAO SIAN -OW

CHAPTER 6- GENITALIA

Retraction of Penis-the remedy is seen in Chapter 14 under "fevers-the Yin type of fever".

Yin-yan transposition- this arises when after a fever, the poisonous heat remains in the sperm and the marrow, and cannot be discharged. If intercourse is performed with a healthy person, the illness of the man will be passed on to the woman, and vice versa, hence it is called 'Yin-yan transposition'. The patient feels heavy and short of breath, the lower abdomen is tense, the genitalia may be affected by spasm and retraction, the heat rises in the chest, the head is too heavy to be lifted up, the eyes are blurred, and the knees and calves are tight. The powder made of burnt panties is valuable.

CHAPTER 14-

Yin-type of fever- after an intercourse between the male and female, may be arising of exposure to wind and cold, or the ingestion of raw or cold food, the result is pain in the abdomen, the scrotum in the male or the nipples in the female are retracted. May be the limbs will be flexed and of a dark purplish hue, and when severe, there is trismus, and cessation of breathing. This is called Yin -type of fever ...

Another remedy-After intercourse between the male and the female, the penis retracts with severe pain and feeling of death ... this is a good emergency remedy, and one should not miss the chance of cure because the remedy is dirty. Speed is essential, for delay will mean the case cannot be saved.

Fig. 1.1 English translation of Pao Sian-Ow (Adopted from Gwee, 1968, p. 5)

format between the Emperor and his court physician Ch'I Po. This is an ancient medical treatise written by a semi-mythical Chinese emperor Huangdi around 2600 BC. The book probably contains a compilation of several authors' writings (Curran, 2008) and the authorship of the book was perhaps between 476 and 221 B.C. (Fig. 1.2). The book was based on Taoist philosophy. The early physicians implicated dysfunctions of

When the pulse corresponding to the liver is slightly big there is numbness of the liver. The penis will shrink and there is persistent cough which causes abdominal pain. Illness due to internal pathogenic factors causes impotence ... illness due to cold causes retraction of the penis. In the case of the liver, grief moves the innermost self and causes harm to the mind resulting in madness, amnesia and lack of sperm. Without sperm, a person will not be well, and the manifestation is one of retraction of the genitals with spasm of muscles, the bones of the chest are depressed, and the hair colour poor. Death usually occurs in Autumn.

肝脉 …… 微大为肝痹，阴缩，咳引小腹。

《灵枢 · 邪气藏府病形》

足厥阴之筋 … 其病 … 阴器不用，伤于内则不起，伤于寒则阴缩入 ………

《灵枢 · 经筋篇》

肝悲哀动中则伤魂，魂伤则狂忘不精，不精则不正当人阴缩而挛缩，两胁骨不举，毛悴色，夭死于秋。

Fig. 1.2 Record of Suo-Yang from yellow emperor's classic of internal medicine (Adopted from Ng & Kua, 1996, p. 565)

the liver and or kidney may precipitate Suo-yang. The concept was that chronic anxiety could hurt the kidney to cause Suo-yang.

European references: It is also a matter of great surprise that Hippocrates (about 370 BC) also mentioned penile retraction and death in his medical writings: "A retraction of the testes and scrotum and penis are significative of severe pain and danger of death" (Coxe, 1846). Aristotle (384–322 BC) also wrote about the relation between contractions of genitals and heat, cold, and fear of death (Bandinelli et al., 2011).

Analysis of the world Koro literature shows that the first available report of a genital retraction or Shook yang cases (in the epidemic form) is found as early as 1865 in the Guangdong province of South China (Jilek, 1986). There are reports of over 250 sporadic Koro cases and at least 20 Koro epidemics involving countries like China, Indonesia, Singapore, Thailand, and India. The term "Koro" designating this malady appeared in 1874 in the Buginese dictionary (Matthes, 1874). Since the last 128 years, though sporadic Koro cases have been reported with diverse comorbidity (medical, neurological, urological, and psychiatric) from many countries, the epidemic form is restricted mainly to the South-East Asia region, including India.

Linguistic Origin of the Term "Koro"/"Suo Yang" or "Shook Yang"

Koro is a Malay term. B. F. Matthe's 1874 publication of a Buginese dictionary contains the first known reference of the name *Koro* (Edwards, 1984), which means "to shrink" and *lassa koro* is defined as "a shrinking of the penis, a sort of disease that is not unusual amongst the natives and must be very dangerous" (Palthe, 1936a). The term Koro is used by the Buginese and Macassarese people of Southern Sulawesi, although the corresponding exact Macassaran term is *garring Koro.* The term's exact origin is uncertain as the Macassaran and Buginese dialects have no corresponding cognate in Malay and Bahasa Indonesia's speech. In Bugis and Makassar culture, the word *koroq* means that the "penis is actually shrinking, or retracting," and the Dutch physicians "adopted the word *koroq*, leaving out the glottal stop at the end of the word" (Mitchell, 2018). Gwee (1968) traced several Malay lexical terms as a possible origin, e.g., *Kuru, Kerukul, Keroh,* and *Keruk.* In Malay and Indonesian dialects, the tortoise is known by *Kura* or *Kura-Kura* (Wilkinson, 1932) and in Macassarese by *Koero* (Slot, 1935). Both the Malay and Chinese use the tortoise head symbolically for the glans penis, and coitus reservatus is linked in ancient Chinese writings to retracting a tortoise's head (Rubin, 1982). The similarity between the tortoise withdrawing head under its wrinkled neck (Fig. 1.3) and ultimately within the body with that done by the shrinking penis may have given rise to the term's folk-etymological expression *Kuro* or *Kura* and eventually by corruption to Koro.

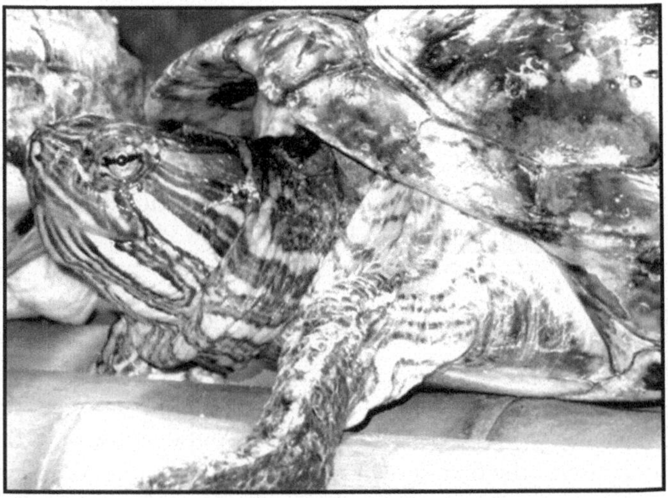

Fig. 1.3 Retracting head—neck of tortoise (Photographed by the author at Singapore Zoo)

Some ethnographic researchers suggested different probable origins for the name Koro. Adriani and Kruijt (1912) and LeBar (1972) proposed that the name of the illness is derived from the same name for a river and its surrounding valley and a local tribe (Toraja) in the northwestern part of Sulawesi (Celebes). Toraja is an Indonesian ethnic group that speaks the Baree dialect in Sulawesi.

The Chinese equivalent of "to shrink" is "shook." The ordinary Chinese word for glans penis is "yong tho" and the term "kwee tho" means both heads of the tortoise and the glans penis (Fig. 1.4) (Plathe, 1936b). Based on these cultural cognates, at least two orthography sets in Chinese to designate the disease, namely in Mandarin—"**Suo Yang**" and in Cantonese—"**Suk Yang**." Suo or Suk (shook) denotes "shrinking, contracting, shortening, reducing, decreasing, retracting, and drawing back" (Werner, 1961), and Yang is the male principle, i.e., genitals or penis. In Chinese, the penis is called "yin jing," the scrotum "yin nang," and the vagina as "yin dao." The penis is a protruding body part, it is rich in yang elements, so the disorder is known as Suo-yang (Ng & Kua, 1996).

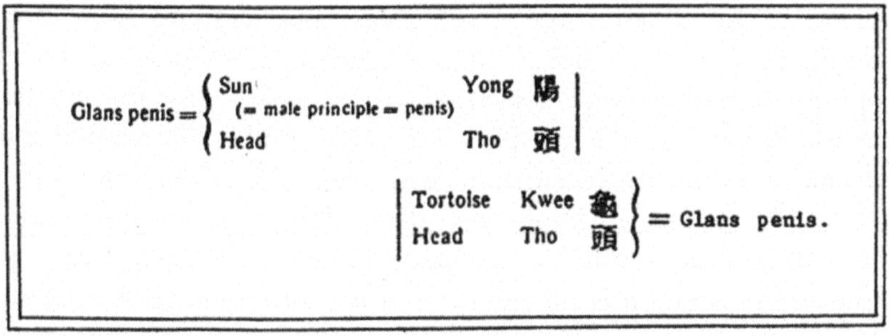

Fig. 1.4 Chinese folk etymology of Koro (Adopted from Palthe [1934, p. 1718])

Over the years, Koro was reported mainly in its epidemic form from the different South-East Asian countries, and that too is in "Classical form." The Classical form should qualify the following clinical symptom criteria: (1) Cognitive: perception of acute retraction of the penis (or breast or vulva in female); (2) Psychological: acute panic-like reaction (with both psychological and somatic manifestations); (3) Emotional: acute fear of impending danger, most commonly death (or sexual disability) from this disorder. The whole episode lasts from a few minutes to an hour; (4) Behavioral: This episode is accompanied by a preventive maneuver (by self or others) either by manual or mechanical means of pulling the penis (or breast) outward to prevent retraction; (5) Commonly, there is a myth or community folk belief of this Koro illness prevailing in the background. The suddenness of the episode and the clinical picture described above constitute the culture-bound classical Koro.

Sporadic cases are reported from many countries across the globe, mainly secondary to some other pathology. There is a wide-conceptual confusion observed in these reports of sporadic Koro cases. When the nature of the retraction is chronic for days or weeks (or months or years) with extraordinary health concern (sexual or somatic) but without fear of impending death and acute anxiety and commonly present with other medical or psychiatric or substance abuse disorder—then it is more logical to designate them as Koro-like symptom (KLS) (Chowdhury, 2008). There should be semantic clarity while defining any penile sign as Koro: In Koro, retraction of the penis (and scrotum) from intra-abdominal pull is the hallmark. It is a dynamic morphological sudden symptom formation (with associated acute anxiety episodes and fear of death). There are many reports where we find a long-standing or recurrent obsessional preoccupation with penis size or hypochondriacal penis-health concern or simply overvalued ideas about the smallness of penis—all these are not Koro presentation in the correct sense. Another confusing presentation is the delusion of penis shortening or smallness and even vanishing of the genitals in association with schizophrenic or paranoid illness—these are not Koro presentations, and new terminology is evolving like "Koro delusion" or part of Cotards syndrome (Alvarez et al., 2012). Vanishing genitals is not a Koro symptom. In Koro, the penile dissolution or disappearance occurs (but is visible) because of intra-abdominal pull.

In some cases, proper Koro features (retraction of the penis with acute anxiety attacks and fear of death or sexual disability) are present in a recurrent fashion over a long period—in these cases, the term Chronic Koro may be applicable. Such a presentation is more sub-acute rather than an acute dramatic presentation. And many of these cases had a history of intense sex-related guilt because of masturbation habits or prostitute visits, etc. It is also noted that a variety of topics are reported as a conceptual component of retracting—anxiety in addition to death-fear, like sexual disability, sex change, loss of masculinity, infertility, or even madness. Many KLS is being reported secondary to diverse medical, neurological, urological, and psychiatric pathology in recent years. In addition to that, the DSM-5 classification of Koro under ORCD—"Other specified Obsessive–Compulsive and Related Disorders" (300.3) opens up a new horizon of research on Koro psychopathology. So in the future, any perceptual abnormality about penis size, shape, or morphological change (with obsessional, hypochondriacal, or dysmorphophobic color) or psychotic genital delusional projection, including nihilistic perception (El-Tantawy, 2017) of "no penis"—all to be screened under ORCD lens.

The female expression of Koro is mainly evident in the epidemic form (Total reported 174 cases). Sporadic female Koro is rare. Palthe (1935) reported a female case: "The disease was also observed in females, in chief complaints being that the labia "shoot within". It was noted that a woman in Mandomai village died from Koro. The local law forbade men to help female illnesses relating to genitalia." Linton (1956) cited an example of female Koro patients in Borneo ("feel that their breasts are shriveling up and that their labia are being sucked inward"). But since then till 2019, only three sporadic female Koro is reported in the literature: from Hungary (Kovács & Osváth, 1998), from India (Srivastava & Pandit, 2013), and England (Chowdhury & Chawla, 2019).

The disease is, however, known by different syntaxes in different cultures. Table 1.1 illustrates the various ethnolinguistic expressions of the illness in different geocultural groups and regions and countries.

Changing Nosology and Concept of KORO: A Brief Outline

1859: The retraction of penis illness (*koroq*) occurred in several regions in Indonesia. The first records are from South Sulawesi where *Koro* was described in 1859 (Mitchell, 2018).
1895: Blonk used the term "Koro" first to address the clinical phenomenon of penile retraction. He provided a theory of compulsive-obsessive ideas behind Koro.
1896: van Berero described Koro as "a strange compulsive idea."
1908: "Asiatic psychoses" by Legendre (reported an epidemic in China).
1912: Adrian and Kruyt proposed that the name of the illness was derived from a tribe in the Sulawesi region, bearing the name *Koro.*
1934: Palthe stated Koro as an unusual form of anxiety neurosis, and he also provided the concept of castration anxiety in Koro.
1935: Mulder defined Koro as a form of anxiety neurosis.
1943: Bychowski reported the concept of disorder of body image concerning "penis loss perception."
1948: Kobler stressed the psychoanalytical concept of acute castration anxiety in Koro.

Table 1.1 Various ethno-linguistic expressions of genital retraction morbidity in different countries

A. China	a. Mandarin: Suyang, suo yang, shu-yang, showyang, shoojang b. Shanghi: Shook Yang or Shuk yang c. Cantonese: Shook yang; Shook yong; Shook jong; Seon-Ma Funn—in simplified Chinese 缩阳 and traditional Chinese 縮陽 d. Kong-suo (penis shrink)—villagers of Fuhu in Yangxi County of Guandong Province, China (Jie, 2010) e. Sio iong—Hokkien [Suo meaning 'to contract or constrict; "to retract" or "to reduce"]
B. South-East Asia	a. Koro—Singapore, Indonesia, Malaca, South-Central Mindano of Philippines, Macassaran area of Sulawesi, Kalimantan b. Lannuk-e-laso—South-Central Philippines c. Bang-Utott—Philippines d. Rok Joo—Thailand e. Tira—Mangaia, Cook group of Islands (due to overindulgence in coitus) (Marshall, 1980) f. Indonesia: Bangka—in Palembang; Mitchell (2018) provided many local names in Indonesia: Kerut, Koro laso (shrunken penis); Mbaze (in Ande language in South Sulawesi and Flores); Hidu—going inside disease or Hei lulu—everything pulled up (in Sumba island); In the west and central Flores the retraction panic syndrome is known as *ru'u pota*, "shrinking magic" g. Timor: In the Belu district, Koro is known as *lulik oan subaran*, "the little sacred thing is hiding itself" (Mitchell, 2010)

C. India	a. Jha-Jha—Lower-Assam b. Jhin-Jhinia—Assam and North Bengal region of West Bengal c. Beriberi—Darjeeling district (Kharibari block) of West Bengal d. Kattaow (small tortoise/"cut off")—Koch Behar district of West Bengal e. Disco, Disco fever—South Bengal and Calcutta of West Bengal and Baleswar district of Orissa f. Disco virus—South 24 Pargana district of West Bengal

Countries from where Koro/Koro-like illness reported

South-East Asia	Indian Sub-Continent	Middle East & Africa	Europe, Americas, & Others
China, Taiwan, Singapore, Hong Kong, Malaysia, Indonesia, Japan, Thailand, Philippines, South Korea	India, Pakistan, Sri Lanka, Nepal, Bangladesh[a]	Jordon, Israel, Saudi Arabia, Egypt, Qatar, Iran, Oman, South Africa, Nigeria, Sudan, Tanzania	United Kingdom, Ireland, Greece, France, Hungary, Portugal, Spain, Austria, Poland, Check Republic, Italy, Malta, Turkey, Russia, North America, Canada, Mexico, Brazil, New Zealand, Australia

[a]The author, during his field trip to North-Eastern Indian states in 2011, met Prof. H. R. Phookun, a researcher of the 1982 Assam Koro epidemic. He said that there were quite a few good numbers of Bangladeshi Muslim Koro patients seen in Gauhati Medical College. He traced a link with a pocket in Bangladesh where people have frequently suffered Koro attacks, and they linked it with persons who visited Bangladesh from neighboring Myanmar. In Assam, it is popularly called "*Mian Syndrome*" (*Mian* is an Urdu syntax used to address a male person as "Mr." in Muslim culture). Though there is no published report on Koro from Bangladesh, there are cases who avail treatment from neighboring Indian states like Assam or Tripura

1965: Yap reported from Hong Kong: It is a landmark year since then Koro was regarded as a culture-bound depersonalization syndrome. Subsequently, Koro was mentioned as a "Culture-bound syndrome."
1965: Rin reported from Taiwan—stressed the importance of the Chinese Yin-Yang concept in Koro.
1968: Gwee (from Singapore) identified Singapore's Koro epidemic as an "acute hysterical panic reaction."
1968: Ngui (from Singapore) identified Koro in Singapore's epidemic as "culture-bound syndrome."
1972: Lapierre reported Koro's first case associated with a general medical condition (left frontotemporal cerebral tumor) from Canada.
1983: Hughes (from Montreal) introduced the concept of "Genital retraction taxon" model to explain genital retraction in Koro.
1984: Edwards (USA) proposed the term "genital retraction syndrome" (GRS), to replace Koro.
1984: Berrios and Morley (from the UK) first used the term "Koro-like symptoms" (KLS).
1987: Money and Annecillo (USA) reported body image pathology in shrinking-penis syndrome.
1989: Chowdhury (India) reported dysmorphic penis image in Koro (epidemic cases).
1990: Bernstein and Gaw (USA) proposed a new classification scheme of Koro for DSM IV.
1992: ICD-10 Included Koro under the category F 48.8—"Other specified Neurotic Disorders" along with Latah and Dhat syndrome—all of which have culture-specific etiologies.
1994: Chowdhury proposed the term "Chronic Koro" for stereotyped recurrent attacks over a considerable period.
1994: DSM IV, APA included Koro as one of the entries in the Glossary of Culture-Bound Syndromes in Appendix I.
1996: Chowdhury proposed Primary (culture-bound expression) and Secondary (with other disorders) forms of Koro.
1998: Bartholomew (New Zealand) argued against the medical perspective of Koro and provided a sociological construct of epidemic Koro.

2000: DSM IV, T.R., APA, listed Koro in the Glossary of Culture-bound Syndromes of Appendix I without any diagnostic code.
2001: The Chinese Classification of Mental Disorders (CCMD 3) includes Koro, among other 40 culturally related diagnoses (CSP, 2001).
2008: Chowdhury described different criteria for the clinical use of the term Koro and Koro-like symptom (KLS).
2013: DSM-5: the "cultural tag" from Koro is withdrawn and is brought under "Other specified Obsessive-Compulsive and Related Disorders" with a diagnostic code—300.3.

Global Distribution of Koro or Genital Retraction Epidemics

1908: Koro epidemic in Szechwan, China
1952: *Suo-yang* epidemic in Guangdong, China
1962: *Suo-yang* epidemic in Guangdong, China
1966: *Suo-yang* epidemic in Guangdong, China
1967: Singapore Koro epidemic
1972: Koro epidemic in Thailand
1974: Koro epidemic in Guangdong, China
1975: Koro epidemic in Palembang, Indonesia
1976: Koro epidemic in Thailand
1979: Koro-like epidemic in Lagos, Nigeria, Africa
1982: Koro epidemic in Thailand
1982: Koro epidemic in North-East India (Assam and West Bengal state)
1984–1985: Koro epidemic in Guangdong, China
1987: Koro epidemic in Guangdong, China
1988: Koro epidemic in Tripura, India
1988: *Suo-yang* epidemic in Warring County, Hainan, Guangdong, China
1992: Ilechukwu reported a "magical penis loss" epidemic from Nigeria

1993: A mini Koro epidemic in South 24 Parganas district of West Bengal, India
1999: Koro epidemic in Ende city of Flores, Indonesia
2010: Koro epidemic in India (West Bengal, Assam, Tripura, Mumbai, Kerala states)
2015: Koro epidemic in Tripura, India.

Changing Spectrum of Koro Symptomatology

It is interesting to note that Koro's concept has expanded considerably over the years, and new clinical issues are gradually incorporated into its symptomatology. The classical presentation, to recall, for the male, is the perception of retraction of the penis from an intra-abdominal pull and accompanied by extreme anxiety and panic with the fear of death. For females: retraction of nipple or breast into the chest and/or retraction of vaginal vulva inside because of inner pull with anxiety and fear of death —are the cardinal presentation. The last 126 years of literature review have shown that there are considerable addition of symptoms in the original clinical construct (Tables 1.2 and 1.3).

Some reports very precisely reported the precipitating or triggering events or situations immediately before the Koro attack. The following summary table (Table 1.4) shows this variety of events preceding the Koro attack.

Some reports of Koro indicated the possible role of some drugs—both therapeutic and abusive, in the perception of Koro symptoms. Following is a summary table of such associations (Table 1.5).

Nosological debate and diagnostic confusion regarding Koro over the years is astonishing. The following table will speak for these varied diagnostic concepts and clinical constructs attached to Koro (Table 1.6).

Africa in the Koro Map

It is of much interest to cultural psychiatry that since the mid-1990s, some epidemics concerning "penis vanishing or genital theft"

Table 1.2 Variations of genital symptom

Male	Female
Itching of the external genitals (Jilek & Jilek-Aal, 1977a)	Frigidity (Jilek & Jilek-Aal, 1977a)
Feeling of crawling, pinching, burning, and irritation in the tip of the penis (Anumonye & Adaranijo, 1978)	Breast "withdrawal" into the thoracic cavity and chest pain (Moekti & Denin, 1978)
Insensitive penis (Cai, 1982)	Vaginal dilatation (Suwanlert & Coates, 1979)
Feeling of numbness or coldness in the penis (Lucieer, 1984–1985; Yap, 1964b)	Breast pain, flattening of breast mass on the chest wall, pricking sensation in the breast, retraction of a single nipple, vaginal pain (Chowdhury, 1994)
Retraction of both—testes and penis (Kar, 2005; Leo et al., 1989; Mukherjee, 1987; Scher, 1987; Westermeyer, 1989)	
Complete loss of penile sensation only and shortening of the penis without retraction, alteration of penis morphology (reduced glans size, reduced penis-shaft girth), and loss of penile muscular tone (Chowdhury, 1992b)	
Inability to feel the penis (Atalay, 2007)	
The penis is melting in the heat (like ice) and would disappear (Stip et al., 2007)/penis is fading as the abdominal heat made it melt (Alvarez et al., 2012)	

Table 1.3 Ideational component of fear other than death

1	Worry about being "a man without a penis" (Ede, 1976)
2	Fear of turning into a female (Ang & Weller, 1984; Moodley, 1985)
3	Sexual invalidism and losing his wife (Ifabumuyi & Rwegellera, 1979)
4	Fear of "insanity" in male (Zain & Subramanian, 1991)
5	Fear of turning into a eunuch in female, bewitched feeling (Chowdhury, 1994)
6	Fear of "damage to sex organ" (loss of sexual power) (Chowdhury, 1992a)
7	Fear of "complete impotence" (Chowdhury, 1992c)
8	Fear of "penis loss," not death (Chowdhury & Rajbhandari, 1995)
9	Fear of sexual dysfunction (Kennedy & McDonough, 2002)
10	Fear of impotence and change of gender (Bandinelli et al., 2011)
11	Fear of disfiguration of their body and fear of some severe future health malady (Female case) (Ghosh et al., 2013)
12	Fear of loss of child-bearing and breast-feeding capacity in females (Banerjee et al., 2020)

(breast/vagina vanishing also) were reported from West-African nations, viz. Ghana (1997), Senegal (1997), Benin (2001), Gambia (2003), Sudan (2003), Nigeria (2001–2010), Cameroon (2008), and Congo (2008). The victims explained the experience as genital theft and accused someone (who is a part of a covert agency) of stealing the penis to inflict impotence. There is a strong cultural belief in occultism, witchcraft, and juju, which is operative in the background and some financial motive of an antisocial gang, as evident from the fact that the alleged accused person (who steals the organ) is demanded money for ransom. These are not examples of Koro but may be seen as a variant of Koro or genital neurosis (the core symptom is centering with the penis). This genital loss/disappearance phenomenon also involves magical stealing or witchcraft and sorcery with underlying cultural belief, which is expressed as Mass Psychogenic Illness (Dzokoto & Adams, 2005) or within the framework of "mutual constitution" as defined by Adams and Dzokoto (2007).

[**Koro Plant:** Interesting to note that there is a plant named KORO (*M. Pruriens*), a type of legumes, which grows abundantly in various regions of Indonesia, especially in Central Java. There are 23 types of koro, but only a few varieties are consumed by the public. Nutritional

Table 1.4 Precipitating event or factor before Koro attack (perception)

Sl.No	Author (year)/precipitating or triggering event or situation	Country of reporting
1	Gwee (1963): insect bite on the penis/while passing urine	Singapore
2	Yap (1965a): 4 patients after masturbation; 4 patients after coitus; 4 patients after sexual arousal; 3 patients after hearing about Koro news; 2 patients after a cold bath; 1 patient during urination in the cold wind; 1 patient when frightened	Hong Kong
3	Rin (1963): after a day of intercourse with a prostitute	Taiwan
4	Garg (1968): during the passing of urine	U.K. (Durham)
5	Ngui (1969): Singapore epidemic—226 cases (220 males and 6 females)—1 after masturbation, 1 following sexual intercourse; 25.9% had the attack during micturition, 1.2% after defecation; 17.3% after exposure to chill or cold weather or air-conditioning and in 15.9% cases during or soon after the bath. In total, in about 61% of cases, their attacks were precipitated by activity or conditions that were focused on their genital organ	Singapore[a]
6	Sachdev and Shukla (1982): a tingling sensation in the legs	India (Assam)[a]
7	Cai (1982): intercourse with a menstruating woman—3 cases/genital injury-1 case	China (Guangdong)
8	Malinick et al. (1985): after an attempt of oral sex with a prostitute	USA (Chicago)
9	Lucieer (1984–1985): following intercourse	Africa (Tanzania)
10	Emsley (1985): after a failed attempt at coitus	S. Africa (Cape)
11	Moodley (1985): withdrawal state from Lorazepam	U.K. (London)
12	Oyebode et al. (1986): after eating a banana	Singapore
13	Tseng et al. (1988): Guangdong epidemic—69% of men had a prodromal chill phase	China (Guangdong)[a]
14	Kuruppuarachchi et al. (2000): penile injury during masturbation	Sri Lanka

(continued)

Table 1.4 (continued)

Sl.No	Author (year)/precipitating or triggering event or situation	Country of reporting
15	Roy et al. (2011): In 1 case triggered after receiving a mobile phone call from his brother/One case after observing the television report of "penis retraction disease" in the locality	India (Assam)[a]

[a]Epidemic cases

Table 1.5 Association of drugs with Koro

Sl. No	Therapeutic drugs	Author (year)
1	After consumption of Ludiomil tablet (100 mg) each for eight preceding nights	Walenberg (1981)
2	Withdrawal state from Lorazepam	Moodley (1985)
3	Psychosis (depression with auditory and visual hallucination) caused by L-dopa therapy with a delusion of genital shrinkage	Chen (1991)
4	After abrupt cessation of olanzapine	Ramos and Budman (1998)
Abusive drugs		
1	Heroin withdrawal	Yap (1965a) and Chowdhury and Bagchi (1993)
2	Amphetamine	Yap (1965b) and Bloor (2004)
3	Amphetamine, cannabis, methadone, LSD (Lysergic acid diethylamide)	Dow and Silver (1973)
4	Buprenorphine withdrawal	Chowdhury and Banerjee (1996)
5	Cannabis smoking	Chowdhury and Bera (1994), Earleywine (2001), Kalaitzi and Kalantzis (2006) and El-Tantawy (2017)
6	Steroid (Dexamethasone)	Praharaj (2004)
7	Solvents inhalation	Stip et al. (2007)
8	Poly-substance abuse with alcohol	Marques (2015)

Table 1.6 Different diagnostic terms used to describe Koro (1886–2020)

Sl No	Author (year)/reported from	Diagnostic term
1	Raven (1886)/UK	Retraction of the penis
2	Blonk (1895)/Dutch-Indies	An irresistible compulsion or an acute anxiety neurosis
3	Brero (1896)/Dutch-Indies	A strange compulsive idea
4	Vorstman (1897)/Dutch-Indies	Delusion
5	Kraepelin (1904)/Germany	Obsessive-compulsive disorder
6	Legendre (1908)/China	Asiatic psychosis
7	Slot (1935)/Dutch-Indies	Nerve contracting disease
8	Palthe (1934)/Dutch-Indies	An unusual form of anxiety neurosis
9	Mulder (1935)/Dutch-Indies	Anxiety neurosis
10	Baasher (1963)/Africa	Anxiety state
11	Gwee (1963)/Singapore	Acute hysterical panic reaction
12	Yap (1964a)/Hong Kong	Culture-bound depersonalization syndrome
13	Rin (1965)/Taiwan	Panic state
14	Gwee (1968)/Singapore[a]	Acute panic reaction with the delusion of penile retraction (may be hysterical delusion affected by cultural suggestion)
15	Ngui (1969)/Singapore[a]	Culture-bound psychogenic illness
16	Koro Study Team (1969)/Singapore[a]	A panic syndrome, linked with cultural indoctrination
17	Edwards (1970)/USA	Koro pattern of depersonalization
18	Lappierre (1972)/Canada	Psychogenic localized depersonalization due to post-operative stress
19	Marks and Lader (1973)/UK	Acute anxiety with cultural specificity
20	Jilin and Jilek-Aall (1977b)/Thailand[a]	Mass hysteria
21	Moekti and Denin (1978)/Indonesia[a]	Nonrational dissemination of castration anxiety
22	Ifabumuyi and Rwegellera (1979)/Nigeria	Recurrent anxiety with multiple hypochondriacal symptoms
23	Constable (1979)/UK	Acute anxiety (shared by his wife also)
24	Rosenthal and Rosenthal (1982)/USA	Hypochondriasis
25	Chakraborty et al. (1982)/India	Anxiety neurosis

(continued)

Table 1.6 (continued)

Sl No	Author (year)/reported from	Diagnostic term
26	Nandi et al. (1983)/India[a]	Acute anxiety reaction
27	Hughes (1983)/Canada	Atypical somatoform disorder, panic disorder, and/or sexual disorder not otherwise specified
28	Ang and Weller (1984)/UK	Hyperacute anxiety with a delusional belief occurring in a psychotic setting
29	Edwards (1984)/USA	Genital Retraction Syndrome
30	Fernando (1988)/NZ	Monosymptomatic hypochondriasis
31	Kaplan and Sadock (1988)/USA	Atypical psychosis
32	Maslowski (1988)/Malta	Hypochondriacal delusions
33	Tseng et al. (1988)/USA[a]	Genital retraction panic disorder
34	Chowdhury (1989)/India[a]	Penile dysmorphophobia
35	Amering and Katschnig (1990)/Austria	Culture-specific form of panic disorder
36	Stein et al. (1991)/USA	Body dysmorphic disorder or somatic type delusional disorder
37	Fishbain (1991)/ USA	Somatoform disorder
38	Chen (1991)/UK	A delusion of genital shrinkage
39	Sheeley (1991)/USA	A cultural variant of hysteria
40	Chaturvedi (1993)/India	Transcultural variation of anxiety
41	Goetz and Price (1994)/USA	A variant of body dysmorphic disorder
42	Ungvari and Mullen (1994)/NZ	A delusion of penile retraction
43	Chiniwala et al. (1996)/USA	A delusion of genital retraction
44	Wilson and Agin (1997)/USA	Anxiety Disorder
45	Al-Hmoud (1999)/Jordan	Anxiety disorder and panic
46	Saman et al. (2007)/Pakistan	Somatization of the castration fear
47	Atalay (2007)/Turkey	Anxiety disorder NOS
48	Kondan (2008)/UK	Generalized anxiety disorder with panic disorder
49	Roy et al. (2011)/India[a]	Mass Psychogenic Illness
50	Alvarez et al. (2012)/Spain	A subtype of Cotard syndrome (in psychotic depression)
51	Kumar et al. (2013)/India[a]	Acute Anxiety state
52	Garg et al. (2017)/India	Hypochondriacal delusion
53	Tau and Masukar (2020)/USA	Koro delusion (in Alzheimer's disease)

[a]Epidemic cases

content in various kinds of koro is relatively good. Though no research has shown its association with Koro illness, yet it is a matter of further observation whether this name has anything to do with the naming of the disease.]

References

Adams, G., & Dzokoto, V. A. (2007). Genital-shrinking in Ghana: A cultural-psychological analysis. *Culture & Psychology, 13*, 83–104.

Adriani, N., & Kruijt, A. C. (1912). *De Bare'e - Sprekende Toradja's van Midden-Celebes*. Landsdrukkerij.

Al-Hmoud, N. (1999). Koro-like syndrome in a Jordanian male. *Eastern Mediterranean Health Journal, 5*, 611–613.

Alvarez, P., Puente, V. M., Blasco, M. J., Salgado, P., Merino, A., & Bulbena, A. (2012). Concurrent Koro and Cotard syndromes in a Spanish male patient with a psychotic depression and cerebrovascular disease. *Psychopathology, 45*(2), 126–129.

Amering, M., & Katschnig, H. (1990). Panic attacks and panic disorder in cross-cultural perspective. *Psychiatric Annals, 20*(9), 511–516.

Ang, P. C., & Weller, M. P. I. (1984). Koro and psychosis. *British Journal of Psychiatry, 145*, 335.

Anumonye, A., & Adaranijo, H. (1978). Chronic nonspecific urethrities as psychological reaction among Nigerian neurotic patients. *Nigerian Medical Journal, 8*, 3–5.

Atalay, H. (2007). Two cases of Koro syndrome or anxiety disorder associated with genital retraction fear. *Türk Psikiyatri Dergisi, 18*(3), 282–285.

Baasher, T. A. (1963). The influence of culture on psychiatric manifestation. *Transcultural Psychiatric Research Review, 15*, 51–52.

Bandinelli, M., Trevisi, M., Kotzalidis, G. D., Manfredi, G., Rapinesi, C., & Ducci, G. (2011). Chronic Koro-like syndrome (KLS) in recurrent depressive disorder as a variant of Cotard's delusion in an Italian male patient. A case report and historical review. *Rivista di Psychiatria, 46*(3), 220–226.

Banerjee, D., Sharma, S., & Antony, S. (2020). Koro and migration: Observational study of an outbreak of Koro in a migrant population working in South India. *Journal of Psychosexual Health, 2*(2), 174–178.

Blonk, J. C. (1895). Koro. *Geneeskunding Tijaschrift voor Nederlandsch-Indie, 35*, 562–563.
Bloor, R. N. (2004). Whizz-dick: Side effect, urban myth or amphetamine-related Koro-like syndrome? *International Journal of Clinical Practice, 58*(7), 717–719.
Cai, J. B. (1982). Five case reports of Suo-Yang Zen. *Chinese Journal of Neuropsychiatry, 4*, 206–288.
Chakraborty, A., Das, S., & Mukherjee, A. (1982, December 3–4). Koro makes an epidemic appearance in India. *Transcultural Newsletter, III.*
Chaturvedi, S. K. (1993). Neurosis across cultures. *International Review of Psychiatry, 5*(2–3), 179–191.
Chen, E. (1991). Drug induced Koro in a non-Chinese man. *British Journal of Psychiatry, 158*, 721.
Chinese Society of Psychiatry. (2001). *The Chinese classification and diagnostic criteria of mental disorders—Version 3 (CCMD-3)*. Chinese Society of Psychiatry.
Chiniwala, M., Alfonso, C. A., Torres, J. R., & Lefer, J. (1996). Koro in an immigrant from Guinea with brief psychotic disorder. *American Journal of Psychiatry, 153*(5), 736.
Chowdhury, A. N. (1989). Penile perception of Koro patients. *Acta Psychiatrica Scandinavica, 80*, 183–186.
Chowdhury, A. N. (1992a). Koro social response (*urban*): A longitudinal study of North Bengal Koro epidemic. *Indian Journal of Psychiatry, 34*, 46–52.
Chowdhury, A. N. (1992b). Clinical analysis of 101 Koro cases. *Indian Journal of Social Psychiatry, 7*, 67–70.
Chowdhury, A. N. (1992c). Koro in affective disorder with a case report from industrial setup. *Industrial Psychiatry Journal , 5*(2), 71–83.
Chowdhury, A. N. (1994). Koro in females: An analysis of 48 cases. *Transcultural Psychiatric Research Review, 31*, 369–380.
Chowdhury, A. N. (2008). Cultural Koro and Koro-like symptom (KLS). *German Journal of Psychiatry, 11*, 81–82.
Chowdhury, A. N., & Banerjee, G. (1996). Recurrent Koro in repeated IV buprenorphine withdrawal. *Addiction, 91*, 145–146.
Chowdhury, A. N., & Bagchi, D. (1993). Koro in heroin withdrawal. *Journal of Psychoactive Drugs, 25*, 257–258.
Chowdhury, A. N., & Bera, N. K. (1994). Koro following cannabis smoking. *Addiction, 89*, 1017–1020.
Chowdhury, A. N., & Rajbhandari, K. C. (1995). Koro with depression from Nepal. *Transcultural Psychiatric Research Review, 32*, 87–90.

Chowdhury, A. N., & Chawla, M. (2019). Koro in female: A case report and a mini review. *European J Psychiatry, 33*(4), 182–185.
Constable, P. L. (1979). Koro in Hertfordshire. *Lancet, 1*, 163.
Coxe, J. R. (1846). *The book of prognostics. The writings of Hippocrates and Galen. Epitomised from the original Latin translations. Section IIa.* Lindsay and Blackston.
Curran, J. (2008). The yellow emperor's classic of internal medicine. *British Medical Journal, 5*(336 [7647]), 777.
Diagnostic Criteria from DSM-IV. (1994). *American Psychiatric Association.* American Psychiatric Press Inc.
Diagnostic and Statistical Manual of Mental Disorders. (2000). *Fourth Edition: DSM-IV-TR.* American Psychiatric Association.
Diagnostic and Statistical Manual of Mental Disorder. (2013). *Fifth edition.* American Psychiatric Association.
Dow, T. W., & Silver, D. A. (1973). Drug induced Koro syndrome. *Journal of the Florida Medical Association, 60*, 32.
Dzokoto, V. A., & Adams, G. (2005). Understanding genital-shrinking epidemics in West Africa: Koro, juju, or mass psychogenic illness? *Culture, Medicine & Psychiatry, 29*(1), 53–78.
Earleywine, M. (2001). Cannabis induced Koro in Americans. *Addiction, 96*(11), 1663–1666.
Ede, A. (1976). Koro in an Anglo Saxon Canadian. *Canadian Psychiatric Association Journal, 21*, 389–391.
Edwards, J. G. (1970). The Koro pattern of depersonalization in an American schizophrenic patient. *American Journal of Psychiatry, 126*, 1171–1173.
Edwards, J. W. (1984). Indigenous Koro: A genital retraction syndrome of insular South East Asia: A critical review. *Culture, Medicine & Psychiatry, 8*, 1–24.
El-Tantawy, A. M. M. A. (2017). Chronic Koro-like syndrome co-morbid with schizophrenia and history of cannabis abuse in an Egyptian patient: Case report. *Arab Journal of Psychiatry, 28*(1), 92–96.
Emsley, R. A. (1985). Koro in non-Chinese subjects. *British Journal of Psychiatry, 146*(1), 102.
Fernando, N. (1988). Monosymptomatic hypochondriasis treated with a tricyclic antidepressant. *British Journal of Psychiatry, 152*, 851–852.
Fishbain, D. A. (1991). Koro classification and case reports. *American Journal of Psychiatry, 148*(12), 1765–1767.
Garg, B. K. (1968, June 15). Koro in Britain. *British Medical Journal*, 700.

Garg, K., Kumar, C. N., & Sharadhi, C. (2017). Koro: Much more than just a culture bound syndrome. *Asian Journal of Psychiatry, 29*, 146–147.

Ghosh, S., Nath, S., Brahma, A., & Chowdhury, A. N. (2013). Fifth Koro epidemic in India: A review report. *World Cultural Psychiatry Research Review, 8*(1), 8–20.

Goetz, K. L., & Price, T. R. (1994). A case of Koro: Treatment response and implications for diagnostic classification. *Journal of Nervous & Mental Disease, 182*(10), 590–591.

Gwee, A. L. (1963). Koro—A cultural disease. *Singapore Medical Journal, 4*, 119–122.

Gwee, A. L. (1968). Koro—Its origin and nature as a disease entity. *Singapore Medical Journal, 9*, 3–6.

Hughes, C. C. (1983). The genital retraction taxon. In R. C. Simons & C. C. Hughes (Eds.), *The culture-bound syndromes. culture, illness, and healing* (Vol. 7) (Studies in Comparative Cross-Cultural Research). Springer.

ICD-10. (1992). Classification of mental and behavioural disorders. In *Clinical description and diagnostic guidelines*. World Health Organization, Geneva. Oxford University Press.

Ifabumuyi, O. I., & Rwegellera, G. G. C. (1979). Koro in a Nigerian male patient: A case report. *African Journal of Psychiatry, 5*, 103–105.

Jie, L. (2010). Koro epidemic among school children in Guangdong, China. *World Cultural Psychiatric Research Review*, 102–105.

Jilek, W. G. (1986). Epidemic of "Genital Shrinking" (Koro): Historical review and report of a recent outbreak in South China. *Curare, 9*, 269–282.

Jilek, W., & Jilek-Aall, L. (1977a). A Koro epidemic in Thailand. *Transcultural Psychiatric Research Review, 14*, 57–59.

Jilek, W., & Jilek-Aall, L. (1977b). Mass Hysteria with Koro symptom in Thailand. Schweizer *Archieve Neurologic Neurochirurgie und Psychiatrie, 120*, 257–259.

Kalaitzi, C. K., & Kalantzis, A. (2006). Cannabis-induced koro-like syndrome. A case report and mini review. *Urologia Internationalis, 76*(3), 278–280.

Kaplan, H. I., & Sadock, B. J. (1988). *Clinical psychiatry, in synopsis of psychiatry* (5th ed.). Williams & Wilkins.

Kar, N. (2005, October 12). Chronic Koro-like symptoms—Two case reports. *BMC Psychiatry, 5*, 34.

Kennedy, N., & McDonough, M. (2002). Koro: A case in an Eastern European asylum seeker in Ireland. *Irish Journal of Psychological Medicine, 19*(4), 130–131.

Kondan, V. R. J. (2008). A case of Koro in a Caucasian man. *Progress in Neurology & Psychiatry, 12*(4), 25–27.
Koro Study Team (Chairman: AL Gwee). (1969). The Koro epidemic in Singapore. *Singapore Medical Journal, 10*, 234–242.
Kovács, A., & Osváth, P. (1998). Genital retraction syndrome in a Korean women. A case of Koro in Hungary. *Psychopathology, 31*, 220–224.
Kraepelin, E. (1904). Psychiatrisches aus Java. *Centralblad fur Nervenheilkunde und Psychiatrie, 27*, 468–469.
Kumar R, Phookun H R, Datta, A. (2013). Koro: A culture bound syndrome: An anxiety disorder. *Indian Journal of Psychiatry, 55*(Sup.1), S131–S132.
Kuruppuarachchi, K. A., Ratnayake, J. A., Dasanayake, N. A., & Rajakuruna, R. R. (2000). The Koro syndrome. *Ceylon Medical Journal, 45*(4), 182–183.
Lappierre, Y. D. (1972). Koro in a French Canadian. *Canadian Psychiatric Association Journal, 17*, 333–334.
LeBar, F. M. (1972). *Ethnic groups of Insular Southeast Asia* (Vol. I) Human Relations Area Files Press.
Legendre, J. (1908). Une curieuse epidemic. *Annales de Medicine Coloniale, 11*(2), 280–281.
Leo, D. D., Mauro, P., & Pellegrini, C. (1989). An organic triggering factor in Koro syndrome? A case report. *European Journal of Psychiatry, 3*(2), 77–81.
Linton, R. (1956). *Culture and mental disorders.* Charles C. Thomas.
Lucieer, W. M. (1984–1985). The bitter taste of liberty. *Psychopathologic Africaine, 20*, 17–40.
Malinick, C., Flaherty, J. A., & Jobe, T. (1985). Koro: How culturally specific? *International Journal of Social Psychiatry, 31*, 67–63.
Marks, I., & Lader, M. (1973). Anxiety states (anxiety neurosis): A review. *Journal of Nervous & Mental Disease, 156*, 3–18.
Matthes, B. F. (1874). *Over de Bissoe's of Heidensche Priesters en Priesteressen de Boeginezen* (p. 31). C. G. Vander Post.
Marshall, D. S. (1980). Too much in Mangaia. In C. Gordon & G. Johnson (Eds.), *Readings in human sexuality: Comparative perspectives* (pp. 236–240). Harper & Row.
Marques, J. G. (2015). Koro, Othello and capgras syndromes in one patient with drug induced psychosis. *Psychiatrica Danubina, 27*(4), 429–430.
Maslowski, J. (1988). Koro-like syndrome in Maltese subject on the basis of chronic schizophrenia. *Bulletin of Maritime & Tropical Medicine in Gdynia, 39*(1–2), 108–110.
Mitchell, D. (2010). Koro in Eastern Indonesia 1999 to 2010. *Asia-Pacific Psychiatry, 2*(3), A7.

Mitchell, D. (2018). *Is shrinking penis syndrome a delusion or real thing?* Paper presented at the 'History of Medicine in Southeast Asia Symposium' at the Indonesian Academy of Sciences, 27–30 June 2018.

Moekti, S., & Denin, S. K. (1978). *A non-rational dissemination of castration anxiety in Palembang, 1975*. Paper presented at the First Asian Teaching Workshop on Mental Health and Culture, Jakarta, July. (Personal Communication).

Moodley, P. (1985). Koro in non-Chinese subjects. *British Journal of Psychiatry, 146*, 102–103.

Mukherjee, T. (1987). Koro-like states. *British Journal of Psychiatry, 150*(6), 881.

Mulder, J. G. A. (1935). Over Koro. *GeneesKundig Tijdschrift voor Nederlandsch-Indie, 75*, 837–838.

Nandi, D. N., Banerjee, G., Saha, H., & Boral, G. C. (1983). Epidemic Koro in West Bengal, India. *International J Social Psychiatry, 29*(4), 265–268.

Ng, B. Y., & Kua, E. E. H. (1996). Koro in ancient Chinese history. *History of Psychiatry, 7*, 563–570.

Ngui, P. W. (1969). The Koro epidemic in Singapore. *Australian & New Zealand Journal of Psychiatry, 3*, 263–266.

Ngui, P. W. (1984). Personal communication.

Oyebode, F., Jamieson, R., Mullaney, J., & Davison, K. (1986). Koro—A psychophysiological dysfunction? *British Journal of Psychiatry, 148*, 212–214.

van Palthe, P. M. W. (1934). Koro-Een Eigenaardige Angstneurose. *Geneeskundig Tijdschrift voor Nederlandsch-Indie, 74*, 1713–1720.

van Palthe, P. M. W. (1935). Anauvulling op Het Artikel "Koro", een Eigenaardige Angstneurose. *Geneeskundig Tijdschrift voor Nederlandsch-Indie, 75*, 836–837.

van Palthe, P. M. W. (1936a). "Koro". Une Maladie Imaginaire et Une Phobie Orientale. *La Presse Medicale, 44*(67), 1331–1332.

van Palthe, P. M. W. (1936b). Psychiatry and neurology in the tropics. In C. D. de Langen & A. Lichtenstein (Eds.), A clinical textbook of tropical medicine (pp. 525–547). G. Kolff and Company.

Phookun, H. R. (2011). Personal communication.

Praharaj, S. K. (2004). Koro and psychosis following steroid abuse. *German Journal of Psychiatry, 7*(3), 49–50.

Ramos, R. H., & Budman, C. L. (1998). Emergence of Koro after abrupt cessation of olanzapine. *Journal of Clinical Psychiatry, 59*(2), 86–87.

Raven, T. (1886). Retraction of the penis. *Lancet, 2*, 205.

Rin, H. (1963). Koro: A consideration on Chinese concepts of illness and case illustrations. *Transcultural Psychiatric Research Review, 15*, 23–30.

Rin, H. (1965). A study of the aetiology of Koro in respect to the Chinese concept of illness. *International Journal of Social Psychiatry, 11*, 7–13.

Rosenthal, S., & Rosenthal, P. A. (1982). Koro in an adolescent: Hypochondriasis as a stress response. *Adolescent Psychiatry, 10*, 523–531.

Roy, D., Hazarika, S., Bhattacharya, A., Das, S., Nath, K., & Saddichha, S. (2011). Koro: Culture bound or mass hysteria? *Australian & New Zealand J Psychiatry, 45*(8), 683.

Rubin, R. T. (1982). Koro (Shook Yang): A Culture-bound psychogenic syndrome. In C. T. H. Friedmann & R. A. Faguet (Eds.), *Extraordinary disorders of human behavior* (pp. 155–172). Plenum Press.

Sachdev, P. S., & Shukla, A. (1982). Epidemic Koro syndrome in India. *Lancet, ii*, 1161.

Saman, I., Siddiqui, N., & Yosafzai, W. (2007). Koro in a 13 years old boy of interior Sindh—A mistreated cultural syndrome. *Journal of College of Physicians & Surgeons of Pakistan, 17*(1), 60.

Scher, M. (1987). Koro in a native born citizen of the U.S. *International Journal of Social Psychiatry, 33*, 42–45.

Sheeley, W. F. (1991). Mechanism and classification of Koro. *American Journal of Psychiatry, 148*, 959.

Slot, J. A. (1935). Koro in central Celebes. *Geneeskundig Tijdschrift Voor Nederlandsch-Indie, 75*, 811–820.

Srivastava, M., & Pandit, B. (2013). Koro—A case report and review. *International Journal of Physiology, 1*(1), 37–40.

Stein, D. J., Frenkel, M., & Hollander, E. (1991). Classification of Koro. *American Journal of Psychiatry, 148*, 959.

Stip, E., Bergeron, T., Lavigueur, C., Fabian, J. L., & Bentaleb, A. (2007). Koro syndrome. *Medico Psychological Annals, 165*(3), 147–153.

Suwanlert, S., & Coates, D. (1979). Epidemic Koro in Thailand: Clinical and social aspects. *Transcultural Psychiatric Research Review, 16*, 64–66.

Tau, M., & Masukar, A. V. (2020). Koro delusion in mild cognitive impairment due to Alzheimer's disease. *J Neuropsychiatry & Clinical Neuroscience, 32*(2), 204–206.

Tseng, W. S., Mo, M. K., Hsu, J., Li, L. S., Ou, L. W., Chen, G. Q., & Jiang, D. W. (1988). A socio-cultural study of Koro epidemic in Guangdong, China. *American Journal of Psychiatry, 145*, 1538–1543.

Ungvari, G. S., & Mullen, R. S. (1994). Koro: The delusion of penile retraction. *Urology, 43*(6), 883–885.

van Brero, P. C. J. (1896). Naar Aanleiding van het Opstel Over 'Koro' van den Heer J. C. Blonk-in de Voring Aflevering van dit Tijdschrift. *Geneeskunding Tijdschrrift voor Nederlandsch-Indie, 36*, 48–54.

Vorstman, A. H. (1897). 'Koro' in de Westerafdeeling van Borneo. *Geneeskundig Tijdschrift Voor Nederlandsch-Indie, 37*, 499–505.

Walendberg, S. S. A. (1981). Koro. *Canadian Journal of Psychiatry, 26*, 140–141.

Werner, E. T. C. (1961). *A Dictionary of Chinese mythology*. The Julian Press.

Westermeyer, J. (1989). A case of Koro in a refugee family: Association with depression and folie a deux. *The Journal of Clinical Psychiatry, 50*, 181–183.

Wilkinson, R. L. (1932). *A Malay-English dictionary*. Maytilene.

Wilson, S., & Agin, C. (1997). Genital pain associated with genital retraction: A case of Koro syndrome. *Journal of Pain & Symptom Management, 13*(3), 176–178.

Yap, P. M. (1964a). Suk-yeong or Koro: A culture-bound depersonalization syndrome. *Bulletin of the Hong Kong Chinese Medical Association, 16*, 31–47.

Yap, P. M. (1964b). Koro or Suk-yeong : An atypical culture-bound psychiatric disorder found in Southern Chinese. *Transcultural Psychiatric Research Review, 1*, 36–38.

Yap, P. M. (1965a). Koro—A culture-bound depersonalization syndrome. *British Journal of Psychiatry, 111*, 43–50.

Yap, P. M. (1965b). Koro in a Briton. *British Journal of Psychiatry, 111*, 774–775.

Zain, A. A. M., & Subramanian, M. (1991). Sporadic Koro and marital disharmony. *Psychopathology, 24*, 49–52.

2

Perceptual Deviation in Penis Image

A perceptual deviation in the penis image is an important issue in the Koro phenomenon. It is seen during North Bengal Koro epidemic that many patients with sexual dysfunction also reported a defective penile perception regarding its morphology or functional capability. This discussion is mainly on faulty penis image, viz. the apprehension of a "small" or "shortening" of the penis. Some patients may attribute intra-abdominal traction (as in Koro) or to reasons other than abdominal pull (as in some impotence or Dhat patients, in persons with extreme penile preoccupation—hypochondriacal or obsessive) to penile abnormality. Variability in penis-image perception among Koro patients is noteworthy. Chadda and Shome (1991) reported a Koro case with episodic and situational penile shortening—only during micturition and exercise. Wilson and Agin (1997) reported a Koro case who perceives retracting penis and scrotum during different physical activities like walking, driving or sitting, hiking, fishing, and micturition. Manson-Bhar (1954) mentioned different organic conditions as Koro precipitator, viz. edema of the lower abdomen, hernia, hydrocele, and elephantiasis of the scrotum.

A. N. Chowdhury, *Koro*,
https://doi.org/10.1007/978-3-030-87962-4_2

In what follows, the subject matter is grouped under four headings. This discussion would help understand and manage alleged sexual dysfunction (including Koro) from male subjects' cognitive perspective. This understanding was the insight gained from the 1982 North Bengal Koro epidemic and thus briefly summarized under the following four headings:

1. *Penis visibility and Visual Axis*: The penis in adolescent or adult males is a draped private organ that is neither visually exhibited like other body parts nor is there any license to be viewed by others. Body parts like the face, arm, hand, finger, or leg can be seen most of the time by the owner himself and others (the rest of the population). That helps develop a stable organ cognition based on reciprocal feedback, scrutiny, criticism, and suggestions regarding the body part. This fundamental process allows an individual to create a consensus opinion about his body parts, which helps him frame a cognitive map of his exposed parts' attitudes. If he should have feelings of inferiority, query, dissatisfaction, or anxiety regarding a particular body part, these reciprocal interactions will usually neutralize such conflicts. However, the picture vis-à-vis the penis organ is altogether different. Firstly, there is customarily no room for such a discussion by other viewers concerning somebody's penis due to obvious privacy reasons. Secondly, unlike other body parts, an individual cannot compare his penis organ with others. This, therefore, excludes the possibility of the penis being the subject of open, reciprocal, and comparative discourse. Hence the penile cognition remains mostly a private cognition of an individual.

   Teenagers may talk about their penis (es) with peers and friends, many of whom have a penis perception full of fantasy with unhealthy overtones. Such ideas and beliefs are in no way helpful for the development of a healthy penis image. These discussions take place most of the time under the veil of shyness and anxiety in the atmosphere. They always involve an unreal construct of masculine strength, prowess, and myth of sexual morality. So, for these social reasons, anatomical situations, and moral aesthetics, the penis remains under the domain of very private scrutiny rather than be an issue of open social discussion. Those who have had the chance of premarital heterosexual relations may also have the probability of having a debate or an opinion about their penis (es) from their partner (s). Still, if negative, this opinion may make the recipient highly vulnerable and may cast a devastating influence on the individual's masculine image. In most cases, each such premarital heterosexual situation is either experimental merely to test "potency" or pleasure-seeking. The sexual performance is crucial there and not the observation of the penile anatomy. The negative criticism about the penile anatomy may generate a bad penis image accompanied by tormenting anxiety, which may also drag the subject toward sexual dysfunction. A similar situation may evolve from a marital relationship as well. Therefore, it is seen that in a prudish society, hardly any opportunity exists for an interested individual could undertake wherein a healthy discussion on the penis and sexuality in the broad sense. As a result, an individual is primarily dependent on two things—his visual examination (of the penis) followed by the corroboration of his ideas and beliefs. As I remarked earlier, most of these ideas and opinions are culturally framed, having little scientific basis, and are associated with many false and magical sexual myths.

Private penile scrutiny is of two types: one, visual, and two, anatomy-sensory-tactile perception. The visual perception of one's penis is different than that of other body parts. The visual field for other body parts is more comprehensive and frontal, or it can be shifted for better visualization toward a preferential position aligned with the optical axis. This visibility factor is vital for the development of body image. If a body part is not seen, it may be a source of fear and anxiety. A typical example is the face and back of our body. Intense concern about the look as often seen in adolescence or dysmorphophobic subjects (regarding the nose or ear configuration) and their frequent mirror-looking behavior is an example of the repeated visual checking-rechecking aspect of body image. The underlying anxiety is the driving force for seeking cosmetic surgery or the unusual use of decorative soaps or lotions. The "unseen" character of the back is a source of fear, anxiety, and threat of a different dimension. So a sufficient visual clarity is crucial for the process of body/organ image perception. There is a complete option of viewing other body parts like the arm, finger, leg, and front of the trunk. Outer movable body parts can be seen through a full solid angle by shifting the position appropriately aligned with the visual axis by maximizing the vector projection of the optical image of the organ.

In contrast, for viewing the penis, the picture is entirely different because: (1) the anatomical location of the organ itself only permits an oblique view in acute solid angle; (2) fixity of the organ dose prevents its shifting from the standard anatomical position toward the visual axis; and (3) the view from the top in a vertical line of the penis and scrotum allows a very narrow vector projection of the optical image (Fig. 2.1). This anatomic-optical specificity for penis viewing hinders the perception of the penis organ in its dimensional totality. So, usually, there remains a perceptual gap or deficit so far as the details of the size, shape, volume, and general appearance of the penis are concerned. This narrow visual perception does not warrant a complete cognition of the penis image than that for other body parts.

An individual may have variation in penile morphology due to sexual arousal (other than the situation of frank intercourses). In those cases, this change of penis size and shape is merely experienced by anatomic-sensory-tactile perception rather than viewing. So erection mostly remains a matter of sensory-tactile perception compared to the usual visual perception of other body parts.

The penis-image perception that individuals usually have is something like a "go with what you have" type perception or a generalized "working" penile perception. So long as the functional aspect of the penis goes all right, other limitations in the penis image neither surface nor cause any morbid concern about its anatomy. Those who are keen about their penis organ because of some reason (e.g., impotence, sexual conflict, and guilt, or supposed or real sexual organ dysfunction) may show undue penis awareness. They engage themselves in visual scrutiny, which is crucial for such persons because they usually attribute their sexual dysfunction and anxiety to self-alleged anatomic-physiological penis conditions. These conditions ultimately earn a "disease" or "abnormal" character at par with the subject's sexual beliefs and misconceptions. Thus an impotent patient

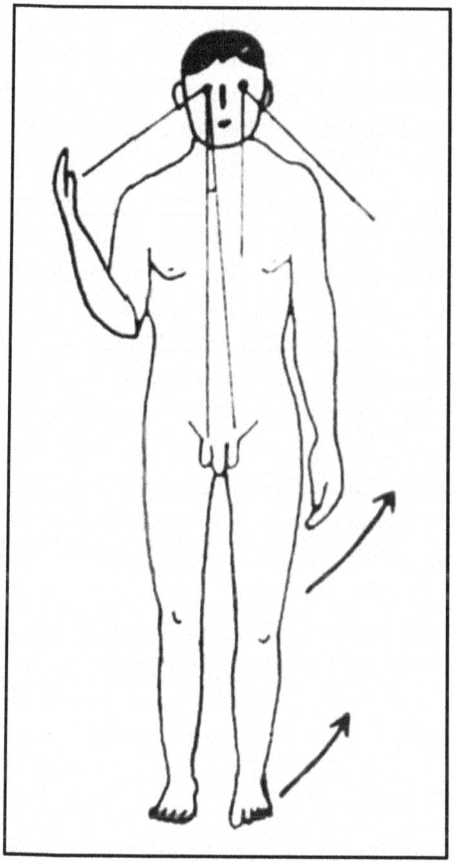

Fig. 2.1 Penis visibility in an acute solid angle: the different frontal variable position of visual axis in which other body parts could be easily aligned

suddenly discovers that his penis is slightly left-titled or the urine flow is not with "enough" expulsive force, or the length of the penis has decreased, etc. Even the cremasteric contractions are viewed with great pathological significance or the "changed palpability" of testicles (hard or soft) carries a definite illness message. These are a few examples where psychosexual anxiety transmits to organ anxiety and makes a firm ground for sexual morbidity. Recently several pieces of research have shown that the SPS (small penis syndrome) (Wylie &

Eardley, 2007) or supposed penile deficiency (Lee & Reiter, 2002; Shamloul, 2005) is quite common in a cohort of men seeking treatment for a short penis. The objective methods of penile size evaluation showed that people harbor false volumetric penile perception despite having a standard penis size. Ghanem et al. (2013) also found similar dysmorphophobic penis perceptions among persons of average size. This pathological or hypersensitive penis awareness and private organ scrutiny are critical primary steps toward the penile symptom-choice in many alleged sexual dysfunctions. The situation, reason, and feeling at the background of this private organ search are decisive because the tendency to attribute sexual misbelieves to the organ is positively correlated. An example may be drawn from the psychopathology of delusional idea where a trivial phenomenon suddenly gains delusional conviction and is interpreted in a new light, "as if the scale had fallen from my eyes" (Slatter & Roth, 1969). Analogously, here also, different penis "abnormalities" is discovered by the individual. Eventually, pathological sexual anxiety will be displaced onto the organ, an organ vital for masculinity's image.

2. *Penile Anatomic-physiological Specificity*: A perception of penile shortening or small penis is a commonly reported clinical finding at urology clinics (Mondaini et al., 2002). The penis has two distinct morphological states: one, the trait penis condition, i.e., the penis during its normal flaccid state, and two, the state penis condition, i.e., the penis during sexual arousal in an extended state. The size and shape of the flaccid penis are not constant or static because many different situations like exposure to cold, fever, and physical exhaustion may cause a shortening of the penis length. The extent of this shortening has no universal standard. Physical conditions like an excessive pad of fat in the lower abdomen or over the pubis region (Buried penis syndrome, Ho & Gelman, 2018) or abdominal swelling as in ascites may cause apparent penile shortening. A similar finding is common in scrotal swelling of orchitis or scrotal filaria (Chowdhury,). Post-masturbation or post-coital penis size is also small because of the obvious reasons for vascular physiology and refractory period (Christ, 1995). There is no standard measurement of this reduction in penis length. The labeling of this shortening as "pathognomonic"

depends entirely on the penile length perception of the individual, i.e., his estimate and bias about penis length, concerning normal and abnormal, influences this observation. As a case in point, an impotent patient suddenly discovers after a bath that his penis is too small, and he attributes his erectile inability to this "organ defect" and consults more than a dozen doctors for two years without any result!

So the smallness or shortening of the flaccid penis generally is not a clinical phenomenon, but it becomes a phenomenon of great significance only when an individual designates his morbid thoughts/cognition on it. In Koro, this cognition believes in a malevolent intra-abdominal pull operative at the penis root (Chowdhury, 1991). So the perception of alteration of penis size and shape is sometimes is entirely a cognitive process. Tonini and Lazzerini (2000) described how the myth of penis size influences many people for a premarital check-up. Why is the "smallness" or "shortening" of the penis a common complaint in penis image disturbances? What is the cognitive clue for this pathoperceptual phenomenon? This concept has a normal cognitive background specific to the penis organ itself. The concept of "smallness" or "shortening" has a standard organ image referential perspective. The size increase of other body parts never contributes to the cognition of smallness. The penis is a dynamic organ having two states: erect and flaccid, and it has a bidirectional morphological character. So the construct of "smallness" or "shortening" is a visuo-sensory reality inherently associated with the penis anatomy and vascular physiology. Scrotum also has this apparent bidirectional volumetric disposition, albeit to a lesser extent. There is no other overt part of the body that has this unique character. So the probability of "smallness" or "shortening" is a natural cognitive component of penis image perception, which retransfers over to the perception of morbidity only in vulnerable subjects. Interestingly, in the context of the Koro epidemic in tapioca plantation workers in Nakhon Ratchasima Province, Indonesia, Keshavan (1983) found the role of suggestible personality with heightened self-scrutiny and over-concern about genitalia as the neurotic background of genital shrinkage symptom genesis. Fernando (1988) reported a Koro case where symptoms were associated with hypochondriacal health concerns of dysmorphophobic nature (asymmetrical body). Joseph (1986) found epileptic body image distortions involving the genitals in two Koro patients. Dantendofer et al. (1996) found Koro symptoms in a case with distinct subcortical and cortical lesions. They thus suggested that the parietal lobe may have some role in body image disturbances, i.e., in Koro perception. Cannabis smoking has been reported to cause depersonalization and penis image distortion and thus generate Koro perception (Chowdhury & Bera, 1994; Earleywine, 2001; Kanwar et al., 2018).

3. *Effect of Cultural Sexual Cognition*: We will now discuss how symptom choice centers on penis perception. Culture influences sexual cognition (both morphology and functional aspect). In this context, one good example is reports of Koro cases from the USA and UK involving immigrant patients (Ang & Weller, 1984; Constable, 1979; Edwards, 1970; Hess & Nassi, 1977). In these situations, the vast difference in the cultural construct of sexuality creates a *cognitive conflict*. The cultural influence on sexual cognition and behavior becomes more predictive in the face of a permissive social environment where sex is more liberal and free mixing is not frowned upon. This is usually very important for those coming in contact with Western culture and of Oriental origin, where sex is generally taboo and has a severe moral overtone. The sexual orientation, heterosexual behavioral custom, and sexual opportunities and exposure in technologically advanced countries are entirely different. This difference may generate some sexual conflict in an individual's sexual behavior in the acculturation process, given the context of his cultural frame of reference. Similar Western (modern)–Oriental (traditional) differential interactions have been reported from other health-related areas also (Sarell & Baider, 1984; Wise & Rosenthal, 1982). As a case in point, a married Indian male had enjoyable sexual contact with a woman ("call girl") during his visit to France. On his return to India, he suffered a failed intercourse at his first attempt with his wife. The subsequent attempts were also unsuccessful. He explained his failures as "I feel deeply guilty because I enjoyed a woman other than my wife, which is an unpardonable sin." A liberal sexual atmosphere, even free access to blue films or pornographic material, may evoke sex guilt

in predisposed individuals (Gerrard & Gibbons, 1982). There are quite a few examples in the literature where Koro precipitated after an encounter with a prostitute (Bernstein & Gaw, 1990; Malinick et al., 1985; Witztum et al., 1998). Interestingly liberalization of sexual social morality and the abundance of sexual outlets in modern Thai society has been implicated in Koro epidemic there (Suwanlert, 1978).

Culture has a significant influence on sexuality at large. Bhurga and Silva (1993) very aptly said: "Sexual behaviour is particularly open to cultural and social influences. Culture affects sexual behaviour, attitudes, and expectations." It is not the place to have a full-length discussion on cultural influence on sex organ perception and its associated myths and beliefs. There are some arbitrary standards of genital shape, size, and features of attractiveness that people held in their minds in every culture. These ideas may influence their perception of normality versus abnormality, both in terms of morphology and functions of sexuality and sexual behavior (Atallah et al., 2016; Stevens, 2015). Socio-cultural influence on penis perception is well documented (Sharp & Oates, 2019). One good example at this point: Salama (2016), in the anthropometric study of penile dimensions among Egyptian men, stated that:

> Since the early medieval times, the Arabic literature emphasizes that penis size is "a sign of honor" and that "a longer penis is preferred." This idea is still imbedded in the minds of many Arabic men. These men believe that good reproductive and sexual function accompanied by the ability to gratify themselves and their partners is associated with a larger penis size. These men also usually look at the penis as an identifier of masculinity.... In Arabic nations, and according to Islamic themes, the loss of one's penis is comparable to losing one's soul and life (Al-Khamees, 2003; Al-Zoaimel, 2012) in what is called *di-ya*, an Arabic word that means the obligatory money paid for crimes involving the loss of life or damage of one's body organs and function. This matching between loss of one's penis and life may indicate to which degree a penile image occupies a big area in the mind of any Arabic man. (p. 220)

Sex guilt has two components: (a) Subjective—psychological, i.e., conflicts, anxiety, depression, self-reproach, and (b) Objective—organic, i.e., concern with the sexual body part, viz. penis and often with scrotum. In many instances, extreme organ awareness thus generated or prompts the individual to check and recheck the sexual organ anatomy and physiology. Several Koro case reports showed that sex guilt after prostitute visits paved the way for Koro perception (Al-Hmoud, 1999; Ntouros et al., 2010; Witztum et al., 1998). This heightened responsiveness at the background of private scrutiny of sex organs paves the way to develop a dysmorphophobic perception (Devis et al., 2012; Silva et al., 2016) accompanied by functional morbidity according to his sexual-cultural cognitive status. A prevalent example in this area is the venerophobia (Oates & Gomez, 1984). There are reports of sex guilt over masturbatory habits or even viewing pornographic material in Koro cases (Khubalkar & Gupta, 1984). So, in every case with subjective penile pathology, the detailed psychosexual history, the evaluation of the sexual-behavioral profile, and the sexual, cultural beliefs may help identify the very morbid penile perception genesis.

4. *Management*: The management of such cases involves carefully eliciting and exploring the history with special stress on the onset point. Questions like how he discovered the defect or abnormality, what difficulty prompted him to visual penile scrutiny etc., have to be asked. If necessary, referral to medical or urological clinics should be done. If no associated organic abnormality is found, then a few cognitive psychotherapy sessions, quite educative in nature (explaining anatomy and physiology of genital organs in a simple language), should be instituted to correct his false perception of penis image. A participatory drawing on the alleged issue may often be helpful. Recently there are many such cases attend adolescent sex-clinics. These patients always have significant false perceptions and health anxiety (Wylie & Eardley, 2007). Hence, in some, anxiolytic medication will be helpful. Depression, reactive in nature, is a ubiquitous accompaniment. Antidepressants in moderate dosage will also be beneficial. All these cases should have a clinical threshold for anxiety or depressive disorder diagnosis. Many patients often crave

vitamin "tonics" or tablets as they believe that these medications will help them revive their "masculine energy." (Many commercial companies produce tonics/tablets/capsules by exploiting and capitalizing this "sexual cognition"!). Judicious prescription of B-Vitamins with appropriate psychotherapy may enhance treatment compliance in some cases. Some patients may express particular faith in specific food items to regain "masculine strength," e.g., meat, egg, etc. These dietary items may well be included in the diet prescription if helpful. The treatment success lies in the skillful exploration of the patient's explanatory framework and utilization of cognitive clues, anxiety reduction, scientific information, and an empathic doctor–patient relationship.

References

AI-Hmoud, N. (1999). Koro-like syndrome in a Jordanian male. *Eastern Mediterranean Health Journal, 5*, 611–613.

Al-Khamees, A. (2003, August 26). *Muslim di-ya assessment in Saudi Ryal*. https://uqu.edu.sa/majalat/shariaramag/mag27/pdf/doc09.pdf

Al-Zoaimel, B. (2012, September 30). *Medical Sharia*. https://www.aleqt.com/2012/09/30/article_697441.html

Ang, P. C., & Weller, M. P. I. (1984). Koro and psychosis. *British Journal of Psychiatry, 145*, 335.

Atallah, S., Crista, J. A., Talli, R., Carmita, A., Byers, E. S., Cynthia, G., Nobre, P., Wylie, K., & Brotto, L. (2016). Ethical and sociocultural aspects of sexual function and dysfunction in both sexes. *Journal of Sexual Medicine, 13*, 591–606.

Berntein, R. L., & Gaw, A. C. (1990). Koro: Proposed classification for DSM-IV. *American Journal of Psychiatry, 147*, 1670–1674.

BhugraD, S. P. D. (1993). Sexual dysfunction across cultures. *International Review of Psychiatry, 5*(2–3), 243–252.

Chadda, R. K., & Shome, S. (1991). Koro classification and case reports. *American Journal of Psychiatry, 148*(12), 1766–1767.

Chowdhury, A. N. (1989). Dysmorphic penis image perception - The root of Koro vulnerability. *Acta Psychiatrica Scandinavica, 80*, 518–520.

Chowdhury, A. N. (1989). Draw-a-penis test (DAPT). *Journal of Personality & Clinical Studies, 5*, 97–100.

Chowdhury, A. N. (1991). Penis root perception of Koro patients. *Acta Psychiatrica Scandinavica, 84*, 12–13.

Chowdhury, A. N., & Bera, N. K. (1994). Koro following cannabis smoking. *Addiction, 89*, 1017–1020.

Christ, G. J. (1995). The penis as a vascular organ. The importance of corporal smooth muscle tone in the control of erection. *Urologic Clinics North America, 22*, 727–745.

Constable, P. L. (1979). Koro in Hertfordshire. *Lancet, 1*, 163.

Dantendorfer, K., Amering, M., Prayer, D., Maierhofer, D., Schnider, P., & Katschnig, H. (1996). Treatment of Koro and panic attacks after stroke. *Anxiety, 2*(1), 53–55.

Devis, D. M., Stever, A. M., Terwilliger, J. M., Williams, M. T. (2012). The relationship between the culture-bound syndrome Koro and obsessive-compulsive disorder. In G. R. Hayes & M. H.Bryant (Eds.), *Psychology of culture* (pp. 213–221). Nova Science Publisher Inc.

Earleywine, M. (2001). Cannabis induced Koro in Americans. *Addiction, 96*(11), 1663–1666.

Edwards, J. G. (1970). The Koro pattern of depersonalization in an American schizophrenic patient. *American Journal of Psychiatry, 126*, 1171–1173.

Fernando, N. (1988). Monosymptomatic hypochondriasis treated with a tricyclic antidepressant. *British Journal of Psychiatry, 152*, 851–852.

Gerrard, M., & Gibbons, F. X. (1982). Sexual experience, sex guilt and sexual moral reasoning. *Journal of Personality, 50*, 345–349.

Ghanem, H., Glina, S., Assalian, P., & Buvat, J. (2013). Position paper: Management of men complaining of a small penis despite an actually normal size. *Journal of Sexual Medicine, 10*, 294–303.

Hess, J. P., & Nassi, G. (1977). Koro in a Yemenite and a Georgian Jewish immigrant. *Confinia Psychiatrica, 20*, 180–184.

Ho, T. S., & Gelman, J. (2018). Evaluation and management of adult acquired buried penis. *Translational Andrology & Urology, 7*(4), 618–627.

Joseph, A. B. (1986). Koro: Computed tomography and brain electrical activity mapping in two patients. *Journal of Clinical Psychiatry, 47*, 430–432.

Kanwar, P., Kumar, R., & Sharma, C. (2018). Cannabis induced koro in a Nepali migrant. *Asian Journal of Psychiatry, 31*, 56–87.

Keshavan, M. S. (1983). Epidemic psychosis or epidemic Koro? *British Journal of Psychiatry, 142*, 100–101.

Khubalkar, R., & Gupta, O. P. (1984). Psychodynamics of Koro (case report). *Indian Journal of Psychiatry, 26*, 180–181.
Lee, P. A., & Reiter, E. O. (2002). Genital size: A common adolescent male concern. *Adolescent Medicine, 13*(1), 171–180.
Malinick, C., Flaherty, J. A., & Jobe, T. (1985). Koro: How culturally specific? *International Journal of Social Psychiatry, 31*, 67–63.
Manson-Bhar, P. H. (1954). Kuru, Latah, Running Amok and Koro. In *Tropical diseases- A manual of the diseases of the warm climate*. Cassell & Company Ltd.
Mondaini, N., Ponchietti, R., Gontero, P., Muir, G. H., Natali, A., Caldarera, E., Biscioni, S., & Rizzo, M. (2002). Penile length is normal in most men seeking penile lengthening procedures. *International Journal of Impotence Research, 14*(4), 283–286.
Ntouros, E., Ntoumanis, A., Bozikas, V. P., Donias, S., Giouzepas, I., Garyfalos, G. (2010, March 15). Koro-like symptoms in two Greek men. *BMJ case report*. https://doi.org/10.1136/bcr.08.2008.0679
Oates, J. K., & Gomez, J. (1984). Venereophobia. *British Journal of Hospital Medicine, 31*, 435–436.
Salama, N. (2016). Consultation for small-sized penis in the Egyptian male: A case control study. *American Journal of Men's Health, 10*(3), 220–227.
Sarell, M., & Baider, L. (1984). The effects of cultural background on communication patterns of Israeli cancer patients. *Psychopathology, 17*, 17–23.
Shamloul, R. (2005). Treatment of men complaining of short penis. *Urology, 65*(6), 1183–1185.
Sharp, G., & Oates, J. (2019). Sociocultural influences on men's penis size perception and decisions to undergo penile augmentation: A qualitative study. *Aesthetic Surgery Journal, 39*(11), 1253–1259.
Silva, L., Rapso-Lima, C., Soares, C., Cerqueira, J. J., Morgado, P. (2016). Koro syndrome in an obsessive compulsive disorder. *European Psychiatry, 33*, Suppl. S618.
Slater, E., & Roth, M. (1969). *Clinical p* (3rd ed.). Bailliere, Tindall & Cassell.
Stevens, P. Jr (2015). Culture and sexuality. In *The international encyclopedia of human sexuality* (pp. 1–8). Wiley.
Suwanlert, S. (1978). Thai cultural concepts related to koro syndrome. *Journal of Psychiatric Association of Thailand, 23*(3), 261–275.
Tonini, G., & Lazzerini, M. (2000). The adolescent and sexual dysfunction: Real or imagined. *Minerva Pediatrica, 52*(10), 593–601.

Wilson, S., & Agin, C. (1997). Genital pain associated with genital retraction: A case of Koro syndrome. *Journal of Pain & Symptom Management, 13*(3), 176–178.

Wise, T. N., & Rosenthal, J. B. (1982). Depression, illness beliefs and severity of illness. *Journal of Psychological Research, 26*, 247–253.

Witztum, E., Bersudsky, Y., Mayodovnik, H., & Kotler, M. (1998). Koro-like syndrome in a Bedouin man. *Psychopathology, 31*(4), 174–177.

Wylie, K. R., & Eardley, I. (2007). Penile size and the 'small penis syndrome.' *BJU International, 99*(6), 1449–1455.

Part II

Historical Perspective

3

Culture-Boundness of Koro: Yin-Yang Dualism and Sexuality in Chinese Culture—A Psycho-Historical Note

Suo-Yang: A Millennium-Old Traditional Belief

The concept of *Suo-yang* or genital retraction as severe sexual morbidity has its origin in the century-old Chinese Taoist medical philosophy. The idea and the clinical presentation of genital retraction illness have been documented under various names in many of the ancient Chinese medical texts: like *yin-yan transposition; yin type fever; yin yang yih;* and *Kaih She Shang Han.* It is presumed that this concept of genital morbidity, as depicted in traditional Chinese philosophy and medical classics, heavily influenced the Chinese social cognition of sexuality, which is still operative today. It is believed that in due course of time, the illness has been transported by the migrant Chinese to certain adjoining geographical regions, namely Indonesia and other Southeast Asian countries.

This analysis very interestingly shows a highly sensitive cultural matrix in Chinese society insofar as male sexuality is concerned. The theme of male–female sexual union, male potency, semen value, and interrelation between the sexual act and disability/death is elaborately described in most accounts. The female role is also remarkably compromised. Various

A. N. Chowdhury, *Koro*,
https://doi.org/10.1007/978-3-030-87962-4_3

sexual myths, folklores, and symbols are abundant, depicting mainly a negative aspect of sexuality in general. This cultural reference probably has a deep link with male sexual anxiety in Chinese society, hence the concept of dreadful genital retraction morbidity, often mortality (Chowdhury, 1995).

Taoism (also known as Daoism) is both a philosophy and a religion attributed to the semi-legendary figure Lao Tzu (? 500 BCE or 480–390 B.C.). Tao or "the way" or "teaching" indicates Taoism's inherent aim, the most influential and original Chinese religion system, philosophy, and inner alchemy that strongly influenced the Chinese culture and various social customs. Taoism has two major divisions. *Tao-Chia,* represents the philosophical and mystical branch, and the other, *Tao-chiao*, is the more religious, magical, and alchemical one. *Tao-chia* is based on the classical texts of *Tao-te ching* of Lao Tzu. Lao-tzu, meaning "old master," was a Chinese sage who was an archive-keeper in the royal court of king Zhous in his early life. He wrote "Tao-te Ching," an introductory text of Taoism. *Tao-Chiao* combined the Taoist doctrines with the existing Chinese alchemy schools (350–250 B.C.) and taught the philosophy of immortality, breathing exercises, and yogic and sexual practices like *fang-chung shu* in the text, titled *Huang-t'intg Ching* or "The Classic Treatise of the Yellow Castle."

The theoretical system of Chinese philosophy and medicine is based primarily on the concept of *yin* and *yang*, the theory of five elements, and the construct of eternal correspondence between the microcosm and the macrocosm. These interactions constitute the physical universe in Chinese "Wu Xing." The construct of yin-yang indicates the function and relationship of these aspects as part of a continuous transformation process and change in the universe (Lozano, 2014). Two complementary systems maintain balance and harmony: the supportive (the generating cycle) and the negative (the controlling cycle). When applied to medicine, the human body, like the universe, is composed of positive and negative forces that confront and complement each other. Each of the five elements is associated with Yin or Yang organ of the body. This duality of positive–negative interconnections and interactions is thought to be operative in the human body's structural anatomy and functional physiology and the symptom manifestations of illness and their treatments. Health has equated a perfect balance in harmony between yin and yang, while illness is perceived as an imbalance (Read, 1926).

The Five Elements theory proposes that all the human body elements as also of nature belong to one of the five categories, viz. wood, fire, earth, metal, and water. Each of these elements, as a concept, represents a specific bodily structure and function. The human body's corresponding visceral components are the liver, heart, spleen, lungs, and kidneys; the emotions are anger, joy, worry, sorrow, and fear; while the five natural conditions are wind, heat, humidity, dryness, and cold. The Five Elements theory attempts to view the natural world and the human body to express individual orderly relationships among these elements. For example, wood creates fire, and fire creates the earth, earth creates metal, metal creates water, water creates wood (Tseng, 1973). Concurrently, there is an antagonism between fire and metal, metal and wood, between wood and earth, and between earth and water.

The idea of continuous intercommunication between the microcosm and the macrocosm holds that nature's principles govern human beings. Like the four seasons and five elements (cold, heat, dryness, humidity, and wind) change in nature, so also there is a change in the five viscera and five spirits (five emotions—joy, anger, worry, sorrow, and fear) in the human body. An eternal cosmic communication or influence is advocated between body and nature. The general advice for maintaining good health and long life is to keep the yin and yang in a perfect, orderly balance in the habits of food taking, living, and sexual practices. This balance under the harmonious mutual relations with the five elements and nature keeps things going in excellent form and functioning.

Sexual Dualism: In Chinese tradition, the metaphysical dyad is characterized by the *yang* and *yin*, which are understood as elementary determinations and real forces acting on every plane of being. This yang-yin duality considers that both men and women represent the omnipotent dualism permeating everything of this universe. The yang and yin's inherent dualism and positive–negative or active–passive principles are represented and counted in all cultural-ethical customs of sexuality and its related health practices.

As a symbol of determination, *yang* has Sky's nature and everything active, positive, and male. In contrast, *yin* has the character of Earth, and everything passive, negative, and female. In graphic symbolism, a continuous line corresponds to *yang*_____ whereas a broken line corresponds to *yin*____ ____, indicating the idea of the "two." The trigrams and hexagrams formed with various combinations of those two elementary signs are given by the ***I. Ching***, the Chinese tradition's fundamental text. The inherent forces in yin and yang philosophy direct and govern the different social roles of men and women and the structure and function of male and female sex organs (Ruan, 1991a).

All phenomena, forms, beings, and changes of the universe are considered at the level of various counteractions and combinations of the yin and yang. From their dynamic aspect, yang and yin are opposed and complementary (Maciocia, 2005). The light and the sun have a yang quality, whereas the shadow and the moon have a yin quality. Fire is yang; the waters are yin; mountain tops are yang, the plains are yin; the spirit is yang, the soul and vital force are yin, the pure is yang, the unfathomable is yin, and so on (Fig. 3.1). One such symbolism is the *yun-yu* or "Clouds Rain." The Chinese literary expression for the sexual act (Gulik, 1961). Clouds here are associated with female live juices or vaginal secretions and the rain to male semen. The predominance of yin in women and of yang in men makes them what they are: at this level, the pure yin and pure yang appear as the substances of absolute womanhood and absolute manhood, respectively.

It is worth noting at this point that the attribution of cold, wet, and dark qualities to yin while the dry, clear, and light qualities to yang, both of which play a role in the philosophical world view and sexual symbolism:

> To the *yin*, therefore, belongs shadows and the darkness with regard to elementary powers prior to form, which correspond in the human being to the unconscious and to the vital, nocturnal part of his psyche, … the day is equivalent to the clear, light ("sunny") quality of the *yang*, which is the very quality proper to manifested, definite, and completed forms that are released from the equivocal darkness and form the indeterminate

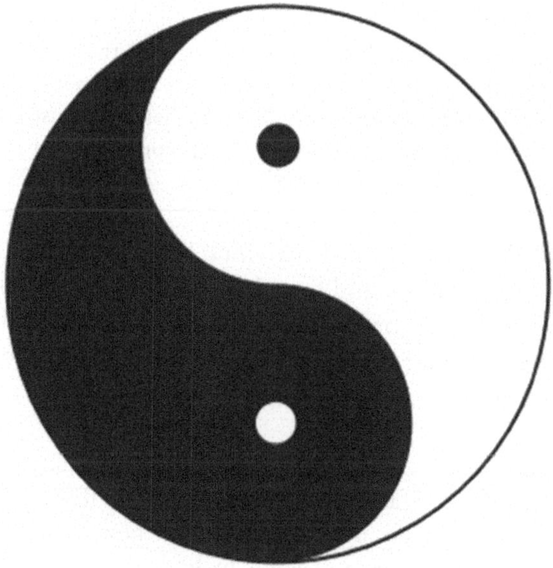

Fig. 3.1 Yin-Yang symbol. *White* is Yang (representing Light or Bright Sun; Strong/Assertive; Dry/Hot/Fire; Male; Positive Charge; Heaven; Spring and Summer) and *Black* is Yin (representing Dark/Moon; Recessive/ Nurturing; Damp/Cool/Water; Female; Negative Charge; Earth; Autumn and Winter [https://en.wikipedia.org/wiki/File:Black_and_White_Yin_Yang_Symbol.png])

> nature of the generative womb and female substance or raw material. (Evola, 1991, p. 121)

This dualism is connected with the ancient social system as reflected in the general belief of "web of Heaven and Earth." That relates to the sexual duties of the Emperor toward his subjects. Guilk (1961) discusses that the Emperor has to or should balance the forces of Heaven (Yang) and Earth (Yin) for the prosperity of his subjects. Camphausen (1991) states this social or community aspect of "sexual duty" as follows:

> That balance, which to the farmers expressed itself in plentiful livestock, abundant harvest, and general conditions such as good weather and the absence of war and other disasters, had to be achieved through the emperor's rituals of sexual union with the empress and with a number

> of other women available for this purpose; Gulik mentions a number of 120. If something nonetheless went wrong and the Emperor seemed unable to keep the forces of Heaven and Earth in harmony, the farming families of villages and countryside came to help. An auspicious night would be chosen, and hundreds of men and women would meet in the fields in a general orgy under the open sky. (p. 207)

Heterosexual Practices: Sexual activities between males and females have profound implications and meaning concerning maintaining health and equilibrium of body or life forces. Kohn (2011) provides the basic principles of male–female union In terms of circulation of sexual energy, a significant form of *qi*, also known as "essence" or *jing*:

> Essence is the key to vitality and health; it easily diminishes through sexual engagements. As a result, Chinese medicine focuses on how to conserve the stock people have originally and how to replenish what is lost. The first- conservation – tends to focus on times and frequencies of intercourse as well as on message techniques that keep the *qi* flowing……The second replenishing – concentrates on the "return" or "reversion" of essence into *qi* with the help of both partner and meditative practices. (p. 13)

Semen Value: Semen is viewed in Taoism as a vital energy source, i.e., *Ching* and/or *Ching-ch'i*, a term used to mean sperm/semen or sexual energy or both ovarian and spermatic sources of energy (Rawson & Legeza, 1973). Taoism emphasizes the loss of this vital energy during male ejaculation because death may ensue once the *ching* energy is used up. So the male should replenish his *Ching* and store it by absorbing as much female yin energy as possible.

Huan-ch'ing Pu-nao is a technical term that means "letting the semen return and strengthen the brain" (Harper, 1987). It describes the method for preserving *Ching* energy as follows: just before ejaculation, the man's penis is sealed off by finger pressure from either partner. With a deep exhalation of breath and grinding of teeth, the *Ching* (semen/energy) is directed upward toward the highest *tan-t'ien* in the brain. It mixes up with the vital energy *ch'i* and offers the individuals a rejuvenating force for immortality (Camphausen, 1991). *Emerald Pillow* is the Chinese technical term for the cranial pump in the brain, storing the sexual energy or *Ching-ch'i*.

Fang-Chung Shu is a Taoist sexual exercise practiced by men to extract women's energy, especially of virgins, to accumulate more energy for his benefit—a practice akin to sexual vampirism. P'eng Tsu, a legendary Chinese sage, is reported: "to have lived more than nine hundred Years" (Levi & Ishihara, 1989) by this method of retention of semen.

Ho-Ch'i is the name of the recurring communal sexual ritual held in ancient China, beginning with the Han dynasty's time, at each new and full moon. These collective sexual orgies were mainly practiced by the adepts of religious Taoism known as the "Way of Supreme Peace" and "Five Peaks of Rice Taoism" until the Sung dynasty. This mass sexual celebration aimed to have intercourse with as many partners as possible to increase sexual energy to achieve immorality (Camphausen, 1991).

Yellow Emperor, the last of the three legendary Chinese emperors, who by name was known as Emperor Huang Ti (2697–2598 BC), is one glorious example who attained immortality by absorbing yin essences of twelve hundred women! It is believed that three legendary females—"Three Lady Immortals"—taught the Emperor the Taoist teachings of sexual yoga or *ho-Chi*. These ladies were Su-nu, the simple girl; Hsuan-nu, the mysterious girl; and Ts'ai-nu, the fancy girl (Blofeld, 1982).

It would be helpful if we have a basic idea about the timeline of different Chinese Dynasties. The following table provides a rough guide about this timeline.

Timeline of Chinese history and dynasties

Ancient period: Archaic Neolithic period	
10,000–2,000 BCE	Neolithic cultures
2,100–1600 BCE	**Xia (Hsia) Dynasty**: First prehistoric dynasty that marked an evolutionary phase between the late Neolithic culture and the Chinese urban culture of the Shang dynasty
1600–1050 BCE	**Shang Dynasty**: Oracle bone writing, Chinese writing develops. Silk weaving is invented, Bronze technology, Use of horse-drawn chariots

(continued)

(continued)

1056–256 BCE	**Zhou (Chou) Dynasty:** Iron casting was invented, large-scale irrigation was introduced, Confucius (551–479 BCE) lived 771- 476 BCE is known as the "Spring and Autumn Period" as per the name of a State (Lu) Chronicle with a traditional association with Confucius
Imperial period	
221–206 BCE	**Qin (Ch'in) Dynasty:** Centralized administration, strict law codes and tax system introduced, standardization of writing script, weights, and measures, the building of the Great Wall began
206 BCE–AD 220	**Han Dynasty:** Buddhism was brought from India; the paper was invented
581–618 AD	**Sui Dynasty:** Great transportation network was built, Gunpowder was invented
618–906 AD	**Tang Dynasty:** Golden age of art and learning, the height of Buddhist influence, and silk-route trade
960–1279 AD	**Song Dynasty:** Age of high culture- printing, poetry, calligraphy, paper money, growth of commerce, and trade
1279–1368 AD	**Yuan Dynasty:** Founded by the Mongols, Beijing was made the capital, visit of Marco Polo (1271–1295 AD)
1368–1644 AD	**Ming Dynasty:** European trade begins, Great Wall was extended
1644–1912 A.D	**Qing (Ch'ing) Dynasty:** Manchu invasion and dynasty
Modern period	
1912–1949 A.D	**Republic period:** Collapse of the dynastic system, domestic revolution
1949 A.D	**People's Republic of China** – PRC was formed (1.10.49)

Adopted from Storozum et al. (2017) and Shih (2017)

Genital Retraction Illness in Chinese Medical Classics

Genital retraction syndrome or Shook Yang was known among the ethnic Chinese because of its multiple references in the Chinese medical texts since ancient times. Following is a brief account of these earliest references of genital retraction.

Nei Ching (Yellow Emperor's Classic of Internal Medicine) is one of the earliest Chinese medical texts of the Pre-Ch'in period (written between 476 and 221 BC) (Veith, 1966). It is believed that this classic was written by Huang Ti, the third legendary emperor of China, though historians hold differing opinions. This book is divided into *su-Wen* (Elementary Questions or treatise on theory) and *Ling Shu* (Ingenious Pivot or treatise on practice). In this book, a reference is made to the shrinking of the penis and spasm of muscles. Nei Ching cosmology and medicine advocated the dual power and interactions between yin and yang. Yin literally means "shady side of the hill" and Yang—"the sunny side of the hill." Men and women have yin and yang, and their good health depends on the yin-yang balance. Sexual excess is one crucial factor that disrupts this balance and may lead to genital retraction or Koro (Leng, 1971). Nei Ching reported genital retraction due to other diseases also (e.g., illness due to cold). (Veith, 1966). Gwee (1968) referred to a translation from the second volume of Nei Ching as follows:

> LIN -CHI ON BASIC ANIMUS: In the case of the liver, grief moves the innermost self and causes harm to the animus. When the animus is injured, the result is madness, amnesia, and lack of sperm. Without sperm, a person will not be well, and the manifestation is one of retraction of genitals with spasm of muscles, the bones of the chest are depressed, and the hair colour poor. Death usually occurs in Autumn. (p. 6)

Zhang Zhong-Jing, a physician of the Han period (206 BC–220 AD) in his book Treatise on Diseases caused by the Cold, wrote that "the penis twisting upon itself…there is shrinkage of the scrotum and coldness of the extremities" (Ng & Kua, 1996).

The five dynasty period was extended from 265 to 960 A.D. The Chin, Sui, and T'ang periods were prominent among them, insofar as their influence on the medical theories and practices is concerned. During the Chin Dynasty, Taoism's rise and in the T'ing dynasty, Buddhism's introduction were notable features. Religious influence in terms of ghost-evil or ghost-bewitched phenomena was noted in mental ill-health conceptualization. The Sui period's well-known book "Treatise on Symptoms of Various illnesses," was written by Chow Yen-Fen. It contains Taoist ideas along with the Yin-Yang theories. In Chapter 10, the genital retraction is described as an aftermath of intercourse in a feverish state.

During the Yuan Dynasty, Chinese medicine was divided into several schools based on treatment principles they adopted to cure illness. A renowned medical school was established by "Four Famous Doctors of Chin Yuan." The concept of the heat-cold theory of disease made its appearance in the text, only during this time. For example, Lu Wan-su believed that diseases were caused by excessive heat in the body, and he advocated using cooling drugs (T'ao et al., 1962).

The Ming Ching period (1368 to 1912 A.D.) was marked with increased recognition and systemic mental disorders classification. Different types of insanities, e.g., excited insanity, stupid insanity, flower insanity, etc., are described in the "Standards for Diagnosis and Treatment" by Wang K'en-t'ang, a notable physician of the early part of this time. The famous medical text, Chin-Yue's Medical Book, contains an elaborate discussion on hysterical neurosis and malingering (Chen, 1937). Interestingly, the psychosexual aspect of sexual impotence is discussed. It was considered the result of emotional disturbances from excessive worry, frustration, depression, and fear or extramarital sexual desire and indulgence in excessive intercourse. Semen is thought to be the essence of energy. Its expulsion causes disability due to the loss of vital life. Nocturnal ejaculation is considered the result of poor mental control over sexual desire (Tseng, 1973). Chang Chi endorsed the clinical entity of genital retraction, and the treatment advocated was the ash produced by the burning of undergarments of the opposite sex (Gwee, 1968). The traditional Chinese medical system of acupuncture relates the genital retraction illness to the middle female meridian (Fig. 3.2), extending to the lower limb's inner side to the genitalia and then to the abdomen's ipsilateral side to the chest (Gwee, 1968). This meridian is governed by the liver, which is believed to be susceptible to emotions like worry, fear, and anger.

In the recent century, the traditional Chinese medical people related Shook Yang or genital retraction illness to the text "New Collection of Remedies of Value," written by Pao Sian-Ow in 1834 (Gwee, 1968). This book describes this disorder's causes and symptoms, including the female manifestations (nipple retraction). This is regarded as a severe medical emergency needing immediate intervention.

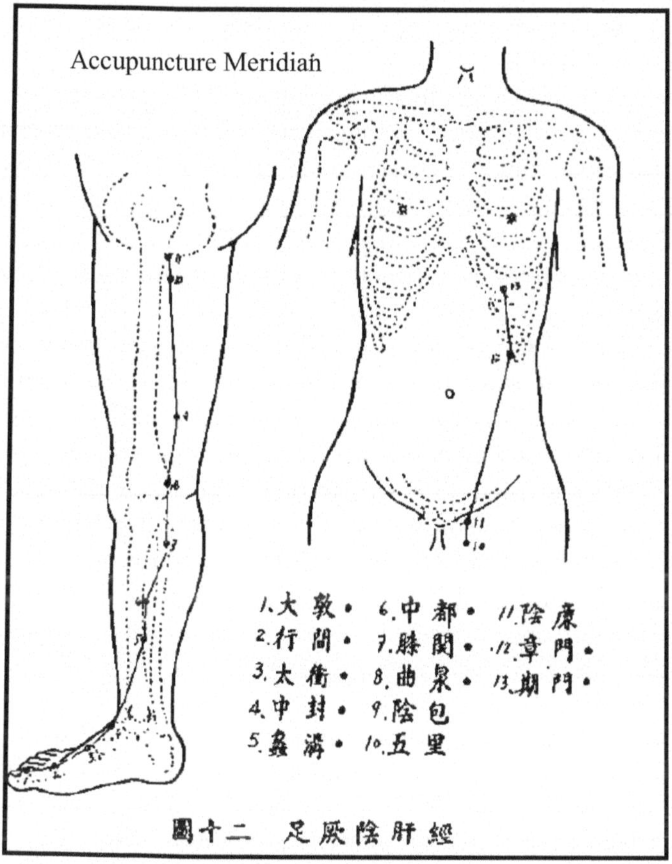

Fig. 3.2 Female meridian (Adopted from Gwee [1968], p. 3)

Disability/Death and Sexuality: A host of precautions and illness potentials are connected with the sexual union between the sexes, so much so that sexual intercourse was perceived in the traditional interpersonal customs of the Chinese society as a very delicate and balance act that has to maintain with specific strictly set up rules, the violation of which may result in grave consequences, even death. In the Taoist handbook on sex, the term *Yin-tao* ("Hidden way") designates sexual intercourse. Taoism lays down the principle that sex may be harmful to those who do not have the requisite knowledge to use sex for spiritual attainment and health.

Henry Maspero (1937), in the section on "The processes of union of yin and yang to nourish the vital principle" discussed several rules relating to sexual union between male and female. The stress is to preserve the Essence—*tsing*. There are many guiding rules relating to time and place of sexual act, some seven prohibitions, and why frequent changing of a partner is essential to obtain "Eternal Life," etc., are described.

In traditional Chinese erotic beliefs and practices, many negative connotations are attached to sexual intercourse. There are a handful of examples concerning the association of various disabilities/illnesses with the act of coitus, even death. It is said that one of the Chinese Emperors died of sook yang (Meth, 1974). Fainting is one such example that is variously related to intercourse, e.g., fainting at the beginning of coitus or "mounting horse wind," fainting at the end of coitus or "dismounting horse wind," or fainting due to profuse and uncontrollable discharge of semen—"incontinence of semen." The account of the management of one such condition is given by Wong (1918):

> The woman should on no account disconnect at once and scream for help. She should retain her presence of mind, clasping the patient tightly in her arms. With a hairpin a puncture should be made on the sacrum. Moxa may be restored to if the puncture proves ineffective.
>
> Dissipated young men, or an old man with a young wife, are said to be especially liable to these attacks. When husband and wife meet again after a long separation incontinence of semen is common. In story books we often read of such cases brought before the court, the woman being charged with murder. (p. 29)

In this context, it is relevant that the Cantonese colloquial term of Koro—"Seon-Ma Fuun" means a "seizure of vapour during the act of mounting a horse," i.e., sexual activity (Gwee, 1963). All the pathological states mentioned above are acute and call for emergency intervention.

Wong (1918) inquired into some common beliefs in sexual diseases in Chinese society and noted a profound influence of the traditional Chinese medical philosophy on the masses' disease cognition. He stated that since ancient times, "sexual intemperance has been regarded as the primary cause of a host of diseases." Sex is so highly pinpointed in Chinese society that "whenever a newly married couple got sick, sexual carelessness is at once set down as the cause." Wong (1918) cites a common illness called *Kiah She Sangh Han*, an acute febrile episode characterized by headache, giddiness, back pain, abdominal colic, retraction of testicles in men and contraction of a nipple in women. It is caused by sexual carelessness or catching a cold, or taking cold food, especially melons or ice cream, immediately after sexual intercourse. Treatment includes hot fomentations (hot, hard-boiled eggs, heated bricks, mud cakes made with urine, roasted garlic, onions or pepper, bottles of hot water, etc.) and medicinal decoctions: ginger, ginseng, aconite, cassia, and cloves.

Yin yang Yih or "male and female exchange" disease is another example that states that if sexual intercourse takes place immediately after recovery from fever (typhoid), the inherent poison would be transmitted to the recovery, then a relapse occurs. This is known as "female relapse." This is considered to be a severe pathology with symptoms like violent colic, retraction of the testicles, and protrusion of the tongue. The popular prescription for remedy consists of an infusion of the root of allium odorum and rat excreta. A woman's fingers and toenails or undergarments are also used for treatment (Wong, 1918).

Death associated with intercourse is an essential theme in many of the Chinese traditional teachings and folktales. Gwee (1968) thus states, "In novels, and folklores, sexual intercourse is regarded as an activity which when improperly conducted, or when indulged in under the wrong set of circumstances, can lead to sudden death, accompanied, or preceded, in many instances by the retraction of penis." Yap (1965a) also noted a high amount of sexual guilt relating to masturbation and nocturnal emission among Chinese Koro patients. Yap traced the humoral theory of yin and yang, which usually maintains a harmonious equilibrium of male (yang) and female (yin) principles. It is believed that during regular intercourse, a healthy exchange of yang and yin humors takes place. But with masturbation and nocturnal emission, this cannot occur, and this unbalanced loss of the yang humor produces Koro.

A sudden catastrophe with the act of intercourse in the form of Shook Yang is termed as "Yin type of cold affliction" and is mentioned in the book "New Collection of remedies of Value" of the Chin period as follows (Gwee, 1963):

> During intercourse, the man may be seized with acute abdominal pain. The limbs become cold and the complexion dusky, the penis retracts into the abdomen. The disease is due to the invasion of cold vapours and the treatment is to employ the 'heaty' drugs. (p. 120)

Gwee (1968) noted a similar belief of genital retraction and death in the Philippines, where genital shrinkage is known as "*Bangutot*." During intercourse, sudden death from penile retraction is also a traditional belief in Singapore and Malaysia (Gwee, 1963). Gwee (1963) traced the necropsy findings of four such postmortem reports of coital death in Singapore and found coronary thrombosis (in three) and cerebral haemorrhage (in one) as the cause of death—not any penile retraction! Edwards (1984) tried to determine the possible cultural clue of this perception of genital retraction as a prodrome of death in China and noted some biophysical changes of penile morphology of left-open corpse's funerary practices of Chinese customs.

All these accounts show that unusual morbid stress has been imparted to the usual act of intercourse, which probably makes people extraordinarily sensitive (and fearful) regarding sexuality, especially about the trivial morphological genital changes of nonclinical significance. The high sensitivity in sexual health creates a mass cognitive facilitative social platform, where any abnormality will quickly gain a supposed sexual etiology. Through the ages, this construct has gained a cultural reality and guided people's behavior accordingly. Wong (1918) thus comments:

> It used to be the custom to impute everything to sexual excess: a death whose cause was not clearly discernible was attributed to sexual excess; of someone became insane, sexual excesses were blamed for it. If a man died suddenly in an ill-famed house, sexual excess were accused… (p. 30)

All these sexual beliefs are still operating in Chinese society as has been evinced in Koro psychodynamics analysis in terms of cultural influence by Rin (1966) and Gwee (1968). Both authors have shown how the deep cultural beliefs about sexuality are operative in causing sexual anxiety and conflicts in Koro patients. The collective thoughts about genital retraction as a fatal disease are noted in the community as well. Ngui (1969) provides the reasons in this context why Koro continues to be endemic among the Chinese:

> Despite having emigrated from China, the overseas Chinese are still very much influenced by Chinese traditional medicinal system. Gwee, in a survey in 1956, found that 90% of Chinese attending the General Hospital in Singapore had also taken Chinese medicine for their complaints. Again many of them used in Chinese traditional medicine have become common household words, such as heat and cold, wind and wetness. It would follow therefore, that belief in penile retraction as a cause of death and in the entity of "Shook Yang" would be a prevalent belief among the Chinese. Against the background of these cultural beliefs, the Chinese population is therefore vulnerable to attacks of Koro. (pp. 263–264)

The recent advances in Chinese society, especially of the educational standards (Gwee, 1984; Ngui, 1984), are the main reason for the decrease of such cultural influences on Singapore's people (and may also be in mainland China). Thus the Koro incidences in recent times show a very minimal occurrence. In a recent study of the psychosocial covariates of the Shen-Kuei and Koro beliefs, Ng and Lui (1992) note that among the 84 randomly selected Chinese males in Hong Kong, 18.7% and 7.7% believed in the Shen-K'uei and Koro myth, respectively. Rin (1986) also noted a decrease in Koro incidence in Taipei, Taiwan, because of education and modern medical care in the recent decade.

Orality and Sexual Anxiety in Chinese Culture

John H Weakland (1956), a Stanford Anthropologist, tried to trace the root of Chinese male's genital anxiety from the traditional dimension of orality observed in Chinese society. He used the concept of psychoanalysis. Orality is used here in a broader perspective, i.e. … "*orality may be latent in symptoms apparently related to something else and that direct references to the mouth may not indicate fundamentally oral phenomena, … any direct imagery of the mouth or eating has some oral significance*" (Bergler, 1949). Weakland (1956) shows the prevalence of orality in the Chinese custom of male-child upbringing and in cultural and erotic conceptualization. All these have a deep relation with the castration fear, sexual anxiety in the males. Rin (1965) also asserts a profound influence of orality in Chinese culture. From his two case reports of Koro, he observed the following:

> A marked emphasis on orality in the Chinese has been noted, and is evidenced by the frequent and prolonged breast-feeding of babies and the prominent and almost exclusive role of the mothers in bringing up children. Eating is a major factor in Chinese social life. Oral features permeate Chinese everyday life; *Chy* (to eat) is the usual word used in greeting instead of "good day"; to nourish well or *parn* (grow fat) indicates one's health; so *parn* and *soon* (become thin) are of great importance in one's perceptions of other people. Also, an indirect form of orality and dependency has been thought to be seen in the high prevalence of opium-smoking and gambling among the Chinese (Muensterberger, 1951). (p. 12)

Weakland (1956), from an in-depth socio-anthropological analysis, asserts a genital phase castration threat in Chinese males, followed by a pleasurable phase with the experience of sexual anxiety and unconscious guilt. In support of this proposition, one may note that guilt over masturbation or illicit sexual contact is a frequent precipitating factor in Chinese Koro patients (Gwee, 1963; Rin, 1963, 1965; Yap, 1965). A cultural metamorphosis of this female threat that may be reflected in recent times is the idea or belief in "penis stealing" by female fox spirits of the Koro patients of Guangdong, China (Prince, 1992a).

Gulik (1951) describes the concept of male gender advantage in the act of sexual union with a female. He stated many examples that show that semen contains the *Chi*—"the universal spirit of life" which the female absorbs through "mysterious vagina" during copulation. A moral restriction thus imposed on intercourse (other than procreation) because of the abuse of *Ching*. That causes loss of sexual energy and the destruction of the body. Therefore intercourse and women are viewed as the "enemy" because woman robs the precious yang essence of man. In sexual union, thus, the man merely seeks a complementary fluid substance for absorbing or for pleasure, thereby strengthening his yang or dragon quality, the principle of his manhood or masculinity, against the yin or tiger quality of the woman (Evola, 1991). The yin-yang sexual philosophy also indicates a higher social status for men than females (Ruan, 1991a). Hence, from the act of coitus "he," not "she," will obtain the benefit, but if semen is ejaculated during coitus, the whole process would be reversed. That is why the woman is called the "foe" because she tends to take away the man's yang. A good woman never makes sexual demands on a man and withdraws his *Ching*, unlike a "fox woman." Here lies the deep-seated psycho-cultural anxiety in male sexual behavior, namely sexual intercourse and related morbidity or mortality.

The theme of female castrator and its consequent male genital anxiety is analyzed by Prince (1992b) at the background of a folk cult of fox spirit in the Koro epidemic of Guangdong, China, in recent years. It is a strong cultural concept in Chinese society. This unconscious fear of castration by the female is well illustrated in different folk projections of females. They are depicted as being dangerous creatures, e.g. "Fox Woman," "Snake woman," or "Tiger girl." In each instance, the orality and its dangerousness are described with the act of sexual union. Here are some examples:

> The fox woman is a common supernatural figure in Chinese folk tales. She appears in many of the stories as 'the entrancing and dangerous woman', who is beautiful and sexually exciting, available sexually, usually even taking the initiative in that type is exhaustion or illness and often death; a man becomes weaker and weaker and finally wastes away. (Heyer, 1953)

> A snake woman may bore a hole in her victim's head and suck out his brains. A proverb says, 'woman's mind is as much as a snake's mouth. (Weakland, 1956)

> Tiger girl would know what she wanted and would know how to get it. …It was not proper wife who awaited him there, but an old bitch possessed of the spirit of the she-wolf who steals at night into the darkened chambers of lonely men and sucks them empty of semen, drinking so deep of their manhood that the well runs dry, and they wonder through the rest of their time staring vacantly at the world about them and mumbling to themselves. (Shaw, 1945)

Gulik (1961) notes different phallic symbols in Chinese culture, viz. turtle, dragon, or snake. The dragon symbolizes the yang and corresponds to the men. It is interesting to observe some special terms for the penis in the Chinese culture, e.g., ambassador, crimson bird, jade flute, jade peak, jade scepter, jade stream (*yu-heng*), ling. In this context, it is relevant that the symbolic expression of coitus in Chinese is the "coiling up of the dragon and the game of the tiger." The dragon symbolizes the yang and corresponds to man (masculine potency), while the tiger for yin is embodied in the woman. The Taoist symbol of Lung-hu also expresses this mixing up of yang and yin energies (with a fusion of corresponding li and K'an forces) mean "dragon and tiger."

Prince (1992b) provided some interesting observations on the concept of coital death. He cites Ueno's (1963) work in Japan, which shows the autopsy report of 5559 cases of "endogenous sudden death" between January 1959 to May 1963 in Tokyo. Of 28 male deaths declared as "coital death," 18 were due to cardiac causes. More than 50% of deaths occurred outside homes. On average, the males were twenty years older than their partners. The time correlation between intercourse and death shows that in eleven cases, death occurred during intercourse, in eight just after intercourse, in eight others between thirty minutes to an hour after intercourse, and in the rest seven between 1 and 18 hours postcoital. Prince (1992b) appropriately interprets these natural occurrences as a cue to the folk myth of malevolent fox spirit prevalent in Chinese and Japanese Cultures:

> These statistics conjure up a picture of illicit sexual relations between an older man away from home and a considerably younger woman. It is possible perhaps to see this scenario as forming the basis of the myth of the beautiful young fox spirit seducing the susceptible male… (p. 130)

Since the second century BC, China has a long traditional history of different codes of sexual behaviors, practices, and philosophical models (Harper, 1987). A wealth of information was recently discovered in silk and bamboo manuscripts from a tomb (tomb three at Ma-wang-tui in Ch'ang-sha, burial dated 168 BC) in Hunan, one of the oldest sex manuals of the world. The role of sexual union is described as a part of general physical activity, while careless action may lead to ill-health, even death. The sexual act is viewed as a technique of absorption of vapor (ch'i) and essence (ching) as like all other Chinese physical cultivation. It also stated the practice of semen retention: ".. in sexual intercourse, the Yin essence of the woman strengthened the Yang essence of the man, who held onto this store of essence through the practice of semen retention" (p. 549).

Yin and Yang's concept has heavily influenced every level of Chinese social life and mentality, thoughts, and cognition, be it art, literature, politics, social custom, science, or sexology (Goldin, 2002). All these sex theories, for centuries, impacted the Chinese psyche and influenced their sexual beliefs and behaviors. Edwards (1976), while discussing health in sexual matters in Old China, provided many examples of social and cultural myth and thus very aptly commented:

> ...Chinese traditional theories on sex constitute an elaborate sexual schema; for centuries a unitary system of sexual misconceptions has been transmitted from generation to generation with such success that the schema still represents a considerable impediment to the adoption of scientifically sound concepts of the role and attributes of sexual functioning in human life. (p. 88)

Another critical question is why so many rules, instructions, proper-improper coital definitions, and death and disability were associated with the regular human sexual act in Chinese medical texts and classics since so many millennia ago! China has a long history since the Twenty-first century BC and has periods of feudal societies and imperial autocracy. Yap (1965) provided one answer to this stress and traditional teachings on sex beliefs and practices as: "importance that was given to sexual hygiene and adequate sexual preferences in the interest of maintaining the classical polygamic household." Gwee (1963), while discussing the cultural aspect of Koro, traced the historical importance of castration for producing eunuchs for Emperor's Court and noted that extraordinary importance was placed on the preservation of semen by traditional Chinese medicine. The social sanction of multiple wives is the factor responsible for developing a cultural psyche impregnated with fears associated with sexual activity. He commented:

> Hence it can be seen that as far as Chinese culture goes, the ground is adequate to give rise to the concept that sexual excesses, apart from being a social and religious taboo, can literally through the loss of the spermatic fluid result in the loss of life. ….
>
> Fatality and retraction of penis seem therefore well correlated in the Chinese mind for many years, and a bit of imagination on the part of a physician can easily conjure up such a condition. Thus it would appear that the disease is probably a result of the free play of imagination of a physician on top of a culture which links fatality with genital retraction and sexual activity with risk to life. (p. 121)

Though this discussion is based on Taoism principles mainly, the mention of Confucius (the conventional name was Master Kong) is also warranted. Confucianism and Taoism were the two most influential ancient philosophies that guided the Chinese social customs and behaviors for many centuries. As one old Chinese proverb says, "If Confucianism is the Chinese's outer garment, Taoism is its soul" (Chang, 1977, p. 19). Confucius (551–479 BC) was a Chinese philosopher, bureaucrat, and politician of the Spring and Autumn period. He was also contemporary to Lao Tsu. *Analects* is an ancient Chinese book believed to contain the sayings and ideas of Confucius. During his time, the socio-political turmoil and chaos prompted Confucius to concentrate on ethics, rules of social conduct, sexual morality, and guideline to maintain discipline and stability in society. He stressed moral values and ritual practice, filial obedience and respect to the family elders, and the state's sound political administration. Confucianism became the Chinese state doctrine during the Han Dynasty in 125 BC. Confucian ethics is a construct of the philosophy of behavior between people within the rigid frame of conduct rules. He mentioned five types of relationships:

emperor and minister, father and son, older brother and younger brother, husband, wife, and friend. He advocated that all these relationships and human interactions should follow a protocol, and each party should obey the rules to maintain the stability of their universe. He advocated a strict control of sexuality between man and woman and stated that marriage is only for procreation and placed high value and importance on a male boy than a girl. Confucianism views sexuality as taboo and forbid open sexual mixing or discussion before marriage. In gender relations, the male was regarded as superior to women. It placed heavy stress on the patriarchal values of traditional society. Gao et al. (2012) put this observation as follows:

> Men and women is expected to have distinct social role that men should go out to work to support family and women stay at home to be caregivers. Besides, a virtuous woman should uphold "three subordinations": be subordinate to her father before marriage, to her husband after marriage, and to her son in widowhood. Confucianism sees sexuality as taboo and forbid discussion about sex. It advocates sex is regulated by formal arrangements (marriage) and culminates in childbirth, so sex outside of marriage is not condoned. Virtue of chastity is particularly supposed to be abided by women, which means remaining virgin before marriage and fidelity to the husbands, alive or dead. In sexual activity, women are also supposed to keep submissive and less sexually aggressive than men. (p. 4)

Hong et al. (1993) described the impact of these two great philosophical doctrines on the Chinese psyche very nicely as follows:

> It seems plausible that the teachings of Confucius and Lao Tsu caused some degree of anxiety over sexual attitudes and practices in ancient China because they were so diametrically opposed. It might be said that Confucian ideas regarding sex were equivalent to Freud's "punitive superego," whereas Taoist attitudes more closely resembled the id. Considerable cognitive dissonance may have been caused by such radically different approaches to sex. (p. 414)

Taoism had significant influence during the Tang Dynasty (618–906 AD), and Emperor Xuanzong (712–756 AD) declared it a state religion. The subsequent development of Buddhism in the Tang dynasty and the work of liberal Chinese intellectuals made a significant change in the Confucian sexual doctrine. That was known as Neo-Confucianism, particularly by the work of Cheng-Zhu school (stressed strongly on ascetic trend), in Song dynasty and beyond (Lo, 1993).

However, recent rapid social changes in China with its political and social market economic reform heavily influence sexual behavioral attitudes and show some critical variation of social cognition and sexual attitudes between urban and rural populations (Higgins & Sun, 2007). Ng and Lau (1990), in a careful analysis of changing patterns of sexual attitudes in Chinese culture, spanning over a century-old long history and "colorful civilization," suggested the importance of balanced research to address the evolution of sexual attitudes in Chinese culture.

Ruan (1991b) provided us a precious historical documentation of the history of sexuality in Chinese culture for the last 2000 years. He presents a comprehensive historical survey of Chinese sexology. It is exquisite documentation of sex in Chinese society, including its historical background, sexual yin-yang philosophy, classical Chinese sexology, Taoist sexual myths and methods, prostitution, classical Chinese erotica, different sexual behaviors, and changing attitudes toward sexuality in present-day China. Lam and Berrios (1992) provided a beneficial account of different psychological concepts and symptomatology, including personality disorders in old Chinese medical texts.

Conclusion

China has undergone a sea-change in the last century, mainly because of its communist revolution. A drastic change is observed in all levels of society—economy, social structure, agriculture, and human behavior. So we can now say "old China" and "new China." A phenomenal transformation and change in Chinese medicine took place (Unschuld, 1999), especially after the globalization era. Traditional Chinese Medicine (TCM) is amalgamated and integrated with Western biomedicine

(Scheid, 1999). It is expected that the social cognition regarding sexuality has also changed a lot, especially among educated middle-class people. The last prominent Koro epidemic occurred in Guandong province in China in 1985–87. After that, only a few sporadic cases of Koro were reported from Chinese ethnicity from different parts of the world. Other than that, there is no report of Koro for the last 30 years from mainland China or Taiwan, Hong Kong, or Singapore. Appropriate to mention here is that cultural psychiatry is also gaining more importance in the academic and administrative mental health area and may help develop a nationwide rational understanding of mental ill-health and related cultural myths and superstition. This hope is being expressed by Zhao and Miao (2007) as:

> The Chinese government has begun to realize the importance of these studies. Some important theoretical and practical suggestions have been accepted by the policy-makers, e.g., to deal with troublesome folk treatments, and to plan mental health services for ethnic minorities. We hope that cross-cultural psychiatry in China will become an explicit science from an implicit one, and play a more important role in the development of Chinese psychiatry as a whole. (p. 109)

Therefore it is expected that the advancement in socio-economic standards, education (including mental health), and technological progress may rationally reorient people about the traditional myths and beliefs about sexuality and sexual behavior (Ng, 1992). It is, of course, a good indication of social progress.

References

Bergler, E. (1949). *The basic neurosis; Oral regression and psychic masochism* (p. 17). Grune and Stratton.

Blofeld, J. (1982). *Taoist mysteries and magic*. Shambhala Publications Inc.

Camphausen, R. C. (1991). *The encyclopedia of Erotic wisdom*. Inner Tradition International.

Chang, J. (1977). *The Tao of love and sex: The ancient Chinese way to ecstasy.* E.P. Dutton.

Chen, P. S. (1937). *The history of Chinese medicine.* Commercial Press.

Chowdhury, A. N. (1995). Yin-yang dualism and sexuality in Chinese culture: A psychohistorical perspective. *J Indian Anthropological Society, 30*, 125–133.

Edwards, J. W. (1976). The concern for health in sexual matters in the "old society" and "new society" in China. *J Sex Research, 12*(2), 88–103.

Edwards, J. W. (1984). Indigenous Koro: A genital retraction syndrome of insular South East Asia: A critical review. *Culture, Medicine & Psychiatry, 8*, 1–24.

Evola, J. (1991). *Eros and the mysteries of love: The metaphysics of sex.* Inner Traditions International.

Gao, E., Zuo, X., Wang, L., Lou, C., Cheng, Y., & Zabin, L. S. (2012). How does traditional Confucian culture influence adolescent' sexual behavior in three Asian cities? *J Adolescent Health, 50*(3 Suppl), S12–S17.

Goldin, P. R. (2002). *The culture of sex in Ancient China.* University of Hawaii Press.

Gwee, A. L. (1963). Koro—A cultural disease. *Singapore Medical J, 4*, 119–122.

Gwee, A. L. (1984). *Personal communication.*

Gwee, A. L. (1968). Koro—Its origin and nature as a disease entity. *Singapore Medical J, 9*, 3–6.

Harper, D. (1987). The sexual arts of ancient China as described in a manuscript of the second century B.C. *Harvard J Asiatic Studies, 47*(2), 539–593.

Heyer, V. (1953). Relations between men and women in Chinese stories. In M. Mead & R. Mentrax (Eds.), *The study of culture at a distance* (pp. 221–234). University of Chicago Press.

Higgins, L. T., & Sun, C. (2007). Gender, social background and sexual attitudes among Chinese students. *Culture Health & Sexuality, 9*(1), 31–42.

Hong, W., Yamamoto, J., Chang, D. S., & Lee, F. (1993). Sex in a Confucian society. *J American Academy of Psychoanalysis, 21*(3), 405–419.

Kohn, L. (2011). Health maintenance in ancient China. *International J Medical Science, 8*, s26–s42.

Lam, C. W., Berrios, G. E. (1992). Historical note. Psychological concepts and psychiatric symptomatology in some ancient Chinese medical texts. *History of Psychiatry, 3*(9), 117–128.

Leng, G. A. (1971). Traditional Chinese methods of mental treatment. In NEST Wagner (Ed.), *Psychological problems and treatment in Malyasia.* University of Malaysia Press.
Lo, P. C. (1993). Zhu Xi and Confucian sexual ethics. *J Chinese Philosophy, 20*(4), 465–477.
Lozano, F. (2014). Basic theories of traditional Chinese Medicine. In Y. C. Lin & E. S. Z. Hsu (Eds.), *Acupuncture for pain management* (pp. 13–43). Springer Science Business Media.
Levi, H. S., & Ishihara, A. (1989). *The Tao of sex* (3rd ed.). Integral Publishing.
Maciocia, G. (2005). *The foundations of Chinese medicine* (2nd ed.). Elsevier Churchill Livingstone.
Maspero, H. (1937, April–June, July–September). *The process of "feeding the vital principle" in old Taoist religion.* (pp. 177–252, 353–430). J Asiatique.
Meth, J. M. (1974). Exotic psychiatric syndromcs. In S. Aricti & E.B.Brody (Eds.), *American handbook of Psychiatry* (Vol. 3, pp. 723–739). Basic Books, Inc.
Muensterberger, W. (1951). Orality and dependence: Characteristics of Southern Chinese. *Psychoanalysis & the Social Sciences, 3*, 37–39.
Ng, M. L. (1992). *Personal communication.*
Ng, B. Y., & Kua, E. E. H. (1996). Koro in ancient Chinese history. *History of Psychiatry, 7*, 563–570.
Ng, M. L., & Lui, P. K. (1992). *The psychological covariates of the Shen-Kuei and Koro beliefs*. Unpublished.
Ng, M. L., & Lau, M. P. (1990). Sexual attitudes in the Chinese. *Archives of Sexual Behaviour, 19*(4), 373–388.
Ngui, P. W. (1969). The Koro epidemic in Singapore. *Australian & New Zealand J Psychiatry, 3*, 263–266.
Ngui, P. W. (1984). *Personal Communication.*
Prince, R. H. (1992a). Koro and the fox sprit on Hainan Island (China). *Transcultural Psychiatric Research Review, 29*, 119–132.
Prince, R. H. (1992b). A symposium on the vulnerable male: Cultural variations on the castration theme. *Transcultural Psychiatric Research Review, 29*, 87–90.
Rawson, P., & Legeza, L. (1973). *Tao: The Chinese philosophy of change.* Thames and Hudson.
Read, B. E. (1926). Gleanings from old Chinese medicine. *Annals of Medical History, 8*, 16–19.
Rin, H. (1963). Koro: A consideration on Chinese concepts of illness and case illustrations. *Transcultural Psychiatric Research Review, 15*, 23–30.

Rin, H. (1965). A study of the aetiology of Koro in respect to the Chinese concept of illness. *International J Social Psychiatry, 11*, 7–13.
Rin, H. (1966). Two forms of vital deficiency syndrome among Chinese male mental patients. *Transcultural Psychiatric Research Review, 3*, 19–21.
Rin, H. (1986). *Personal communication.*
Ruan, F. F. (1991a). The harmony of Yin and Yang. In R.Green (Ed.), *Sex in China: Perspectives in Sexuality. Behavior, Research & Therapy* . (pp. 11–28). Springer.
Ruan, F. F. (1991b). *Sex in China. Studies in sexology in Chinese culture*. Springer Science Business Media.
Scheid, V. (1999, December). The globalization of Chinese medicine. *The Lancet , 354*(4), SIV I0.
Shaw, L. (1945). *Rickshaw boy* (pp. 192–193). Reynal and Hitchcock.
Shih, L. L. (2017). *Timeline of Chinese history*. Available at: https://chinesehistoryandcultureblog.wordpress.com/2017/01/11/first-blog-post/
Storozum, M., Duowen, M., Wang, H., Ren, X., Zhang, Y., & Kidder, T. R. (2017). Anthropogenetic origins of a late Holocene, basin-wide unconformity in the middle reaches of the Yellow river, the Luoyang Basin, Henan province in China. *Quaternary Research*. 1–19. 10.1017.Qua.
T'ao, L., Chi-Fan, C., & Ch'i-Shan, C. (1962). Some early records of nervous and mental diseases in traditional Chinese medicine. *Chinese Medical J, 81*, 55–59.
Tseng, W. S. (1973). The development of psychiatric concepts in traditional Chinese medicine. *Archives of General Psychiatry, 29*, 569–575.
Ueno, M. (1963). The so-called coition death. *Japanese J Legal Medicine, 17*, 330–340.
Unschuld, P. U. (1999, Deccember). The past 1000 years of Chinese medicine. *The Lancet, 354*(4), SIV9.
van Gulik, R. H. (1951). *Erotic colour prints of the ming period*. Tokyo.
van Gulik, R. H. (1961). *Sexual life in Ancient China*. E. J. Brill.
Veith, I. (1966). Huang Ti nei ching su waen. *The yellow emperor' classic of internal medicine*. Translated. University of California Press.
Weakland, J. H. (1956). Orality in Chinese conceptions of male genital anxiety. *Psychiatry, 19*, 237–247.
Wong, K. C. (1918). An enquiry into some Chinese sexual diseases. *National Medical J China, 4*, 26–31.
Yap, P. M. (1965). Koro—A Culture-bound depersonalization syndrome. *British J Psychiatry, 111*, 43–50.
Zhao, X., & Miao, S. (2007). Development of cultural psychiatry in China. *World Cultural Psychiatry Research Review, 2*(4), 104–109.

4

Koro and the Animal Connection

Koro and the Fox-Myth

Without Fox Demons, no Village is Complete.—Chinese Proverb

Fox-spirit Culture: Fox (spirit) has been implicated as a socio-cultural theme in the Koro epidemic in Hainan Island, Guangdong, China (Tseng et al., 1988; Prince, 1992). It was also sadly noted that several girls were believed to be fox-maidens under disguise, and at least one was beaten to death, and others drowned in the sea in the Guangdong epidemic. In many cultures, the fox is regarded as a soul-animal with the power of transformation into human beings, usually with a lousy motif and very rarely with good intention. The implication of fox-spirit in Koro is another example of animal myth causing human disability, and in that sense, it supports the connection of culture-boundness with Koro. A brief transcultural discussion on Fox-connection with Koro is discussed here.

Besides the tortoise, the fox is another animal that is connected with the traditional belief of genital loss in China (Jilek, 1986; Tseng et al.,

A. N. Chowdhury, *Koro*,
https://doi.org/10.1007/978-3-030-87962-4_4

1988). It is believed that the ghost of the dead have no penis or yang element, which is why they cannot return to the material world in human form, which is their intended aim. So the fox spirit or ghost, disguised either as a *Hu-li-jing* or female ghost fox or as a beautiful lady, would come to collect penises (of males) or breasts (of female) for this purpose. This Koro folk-imagery has a long mytho-cultural history and is variously depicted in different Sino-Japanese folktales (Chan, 1998; Prince, 1992).

The Cult of Fox spirit and its association with sex is a long-held mythological tradition in far Eastern countries (Johnson, 1974), mainly in China (Werner, 1922), Japan (Yonebayashi, 1964), Korea (Krappe, 1944), and Vietnam. In all these cultures, the fox spirit is depicted as an erotic figure, a seducer with traits of hypersexuality and seductive nature. The following discussion will focus on some of the characters as evinced in the mytho-cultural folk beliefs in far eastern countries.

China

The fox spirit in China is *Huli Jing*, which literally means "exquisite fox." Huli Jing is immortal by accumulating (by stealing) human life force; they are magical shape-shifters and take human form to seduce human beings. In Mandarin and Cantonese slang, the term *hu li jing* is a derogatory syntax used to describe a woman who seduces a man.

Chinese folk-mythology described at least seven terminologies for different types of fox spirit as follows (Chan, 1998): *Hu:* Fox (general term); *Huli jing:* fox spirit (this form was implicated in the Koro epidemic in Hainan islands); *Hujing*: Fox spirit; *Huxian*: Immortal fox; *Xian:* Immortal or transcendent being—they are worshiped in Chinese folk religion; *Jinwei hu:* Nine-tailed fox and *Laohu*: Old fox.

The character and nature of *Huli jing* show the most common folk concepts that were operative at the background of genital retraction (Koro) in the Hinan island epidemic in Guandong. The Huli jing can change its size, become mist-like, and may disappear and reappear. Huli jing can become either a beautiful woman or a handsome man, unlike the Japanese and Korean beliefs in which the fox usually transforms into a woman. They have different names concerning their age and power. A heavenly or immortal fox is called a *Huxian*. A nine-tailed fox is a *Jiuwei Hu*. An aged fox is *Laohu*. The number of tails is dependent on their age. Aged one would have nine tails when they become *Huxian* and would have the ability to communicate with the heavens.

In Chinese culture, the fox symbolizes longevity, craftiness, power of transformation, and ghosts of dead souls. The fox is one of the twelve animal symbols of Chinese ZODIAC. Foxes have been an essential component of Chinese cosmology for 2300 years. Eroticism, like human quality, is attached to the fox—the dangerously seductive fox is quite common in Chinese folklore. It is believed that fox testicles have high aphrodisiac quality. In China (and among the Eskimos) the fox is a wire animal that appears in the shape of a beautiful woman and seduces the males (Prince, 1992; Rink, 1866). Waida (1987a) provides a fascinating account of this female transformation of the fox:

> Chinese folklore is rich in the motif of the fox that transforms itself into an attractive woman and seduces young men. Foxes are capable of this transformation through the study of Chinese classics or through erotic tricks. Foxes who study the classics acquire first the power to become humans, then immortals, and finally gods. In many stories, young foxes are depicted as sitting in a circle, listening to an old white fox at the center expounding the classics. Foxes can assure human form, if at first only briefly, through the absorption and accumulation of *semen virile* of a male sex partner; by seducing humans, usually young men, and foxes steal life essence and add it to their own. For example, an ambitious young man who has retired to a deserted cottage or temple to prepare for the state examinations is visited at dusk by a beautiful young woman who becomes his mistress. Her erotic skill is such that he becomes exhausted and dies. Fox-women sometimes sincerely love their human paramours and help them with their studies, but they seldom return the life essence they have stolen. Occasionally, the parents or friends become aware of the situation in time and call in either a shaman or a Taoist medicine man, specially trained in fox exorcism and drive her away. (p. 406)

Gulik (1961) provides an exquisite analysis of the fox-spirit theme of the Taoist philosophy in China. The Taoist teaching believes that the earth's "cosmic vital essence" is stored at its center, and the creatures who live in underground holes and caves (e.g., Foxes or badgers or aquatic animals like a tortoise) remain close to this essence. As a result of this cosmic energy's high accumulation, they enjoy long lives and supernatural power. The fox is regarded as an incubus since the period of the T'ang dynasty (618–906 A.D.). Gulik (1961) cities an excellent account of the mystic power of the fox from an author of that period:

> When a fox is fifty years old, in a deserted grave, it will transform itself into a woman of winning mien its hair becomes a chignon. Its snout a powdered face. Its long tail changes into a trailing crimson robe. Then, walking slowly, she'll haunt the lonely village roads and toward nightfall, selecting a secluded place, She'll sing and dance, and alternatively sadly cry, not raising her curved eyebrows, her pretty face kept does that convey! There's hardly a man who is not then beguiled by her… (p. 211)

The concept of the fox spirit also has a long traditional history in Chinese mythology (Stevens, 2013). Kang (2006) from Columbia University published her extensive research on the history of the five centuries shamanistic fox cult in China: "The Cult of the Fox: Power, Gender, and Popular Religion in Late Imperial and Modern China." Even today, this cult impacted the belief system of a wide range of social classes in Chinese society. She describes various folk cult practices, worship activities, and fox spirits' exorcising by extraordinary local healers. She traced the fox worship tradition in Chinese history for thousands of years, researched the spread of fox cult from South to North region of China, domestic fox worship, foxes and spirit mediums in Chinese religious life, fox shrines, and the role of fox cult in daily life and social interactions. She tried to explore the manifold meanings of the fox spirit in Chinese society. "Though by no means a religious figure, the mythological fox spirit has a sizeable presence in Chinese culture that has persisted to the present" (Liao, 2015).

Japan

Folk belief is still alive in Japan; the fox is considered the most skillful of animals in transforming itself into human form, often female (Waida, 1987a). Japanese people regard the fox as a symbol of longevity, magic power for good or evil, and respect it as the messenger of the rice God Inari; Fox-fire is the *ignes fatui*. A black fox stands for good fortune, a white fox for calamity, and three foxes indicate disaster (Cooper, 1993). There are two different categories of foxes—Zenko and Yako. Zenko is friendly and is associated with the God Inari, and Yako are the evil who trick and deceive humans. In Japan, the fox spirit is known by the name *Kitsune*. They are depicted as devoted lovers, friends, and faithful wives, and like the Huli Jing, their wisdom and magic power increase with increasing age. The older and wiser a fox spirit grows more tails- with nine tails, they represent the pinnacle of divinity. Over time, Kitsune's cult became associated with Inari Okami—the Shinto spirit of fertility, agriculture, industry, and worldly success. The Kitsune is regarded as a romantic figure, and there is much folklore about young men unknowingly marrying a Kitsune and having a human child with supernatural power. Fox-spirit possession or Kitsune-tsuki is still a strong folk belief in Japan. Eguchi (1991) provided an exquisite analysis of fox-spirit possession and mental symptoms in two cases (one male and one female) from a mountain village of Western Japan and tried to explain this as a culture-bound syndrome. Japanese shamanism also includes the healing of magical animal possession, including Racoon (Tunuki) and fox (Kitsune) (Blacker, 1999). *Dojo*—a magic exorcism is still existed in modern Japan (Davis, 1980).

Japanese terminology:

- *Kitsune:* Fox. The standard term for a spirit fox.
- *Myobu:* Celestial fox. One of the foxes which are sworn to Inari's service.
- *Nogitsune*: Wild fox (field fox). Nogitsune is not sworn to Inari's service and is therefore capable of evil. They can directly communicate with humans.
- *Youko:* Spirit fox. An uncommon term.

> It is commonly believed that any woman encountered at dark times of the day are likely to be fox women, facial traits that look like fox such as thin eyes and high cheekbones are considered fox like and beautiful. But there had been methods to catch a fox in their carelessness—such as watching out for their shadows (hence why they appear in dark times) or trying to find their tails which they always have difficulty to hide (KingdomKrown, 2013).

Korea

Kumiho is the Korean fox spirit. In Korean folklore, they are female, sexually deviant, malevolent, and act like a demon and a cannibal (Hong, 2012). They can take on human form (always female) at the age of 100 years. Balmain (2017), while discussing the cultural mythology of East Asian countries in Art and Cinema, pointed out about sharing of similar theme due to the cultural proximity of the countries and commented that:

> While the shape and form of the fox differ across mainland China, Hong Kong, Japan and South Korea, it is clear that they function within a shared cultural belief system. As discussed in detail, early tales of fox-spirits across the region are markedly similar, especially in the manner in which the fox-spirit becomes a variant of the femme fatale who threatens the male subject with dissolution through absorption of the life force or jing. (p. 7)

Vietnam

Vietnam's Terrifying Fox Monster is Ho Tinh. It is an enormous nine-tailed fox who inhabited a deep cave. Ho Tinh would disguise himself as a beautiful woman and trick innocent passersby into following her back to the mountain jungle and roads. Like the Korean fox spirit, Ho Tinh is also a cannibal. The evil entity would lead his victims into the cave to trap them and feed on them (Kalmusky, 2018).

Other Cultures

The fox has enjoyed the utmost popularity as a character in the fables of many world cultures. Usually, the fox is taken as a symbol of shyness. It was once believed in Wales and Germany that witches might assume the form of a fox; hence foxes were sometimes burned in midsummer fires (Waida, 1987a).

Fox appears in the folklore of many cultures of the world. Usually, they are depicted as trickery, cunning, and possessed supernatural, magical power, and wisdom (Daniels & Stevens, 2003). In many cultures, they are believed to be a shape-shifter and have the power of transformation into a human form (Carse, 1987). There are many archetypes of the fox cult. Bulgarian folk tales described fox by the name *Kuma Lisa* and in Russian *Patrikeyevna,* and Ukrainian, *Llisichka-sestrichka* and all are depicted in the trickster's role. The Irish fox is *Sionnach* and is believed to foresee events (like weather), and its barking is a sign of rain. There are many folk rituals for the treatment of illness related to fox in Irish culture. In Finnish folk tales, the fox is described as cunning, smart, and careful and the meaning of aurora borealis (revontulet) is "fox fire." Foxes play a variety of roles in Native American mythology from different tribes. Silver Fox is the culture-hero and creator God of many Northern California tribes. Foxes are common clan animals in many Native American cultures. Fox Woman (*Waagoshimi–Mindimooye*) is a minor animal spirit of the Anishinabe and Cree tribes. She is usually portrayed as a wise elder. In the North American California Indians' mythology, the fox plays a prominent role as a trickster. The fox there sometimes appears as a female animal and deceives human companions; Waida (1987a) provides one such description as follows:

> A poor man, living alone, comes home at night to find his house in order and his dinner on the fire. He discovers that every morning a vixen comes to his hut, sheds her skin, and becomes a woman. Having stolen the skin, he makes her his wife. They live in happiness for many years until she discovers the skin, puts it on, and runs away. This scenario of the "mysterious housekeeper" is also found among the Inuit (Eskimos)

> in Greenland and Labrador as well as among the Koriak of northeastern Siberia. (p. 406)

Among Santals, a tribe in India, the fox is called *Toyo,* who possesses a human voice and great supernatural power granted by the Sun god (*Chand*o) and the Moon god (*Ninda Chando*) (Chowdhury, 1993). The theme of "female searching" is also evident in the mythology concerning the fox among the Dogan people of Mali, Africa. *Amma* is the supreme god of the Dogans. Amma created a twin from a primordial egg. Yurugu (or Ogo) was the twin male who was impatient for the female counterpart and broke through the placenta. The torn piece of placenta ultimately becomes the earth. Amma transformed Yurugu into a fox known as the tongueless "*Pale Fox*," who wondered about the world looking for his female counterpart (Thayer, 1987).

Koro and the Tortoise Connection

The term "Koro" comes from the word for "tortoise" in Malay, Indonesian dialects (Wilkinson, 1932). The imagery of genital retraction in Koro is linked with the Chinese's turtle symbolism (Gwee, 1963). In Macassares dialect, *Koero* means tortoise (Slot, 1935). In the Indian context, the symptom of genital retraction was called by the inhabitants of Koch Bihar district, West Bengal, India, as "Kattaw," which in local syntax means tortoise (Chakraborty, 1983, 1990; Chowdhury, 2003).

The turtle or tortoise is one of the most primitive creatures still existing and is connected with the creation myth in many cultures of the world (Wadia, 1987a). It reflects various symbolic meanings, viz. good, bad, or erotic, in different cultures. The unique biological characters, viz., self-defensive retractable head and neck in response to a threat, wide eco-adaptations and long life, the remarkable capability of navigational migration (Lohmann, 1992), profuse power of fecundity, and docile, non-aggressive behavior have been a matter of great wonder, often mystic and magical, for man since early days of the civilization. Its extraordinary capacity to vanish into depths of the endless sea for months or years together prompted the belief in its connection with the other world (world of the dead). Many cultures used the tortoise as a divination vehicle or oracle, making it a psycho-anthropological interest topic. Its extensive reference as a mythical animal in Hinduism is again a matter of great interest in mytho-anthropology. Thus, the turtle or tortoise has earned a specific connotation in religious themes, magical myths, and erotic symbolism in different societies, especially in India and Indo-China. Hes and Nassi (1977) mentioned the statue of *Pietro Barbino* by Valerio Cicolide Settignano (1560) at Fountain of Bacchus in Florence, France concerning the archetype of turtlehead symbolism and penis: a *little fat dwarf seated astride a turtle* (Fig. 4.1), also known as *Fontanella di Nano Morgant*. The author visited the Boboli Garden in Florence in May 1995 and took this photograph of *Fontana Bacchino* (Fountain of Bacchus).

TORTOISE/TURTLE: Zoological Features

In biology, the word tortoise refers to the land-based reptile only, and the term turtle is reserved for the amphibian, marine, or freshwater forms. The zoological name of the tortoise is Testudians or Chelonians. They are mainly amphibious and have adapted to various ways of life. Some live in freshwater, some in muddy habitats, while some have become terrestrial, and some have adapted themselves to the marine way of life, leading a semi-pelagic life. The phylogenetic history of the tortoise shows that it is one of the most primitive species surviving across millions of years of evolution (Pritchard, 1979; Tikader & Sharma, 1985). Throughout this discussion, the words tortoise and turtle are used interchangeably. Throughout this discussion, the words tortoise and turtle are used interchangeably.

Turtle Character of Psycho-anthropological Significance: The tortoise or turtle is one of the most primitive creatures that human civilization has encountered since its inception. The remarkable zoo-specificities of tortoise offer an impressive scope of cognitive categorization so far as the animal's mythical and legendary folk beliefs are concerned (Gubernatis, 1872). The body is boxed by two rigid, unbreakable shields, dorsal (carapace) and ventral (plastron). This great self-protective shelter for

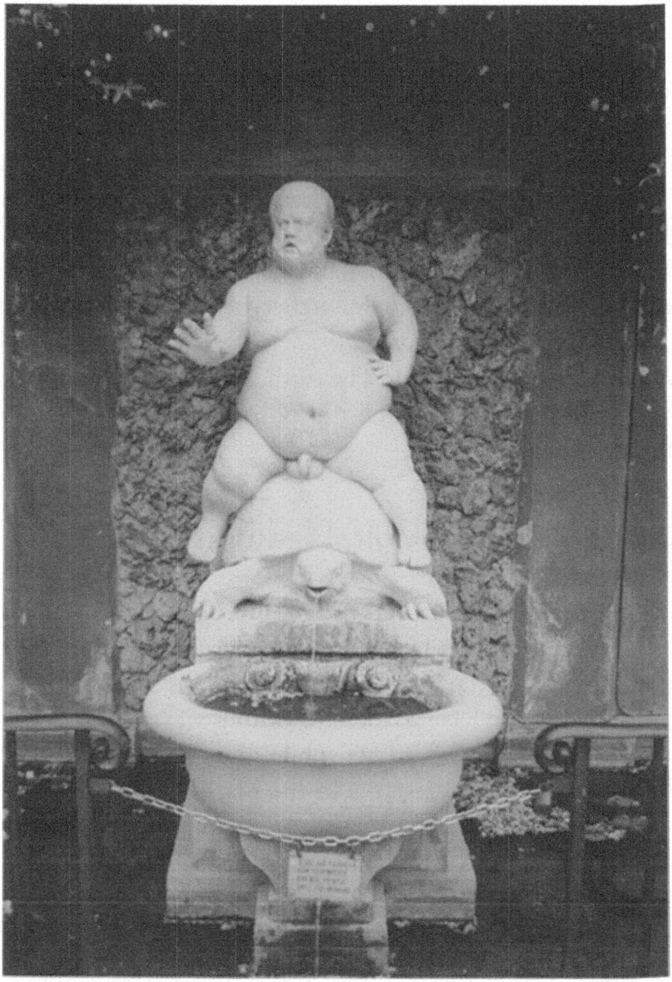

Fig. 4.1 *Fontana Bacchino* (Fountain of Bacchus), Florence (Photographed by the author)

the retractile head, limbs, and tail of the animal offers the basis of the belief in magical energy and its supernatural capacity to withstand the greatest of odds. The encasing of great power and strength within its shell is the cognitive basis for its association with many creation myths of the world. This aspect also acts in the symbolism for wrapping of strength and sacred power of soul within the innermost confidential human body areas, e.g., in *Kundalini Yoga* or *Kurma Asana* of Tantra in Hinduism. The Hindu myth relating to Load Vishnu's incarnation as a "Giant Tortoise" also depicts this aspect of magical strength inherent in the creature.

The varieties of lines with some geometrical designs on the turtle shell called scutes provide a clue to the perception of religious directives or divine meaning within the shell lines. There are many mythological and legendary references of these tri/quadric/hexagonal lines of tortoise-shell, especially in the Chinese culture, e.g., I Ching of Taoism's graphic configuration calligraphy and oracle bone divination. Some specific color arrangement on the shell was regarded as a good omen for the king and his subjects in ancient India. In India, the tortoise is known by the name *Kurma* or *Kachchhap*.

TORTOISE: The Chinese Perspective

In Chinese culture, the tortoise is believed to be a sacred animal and one of the four spiritually endowed creatures (with a dragon, phoenix, and ky-lin). It is also thought that the tortoise possesses oratory power and is also linked with the creation myth. Tortoise in Chinese philosophy represents the watery element, the yin principle (Cooper, 1993). The Taoist philosophy considers the tortoise as the symbol of the universe. Its shape symbolizes the Great Triad or the entire cosmos. The dome-shaped back is the sky, the body in the middle as earth, and the water is under the shell. It's believed that the mythical first emperor of China, Fu His, draws inspiration from a tortoise, who derived the eight primary trigrams of the I Ching from studying the tortoise-shell lines. These lines were regarded as sacred with mystic power. The *Chia-Ku-Wen* or shell and bone script (18th–twelfth century BC) is the earliest recorded Chinese calligraphy. These ideographs were engraved on the shoulder bones of large animals and tortoise shells. Kings of the Shang dynasty (18th–twelfth century B.C.) tried to solve their problems by consulting their ancestral souls and deities through divination (Chavannes, 1911). For perpetual preservation, the sacred answers and directives were engraved on bones and tortoise shells (Needham, 1965). Divination played a considerable role in ancient China. The twenty-four rim plates of the tortoise-shell are correlated with the twenty-four agricultural divisions of the Chinese year (Camphausen, 1991).

Turtle and sexual link in Chinese culture: The tortoise or *Gui* has several sexual associations in Chinese erotic vocabulary. Gulik (1961) states that there are several metaphorical uses of the penis as turtle, dragon, or snake in every Chinese conversation. He further notes that until the Ming Dynasty, the Chinese used the turtle as an artistic and literary symbol for its longevity. The symbolism with genital retraction acts because of the apparent similarity between the head of this creature and the glans penis, precisely the retracting nature of both. Gulik (1961) quoted a passage from a Ming treatise on the art of attaining longevity through coitus reservatus, where the retraction of a tortoise's head is used as a simile. The Chinese term for tortoise "*Gui*" is also used as a secret code for the phallus and in a word for "pimp" (*Wu gui* or "black tortoise") and as a swear-word that roughly equates to "father of a whore" (*gui-gong* or "tortoise master"). "*Gui tou*" ("turtle's head") is a common slang euphemism for a penis. Palthe (1936) also denotes an interesting etymological link between terms used for glans penis and tortoise head: The ordinary Chinese word for glans is *"Yong Tho,"* and the name *Kwee Tho* means both head of a tortoise and glans penis. Gwee (1968) states that there is a tendency to refer to the glans penis as a tortoise head by the Chinese in the usual conversation.

Slot (1935) reported many rituals regarding tortoise and Koro from his study of Macassares people of South Celebes of Dutch-Indies: One had to avoid walking in front of a tortoise. If the animal retracts its head one way, it is a negative sign. Still, if the head is retracted in the opposite direction away from the person, it is a positive sign as far as the chance for the viewer's future Koro attack is concerned. In Macassares dialect, *Koero* means tortoise.

TORTOISE: The Indian Perspective

The tortoise or turtle is a mythical animal and is intimately related to the creation myth in Hinduism. The important tortoise link noted in Hindu mythology is as follows.

Kasyapa or the "tortoise man": He is the primordial sage who appears as North Star in the sky and is the first living creature and progenitor of the human race. He married thirteen daughters of the sage *Daksha* and thence created the living world. Different classes of living creatures were born from these Great Mothers. Other versions of the Hindu creation myth showed the "tortoise sage's" tremendous procreative power (Sarkar, 1990; Zimmer, 1962).

Hindu mythology states that God *Vishnu* is the preserver and maintainer of the order of the creation. He is also the god of love and emotion. There is a canonical list of ten incarnations of *Vishnu* (*dash-avatars*). The different forms of *avatars* are translated as "incarnations," which figuratively means God's unique forms to help humankind at times of great need (Blurton, 1992) and offer an exciting mytho-anthropological perspective. The ten incarnations of Vishnu are: *Matsya* (Fish form); *Kurma* (Tortoise form); *Varaha* (Boar form); *Narasingha* (Half lion-half man form); *Vamana* (Dwarf man form); *Parashuram* (Aggressive man form); *Rama*, *Krishna*, *Buddha*, and *Kalki* (Human form with horse-head). Through this is not the place for a detailed discussion on mythological-anthropological aspects of the various form of incarnations, the most intriguing feature one may note about the association of animal forms from lower to higher class (fish, tortoise, boar, lion, horse) is indicative of the probable Darwinian evolutionary perspective in the creation myth. The different forms have some sociopsychological symbolism too.

Kurma or Tortoise Incarnation of Vishnu: A Reflection of Mighty-Retraction of Energy

Tortoise incarnation's theme is related to the Hindu creation myth. The god-class overpowered the demon-class by achieving immortality by drinking heavenly nectar or *Amrita*, explored from the sea. The legend describes the bringing forth of creation by churning the sea of milk or *khirod sagar*. This cosmic ocean was churned by using the sacred mountain *Mandar* as a churning pole. The snake *Vasuki* was used as the churning rope, coiled around the *Mandar*, and was pulled to and fro by the gods on the tail side (left) and the demons on the snake's mouth side (right). Owing to continued churning friction, the *Mandar* sank into the sea and went down to the nether world or hell (*Patal*). The main difficulty faced then was the non-availability of a suitable fixed object (stable platform). The rotating churning pole should be fixed because such a platform must have immense power to withstand this churning's strong force.

At this point, *Vishnu* took the Tortoise incarnation of the *Kurma* (*Giant Tortoise*) form to provide this robust platform whereby the churning pole was set on his stable back, powered with a divine unbreakable strength (Fig. 4.2). In this form, *Vishnu* assumes the cosmic foundation's role, upon which all things securely rest and without which the world would lack stability. So the most exciting theme inherent in this *Kurma* transformation is the *sankochan* (contraction or retraction) or concentration of great power and strength inside the turtle body. Thus, Kurma symbolizes divine power in a contracted form with immense stress tolerance capacity (Cooper, 1993). The same turtle myth and Lord Vishnu's incarnation is also a part of the creation myth in Indonesia (Java Island) and Cambodia.

Chakraborty and Bag (1989) traced another interesting mythical link of the tortoise transformation of a God, viz. Load *Shiva* in connection with the genesis of Assam's land (from where the 1982 Indian Koro epidemic began). They state:

> Assam is known as the land of the Load Shiva (who is worshipped mainly as the Phallus): the story goes that the union of Shiva with his consort shook the earth so much that it was about to disintegrate. Hearing the urgent plea of the earthlings' Shiva Contracted himself into a tortoise and that is the land of Assam. The tortoise is a revered animal there... (p. 147)

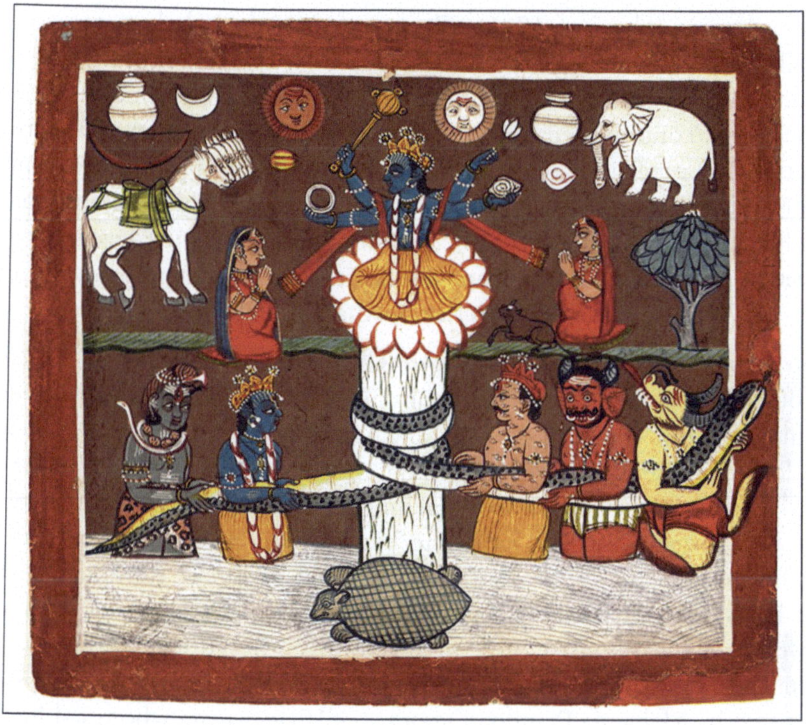

Fig. 4.2 The churning of the ocean of milk—*Vishnu* appears here at the base of the cosmic churning pole as a Giant Tortoise *Kurma* (Ink and opaque watercolor on paper painting of 1780–90; provided by Mr. and Mrs. Alvin N. Haas, 1977: https://www.metmuseum.org/art/collection/search/37989)

Yoga posture: *Kaurmasana* is a yoga posture because it resembles a tortoise with a tucked-in head and limbs. This unique position offers a transcendental experience as has been described in Bhagavad Gita: "When, again as a tortoise draws its limbs in on all sides, he withdraws his senses from the object of senses, and then his understanding is well-poised" (Sinha, 1988).

In the present context of turtle symbolism regarding genital retraction in Koro, one traditional turtle neck use as folk medicine in India is noteworthy. The turtle neck is used in many parts for the treatment of the prolapsed rectum or uterus. The meat is eaten, but the neck is hung up to dry, powered, and applied on the prolapsed organ, then pushed inward again (Shankar, 1991). The tortoise's biological character, especially its "encased" long life and remarkable survival power in the face of extreme odds, relates with its ability as the reservoir of cosmic energy in contracted/concentrated form. This concept of *sankochon* or contractile (retracting) capacity plays a role in the context of "wrapping of the soul" in Kundalini yoga of Hindu Tantra. In different pictorial representations of Kundalini, the emblem of microcosmic energy is depicted as a many-headed serpent emanating from a tortoise, e.g., in Kangra paintings of the eighteenth century (Mookerjee & Khanna, 1989).

Turtle symbolism in Indian Erotic Classics: There are several Indian erotic classics where various symbolisms are drawn from nature (flower, climber, scent, etc.) and animals, including the tortoise in the context of love-making especially the different coital positions. There are several such classics available: The love teachings of Kama Sutra (1967) (written by Mallanaga Vatsayana sometime between second and fifth century AD); the love text of Ananga Ranga (written by a poet Kalyana Malla, probably in the sixteenth century); a love text Panchasayaka or The Five Arrows (composed early in the fourteenth century by Jyotirishvara Kavishekhara); a love text with tantric influence Ratiratnapradipika (written by Maharaja Prandha Devaraya of Vijayanagara who ruled from 1422 to 1466 A.D.); Saaradipika, a love text composed by a man well-versed in erotic wisdom Sri Minanath between thirteenth and fifteenth centuries and Srngararasaprabandhadipika or "The Light of Love" of uncertain date by Harihara who lists 64 coital postures. At least 15 love positions are named after animals like tortoise, cobra, crab, fish, conch, cat, dog, ass, cow, deer, mare, elephant, monkey, crow, and peacock in the texts mentioned above. The following is a brief account of the tortoise position quoted from the English translation of Kama Sutra by Sinha (1988).

Kaurma or Tortoise Love Position

1) Each of you with arms and legs extended in the full *Kaurmasana*,
She below, you above,
Lips, arms and thighs meeting, hands joined;

This is *Kaurma* (The Tortoise).—(Ratiratnapradipika)

2) Seated, mouth to mouth,
Arms against arms, thighs pressed to thighs:
This is *Kaurma* (the tortoise).—(Ananga Ranga)

3) If, seated face to face,
Your toes caress the lovely woman's nipples
Her feet press your chest
And you make love holding each other's hands
It is *Kaurma* (the tortoise).—(Srngararasaprabandhadipika)

The above discussion points to the concept of retracting energy within the tortoise, which may be a psychosocial, cognitive basis of its association or symbolism with genital retraction in Koro. Interestingly, the term "Frighten Turtle Syndrome" (FTS) appears in the urban dictionary in recent times. It utilizes Tortoise symbolism: The act of the male penis retracting back into the pelvis area (often after cold exposure), causing it to look like the head of a frightened turtle.

References

Balmain, C. (2017). East Asian gothic: A definition. *Palgrave Communications, 3*, 31. https://doi.org/10.1057/s41599-017-0038-8

Blacker, C. (1999). *The catalpa bow: A study of Japanese Shamanistic practices.* Routledge, Curzon Press Ltd.

Blurton, T. R. (1992). *Hindu art*. British Museum Press.

Camphausen, R. C. (1991). *The encyclopedia of Erotic wisdom.* Inner Tradition International.

Carse, J. P. (1987). Shape shifting. In M. Eliade (Ed.), *Encyclopedia of religion* (Vol. 13, pp. 225–229). Macmillian Publishing Company.

Chakraborty, A. (1990). *Identity, land and sex*. In C.N. Stefanis (Ed.), *Psychiatry: A world perspective* (Vol. 4, pp. 222–226). Elsevier Science Publishers.

Chakraborty, A. (1983). An epidemic of Koro in West Bengal. *Indian J Psychiatry, 25*, 138–139.

Chakraborty, A., & Bag, D. C. (1989). Genesis of the Koro epidemic in West Bengal and Assam: Implication of turtle cults. *Human Science, 38*, 142–149.

Chan, L. T. H. (1998). *The discourse on foxes and ghosts*. University of Hawaii Press.

Chavannes, E. (1911). Turtle scale divination in Chinese high antiquity (from book By M. Lo Tshen-Yu). *Asian J, 17*, 127–137.

Cooper, J. C. (1993). *An illustrated encyclopedia of traditional symbols*. Thames and Hudson Limited.

Chowdhury, A. N. (1993). Psychiatric morbidity and the fox connection. *Transcultural Psychiatric Research Review, 30*(4), 399–401.

Chowdhury, A. N. (2003). Tortoise: A psycho-anthropological perspective. *Eastern Anthropologist, 56*, 51–59.

Daniels, C. L., & Stevens, C. M. (2003). *Encyclopedia of superstitions, folklore and the occult sciences of the World* (Vol. II). University Press of the Pacific.

Davis, W. (1980). *Dojo: Magic exorcism in modern Japan*. Stanford University Press.

Eguchi, S. (1991). Between folk concepts of illness and psychiatric diagnosis: Kitsune-tsuki (fox possession) in a mountain village of Western Japan. *Culture, Medicine & Psychiatry, 15*, 421–451.

Gubernatis, A. D. (1872). *Zoological mythology*. Trübner & Company.

Gwee, A. L. (1963). Koro—A cultural disease. *Singapore Medical J, 4*, 119–122.

Gwee, A. L. (1968). Koro—Its origin and nature as a disease entity. *Singapore Medical J, 9*, 3–6.

Hess, J. P., & Nassi, G. (1977). Koro in a Yemenite and a Georgian Jewish immigrant. *Confinia Psychiatrica, 20*, 180–184.

Hong, C. J. (2012). *Korean folklore and implications for Korean-American women*. UCLA Thinking Gender Conference. Available at: https://escholarship.org/uc/item/1209m3n1

Jilek, W. G. (1986). Epidemic of "Genital Shrinking" (Koro): Historical review and report of a recent outbreak in South China. *Curare, 9*, 269–282.

Johnson, T. W. (1974). Far eastern fox lore. *Asian Folklore Studies, 33*(1), 35–68.

Kalmusky, K. (2018). *H`ô Tinh: Vietnam's Terrifying Fox Monster*. Available at: https://theculturetrip.com/asia/vietnam/articles/ho-tinh-vietnams-terrifying-fox-monster/

Kang, X. (2006). The cult of the fox. *Power, gender and religion in late imperial and modern China*. Columbia University Press.

KingdomKrown. (2013). *Contextual References—Kitsune*. Available at: https://youseitales.wordpress.com/2013/01/14/contextual-references-kitsune/

Krappe, A. H. (1944). Far Eastern fox lore. *California Folklore Quarterly, 3*(2), 124–147.

Liao, V. (2015). *Tales about nine tails: An overview of Eastern fox spirits*. Available at:https://thespectatorial.wordpress.com/2015/06/16/tales-about-nine-tails-an-overview-of-eastern-fox-spirits/

Lohmann, K. J. (1992, Janauary). How sea turtle navigate. *Scientific American* (pp. 82–88).

Mookerjee, A., & Khanna, M. (1989). *The tantric way: Art, science, ritual* (pp. 59–65). Thames and Hudson Ltd.

Needham, J. (1965). *Science and civilization in China* (Vol. 1). Cambridge University Press.

Palthe, P. M., van W. (1936). Psychiatry and neurology in the tropics. In C.D. de Langen & A. Lichtenstein (Eds.), *A clinical textbook of tropical medicine* (pp. 525–547) G. Kolff and Company.

Prince, R. H. (1992). Koro and the fox spirit on Hainan Island (China). *Transcultural Psychiatric Research Review, 29*, 119–132.

Pritchard, P. C. H. (1979). *Encyclopedia of turtles*. T. F. H. Publications, Inc., Limited.

Rink, H. H. (1866). *Eskimoiske Eventyr og Sagn 1–11 (Tales and legends of Eskimo 1–11)*. Reizels Boghandel.

Sarkar, S. (1990). *Pauranik Abhidhan (Mythological Dictionary)* (6th ed., p. 94). M. C. Sarkar and Sons Private Limited.

Shankar, D. (1991). Indigenous health services—The state of the art. In A. Mukhopadhyay (Ed.), *State of India's Health* (pp. 129–162). Voluntary Health Association of India.

Sinha, I. (1988). *The love teachings of Kama Sutra*. Hamlyn Publishing Group Limited.

Slot, J. A. (1935). Koro in central celebes. *Geneeskundig Tijdschrift Voor Nederlandsch-Indie, 75*, 811–820.

Stevens, K. (2013). Fox spirits (Huli). *J Royal Asiatic Society Hong Kong Branch, 53*, 153–165.

Thayer, J. S. (1987). Amma. In M. Eliade (Ed.), *Encyclopaedia of religion*. (Vol. I, pp. 237–238). Macmillian Publishing Company.

Tikader, B. K., & Sharma, R. C. (1985). *Handbook of Indian Testudines*. Zoological Survey of India.

Tseng, W. S., Mo, M. K., Hsu, J., Li, L. S., Ou, L. W., Chen, G. Q., & Jiang, D. W. (1988). A socio-cultural Study of Koro epidemic in Guangdong, China. *American J Psychiatry, 145*, 1538–1543.

Van Gulik, R. H. (1961). *Sexual life in Ancient China*. E. J. Brill.

Vatsayana's Kama Sutra. (1967). Translated by R.Burton. Diane Publishing Co, Luxor Press.
Wadia, M. (1987a). Foxes. In M. Eliade (Ed.), *Encyclopaedia of religion* (Vol. 5, pp. 406–407). New York: Macmillian Publishing Company.
Wadia, M. (1987b). Turtles and Tortoises. In M. Eliade (Ed.), *The encyclopaedia of religion* (Vol. 15, pp. 96–97). Macmillian Publishing Company.
Werner, E. T. C. (1922). *Myths and legends of China* (pp. 370–385). Dover Publications Inc.
Wilkinson, R. L. (1932). *A Malay-English dictionary*. Maytilene.
Yonebayashi, T. (1964, October). Kitsunetsuki (Possession by Foxes). *Transcultural Psychiatric Research Review, 1*, 95–97.
Zimmer, H. (1962). *Myths and symbols in Indian art and civilization*. Harper.

5

Loss of Cultural Tag of Koro

Introduction

Koro was included under the clinical heading of "Culture-bound Syndromes" in DSM-IIIR in 1987 and retained this berth in DSM-IV in 1994. In DSM-5, 2013, it lost its cultural tag and is placed under "Other specified Obsessive–Compulsive and Related Disorders" (300.3). DSM-5 retained the heading of Culture-bound syndromes under "Glossary of cultural concepts of distress" and included nine culture-bound syndromes, but not Koro. The following is a description of this historical journey over 117 years to explore why and how Koro earned its culture-boundness and carried this nosological tag since 1895 and how it lost this legendry diagnostic association in 2013. Let us follow the timeline of Koro's history since 1895 and references from the literature to explore how this cultural concept was strengthened or challenged over time.

A. N. Chowdhury, *Koro*,
https://doi.org/10.1007/978-3-030-87962-4_5

Methods

Extensive literature search on Koro was done between 1895 and 2020. A total of 394 publications are critically reviewed to make the following discourse on the nature of the historical progress of Koro's concept and nosological construct over the last 126 years.

Late 19th Century: Dutch Credit in the "Birth of Koro"

Though genital shrinkage/retraction symptoms existed for few centuries in Chinese medical texts (by the name *Suo-yang* or *Shook yang*) (Ng & Kua, 1996), the term "Koro" to designate the symptom of genital retraction started from 1874. It is by this name the illness was made known to the Western medical world. Interestingly, Dutch colonial medical inquiry made Indonesia (Dutch-Indies) the country from where Koro made its first appearance in world literature! Quite a handful of Dutch physicians and academic persons made some socio-anthropological investigation of locally prevalent diseases in different indigenous Dutch-Indies populations. Koro was one of them (Bergen et al., 2017). The following brief historical account will highlight this journey.

1874: The first reference of the term "Koro" is found in B. F. Matthes' Dictionary of Buginese Language of South Sulawesi. It said: *Koro* = "to shrink" and *Lasa Koro* = "a shrinking of the penis, a sort of disease that is not unusual amongst the natives and must be very dangerous" (p. 31).

1895: The first report of "Koro" appeared in the Western medical press (Dutch medical journal—Geneeskundig Tijdschrift voor Nederlandsch-Indie) by Dr. J. C. Blonk, a Dutch Physician. He is credited for introducing the concept and name of this folk-illness "Koro" from Makassar in Eastern Indonesia (Nederlandsch-Indie). He reported that this disorder is indigenous among local people, and there is a long history of this illness among the ethnic Chinese there. He thought that Koro might be related to the neurasthenic disposition or sex life of the person.

1896: Dr. P. C. J. van Brero was 2nd physician at the mental hospital in Bogor city (West Java province) and extensively researched "Dementia paralytica." He published (in Dutch) a paper on detailed discussion and interpretation of the Koro case, reported by Blonk (1895). He described Koro as "a strange compulsive idea." He elaborated the Koro or penile retraction perception in terms of "compulsive sensation" and "compulsive perception."

1897: Dr. P. C. J. van Brero published another account (in German) containing a detailed clinical report of Koro and an attempt for its nosological identity concerning the Koro-belief of the South Celebes people. He discusses the Koro anxiety in terms of death anxiety emanating from penile retraction, postulates a theory of compulsive-obsessive ideas, and asserts that this psychopathology has a mass distribution. Dr. A. H. Vorstmann, a Dutch medical officer in Palembang (Borneo), also published two Koro case reports from Kalimantan this year.

The Early Half of 20th Century: Koro's Broader Western Familiarity

The early part of the twentieth century is significant for Koro's reporting in the Western medical press. A series of publications by Dutch, French, and American doctors appeared, including a report of an epidemic in central China.

1908: Dr. J. Legendre, a French military physician, reported an outbreak of genital shrinking syndrome involving 20 male teenage students of a school in Szechwan, China. He refers to the condition as *so-in-tchen*. He viewed this syndrome as an "Asiatic psychosis which can manifest itself collectively as well as individually" and rumor played an important role.

1912: Two Dutch ethnographers Nicolaüs Adriani and Albert Kruyt encountered the genital shrinking phenomenon during their fieldwork in the Dutch East-Indies and reported that the name was derived from a tribe—Toraja in Sulawesi bearing the name *Koro*.

1918: Dr. K. C. Wong, a scholar of Chinese medical history, documented the Chinese cultural myths and beliefs about genital retraction illness. His article on "Sexual Diseases" was a precious medical document from China. He noted *Suo-yang* (retraction of penis and testes) as an acute complication of some sexual disease and locally considered a prodrome of impending death.

1934–1950: Several publications during these 17 years focused on Koro with Chinese and Indonesian (Macassarn ethnicity) cultural endowment. Notable publications were from P. M. van Wulfften Palthe, a Dutch psychiatrist at the hospital for mental diseases at Bongor. He contributed significantly to the clinical understanding of Koro, especially from the Indonesian context. His five papers (1934, 1935a, 1935b, 1936a, 1937) and a chapter in a textbook (1936b) are the most valuable early Koro documents. These provide a piece of rich and elaborate information on the clinical, epidemic, and endemic aspects, the linguistic genesis of the term "Koro," and ethnomedical and cultural perspective of genital retraction syndrome.

Mulder (1935) provided an ethnomedical aspect of Koro's cultural and religious context among the Sulawesi natives. Slot (1935), a government doctor in the South Celebes, provided a comprehensive clinical account of Koro and discussed ethnomedical views and indigenous therapy for Koro. Borrey (1936) described a Koro case, which he saw in Paul-Doumer Hospital in Guangdong. Strong (1945) identified Koro as a particular form of anxiety neurosis and observed a high prevalence among Buginese and Macassarians in the Celebes and North Borneo. From Nanking, Kobler (1948) reported a Koro case and opined Koro as the expression of acute castration fear intermingled with cultural beliefs and superstitions. Chabot (1950), from his fieldwork from South Sulawesi, provided a conceptual frame of Koro psychodynamics about the socio-cultural and sexual construct and Macassarese community codes. All these publications introduced the concept and clinical features of Koro to European psychiatry. The first reference of penile shrinkage in Indian literature was found at the background of Hindu religiosity (asceticism) by Sarkar (1943).

The Decade of 1950–1970: Yap-Rin and Gwee Era

The period from 1950 to 1970 is a very dynamic era in the history of psychiatric classification and the surfacing of Koro as a culture-bound distinct psychiatric entity. Prof. P. M. Yap from Hong Kong relentlessly attempted to provide a suitable nosological berth for Koro as per the International thoughts and classificatory scheme of his time. Dr. Hsien Rin from Taiwan, Dr. A. L. Gwee, and Dr. P. W. Ngui from Singapore contributed to focus Koro as a culture-based pathology to the international audience. The occurrence of the Koro epidemic in Singapore in 1967 further exemplified more clearly the basis of the Chinese cultural background of Koro. This era is a golden era concerning Koro's international acceptance and recognition as a culture-bound illness.

Yap's contribution: P. M. Yap was born in Malaysia, had his academic career in the U.K., and his professional life in Hong Kong. His international educational exposures and firsthand experiences with the cultural manifestation of several psychiatric phenomena in Southeast Asia (like Koro and Latah) and at the same time his exposure to the Western classification system like ICD and DSM prompted his transcultural spirit to understand and make understandable all these culture-related clinical phenomena in terms of current conceptual categories to the world. Yap started his medical career when there was a worldwide renewed interest in the international classification of all medical diseases. In 1949 the sixth revision of the Manual of the International Statistical Classification of Diseases, Injuries, and Causes of death (ICD 6) was published by WHO. The seventh revision of ICD was published in 1955, and the eighth revision in 1965. There was an international compulsion in academic psychiatry to use ICD-codes for indexing mental illness under proper classificatory schemes during these years. At the same time, the American classificatory system—DSM-I was published in 1952 and DSM-II in 1968. At this time, a growing interest was developing in comparative psychiatry. The new academic branch of psychiatry—"Transcultural Psychiatry" was emerging (Wittkower & Rin, 1965), with an attempt to bring different mental manifestations in non-Western cultures within the orbit of the Western classificatory system. In this climate, Prof Yap felt an academic compulsion to develop an acceptable (to Western medics) nosological berth for the far East's culture-bound syndromes, including Koro. His contribution to designate Koro as a culture-bound psychiatric entity was pioneering. Following is the discussion on his eight important academic papers during this era, which made Koro's acceptance to the global academic community as a culture-bound syndrome (with a deep route in Chinese culture).

1951: "*Mental diseases peculiar to certain cultures: A survey of comparative psychiatry.*" This is Yap's first scholarly paper where he tried a comparative analysis of Western psychiatric nosology with the Oriental psychiatric manifestations to bridge the universality of cultural influence on a mental illness over place and time. This is one of the first academic discourses on Koro, pointing toward a viable interface between culture and mental health.

1962: "*Words and things in comparative psychiatry with special reference to the exotic psychoses.*" Here Yap attempted to clarify the term "exotic psychosis" often used by Western academia as a collective term to designate unusual culture-related expressions of psychopathologies. Virtually this paper is a transcultural analysis of the nosological aspects of "exotic psychoses." He proposed a culture-laden term to replace "exotic psychoses" with "atypical culture-bound psychogenic psychosis."

1964a: "*Suk-yeong or Koro: A culture-bound depersonalization syndrome.*" Here he clarified Koro's cultural disposition in a very analytical way. He provided a compelling cultural explanation of Koro: "This is a unique example of a depersonalization syndrome whose form and content, and indeed occurrence and distribution, is determined by cultural factors. The depersonalization is seen as a dissociative mechanism affecting the integrity of the body-image" (p. 45).

1964b: "*Koro or Suk-yeong: An atypical culture-bound psychiatric disorder found in Southern Chinese*". Here he postulated Koro as a culture-dependent anxiety state and defined Koro or *Suo-yang* again as one of the culture-bound psychogenic disorders.

1965a: "*Koro: A culture-bound depersonalization syndrome.*" This is the first clinical report on Koro published in the British Journal of Psychiatry. It contains a detailed clinical description, historical background, etiology, and nosological clarification, based on his study of 19 Koro cases. For the first time since 1895, Koro earned a proper diagnostic label as a "culture-bound depersonalization syndrome" and carried this nosological tag for many years.

1965b: It is a Koro case report from Britain.

1967: "*Classification of the culture-bound reactive syndromes.*" This is a discussion paper with an attempt to classify culture-bound reactive syndromes. He discussed unusual forms of mental illnesses like Amok, Latah, and Koro with their different presentation in different cultures and stressed integrating them under an acceptable classificatory scheme.

1969: "*The culture-bound reactive syndromes.*" Yap provided a nosological proposition for the "culture-bound reactive syndromes," an attempt to balance the German and Scandinavian scientific taxonomies for reactive psychoses to exotic terms (Jilek, 1982). Yap proposed that "reactive syndromes" often present with a mixture of psychotic and neurotic symptoms.

[There is a posthumous publication of Yap on theoretical framework of comparative psychiatry in 1974].

Rin's contribution: Dr. Hsien Rin from National Taiwan University Hospital, Taipei, strengthens the Chinese cultural dynamics in Koro, blended with psychoanalytical thoughts, especially the concept of psychosexual development (orality), symbolism, and castration fear.

1963: His first paper on two Chinese case reports of Koro with a detailed discussion on yin-yang principles' Chinese cultural concept.

1965: Rin published his analysis of two Chinese Koro cases in the International Journal of Social Psychiatry, thus attracting British and Western academia's attention regarding Koro's concept and clinical aspect from the Chinese cultural perspective. He stressed the underlying cultural dynamics in Koro: "The panic state of *suo-yang* can be explained as an extreme form of fear of total castration resulting in death, but beyond this, it is a symbolic manifestation of fear of losing vitality, of becoming sick and weak, and it is deeply related to the fundamental Chinese concepts of sexuality" (p.7).

1966: Rin stressed the relationship between mental symptoms and Chinese culture. Chinese patients present two culture-bound psychiatric syndromes—Suo-yang or Koro and pa-leng or Frigophobia (morbid fear of cold). Both the syndromes were related to the Chinese concept of vitality and believed that its deficiency would have serious health consequences.

His meticulous analysis of the cases showed his sincere attempt to mix the Chinese cultural philosophy with Western psychodynamic theories, probably hoping for its logical acceptance to Western academia. This contention was very nicely put by Chiang (2015) as: "Mirroring the epistemic tension between the Chinese background of the patient and the Western psychodynamic approaches of the physician, koro emerged as a clinical entity on the overlapping geocultural margins of Chineseness and Anglophone psychiatric medicine" (p. 107).

Gwee's contribution: From Singapore, Dr. A. L. Gwee introduced Koro solely as a "Chinese disease." He tried to explain Koro's psychodynamics in terms of Chinese cultures, including tracing the castration theme from Imperial Chinese history. His three publications acted as a confirmatory signal to the global medical audience about Koro's cultural legacy.

1963: "*Koro: A cultural disease.*" It is one of the pioneering descriptions of Koro's cultural aspect of Chinese socio-cultural beliefs and traditional practices. Citations and illustrations of various old Chinese medical texts regarding penile retraction are essential contributions to this paper, strengthening the Chinese cultural link with genital retraction pathology.

1967: **Singapore Koro epidemic**: A landmark year in Koro's modern history because of the massive Koro epidemic in Singapore (started on 29th October 1967). Four publications on this epidemic further strengthen the Chinese cultural basis of Koro.

1. Gwee (1968): "*Koro – its origin and nature as a disease entity.*" It is a discussion paper on Koro with rich information on Chinese cultural beliefs and traditional Chinese medical references on genital retraction pathology. It contains an elegant clinical analysis of Koro, its

definition, an orthography of the term Koro with a citation from ancient Chinese medical texts. He elaborated on how rumor, social belief, and suggestibility worked hand in hand to generate and spread the Koro epidemic among a culturally susceptible population.

2. Mun (1968): *"Epidemic Koro in Singapore."* Mun provided a very valuable description of the role of local psycho-social factors causing the epidemic to the British academia (BMJ).
3. Ngui (1969): "*The Koro epidemic in Singapore.*" It is a detailed report of the Koro epidemic of Singapore. The author discusses Koro illness's historical background (the traditional Chinese medical theories) and Southeast Asian socio-cultural environment. A detailed demographic and clinical analysis of 226 cases (220 males and six females) was provided, and it commented that Koro should be regarded as a culture-bound psychogenic illness because cultural beliefs play a significant role in its genesis.
4. "*The Koro 'epidemic' in Singapore*" (1969) by Koro study team, Chaired by Gwee. It is the third survey report of the Singapore Koro epidemic. It very nicely focused on Koro's Chinese roots: "the disease has a Malay name; it is essentially a Chinese disease." In conclusion, they said Koro is a panic syndrome linked with "cultural indoctrination."

1970: This year is very important because of Koro's first reporting from a non-Chinese ethnicity—an American and secondary to psychotic illness (Edwards, 1970). The author discussed this clinical episode in the light of "subjective ideas of genital change" or "Koro pattern of depersonalization," not through any cultural lens. It marks the deviation of academic thoughts that Koro may not be a culture-dependent localized (in the Far East region) psychopathology. Consequently, Lapierre (1972) reported Koro's case in a French Canadian at the background of an organic illness and suggested that this is an example of psychogenic localized depersonalization due to post-operative stress, which generated distorted penile perception. So the cultural emphasis on Koro is refuted. Interesting to note both the authors adhered to Yap's concept of "depersonalization."

The Decade of 1971–1980: Shifting of Cultural Focus

This decade is significant for shifting the focus of culture-boundness (Chinese) of Koro to universal psychopathology. Reporting of two Koro epidemics from non-Chinese culture (Thailand and Indonesia) weakened its so-called Chinese ethnic–cultural heritage.

Koro epidemics: A strong evidence supporting non-cultural Koro manifestation came from reporting a Koro epidemic from Palembang, Indonesia (Moketi & Denin, 1978), and Thailand in 1976 (Jilek & Jilek-All, 1977a, 1977b; Suwanleart & Coates, 1979). The last authors reported 2000 cases from the Thai epidemic. They surveyed 350 Koro patients (338 males and 12 females) and noted that though Chinese comprise 10% of the population, not a single Chinese was affected.

Several reports of Koro from diverse ethnicities and countries continued to appear as follows: Three Koro reports from Canada shed light on the non-cultural aspect of Koro symptomatology. Dow and Silver (1973) reported drug-induced Koro syndrome in the background of abuse of amphetamine, methadone, cannabis, and LSD. Arbitman (1975) reported a Caucasian case secondary to depression, and marked obsessive–compulsive traits, and a habit of heavy alcohol drinking. This is the first research where the author attempts to explain Koro psychopathology in a non-cultural construct and tried to explore the body image of Koro patients by using a drawing test of the human figure. The author concludes that the patient had a poor self-image that was reflected in the deviation of body image, predominantly in the genital area. So the Koro perception finds another psychological explanation. Ede (1976) reported Koro's case in an Anglo-Saxon Canadian, associated with persecutory delusion. Haslam (1980) refocused the traditional view of Koro as a form of vital kidney deficiency syndrome (Shen k'uie).

Koro reporting from the Non-Eastern world: Hes and Nassi (1977) reported Koro in a Georgian Jewish immigrant from Israel, a faraway country from China. Barret (1978) reported the second case of Koro from England. The first case was reported by Yap (1965b). Most surprisingly, Koro-like case reports appeared from Nigeria, in African culture

(Anumonye & Adaranijo, 1978; Ifabumuyi & Rwegellera, 1979)—they challenged the validity of the "culture-bound" construct of Koro. Constable (1979) reported the third Koro case from Britain. The reporting from non-South Eastern countries shifted the cultural focus of Koro to other functional psychopathologies.

The Decade of 1981–1990: Ethno-Cultural Diversity of Koro

This decade's reports focus more on the generalization of Koro concept toward universal psychopathology, as evidenced by about 83 Koro and related publications during this period! The most important events are: (a) reporting of three epidemics—in Thailand (Suwanlert, 1983), India (Sachdev & Shukla, 1982), and Guangdong, China (Tseng et al., 1988). (2) Reporting more Koro cases secondary to other psychiatric illnesses and from different ethnicities and countries. (3) New waves of thoughts originated from the academic circle for a more modern classification for Koro (Bernstein & Gaw, 1990; Edwards, 1984). Even some researchers opposed the sole culture-bound identity of Koro. On the other hand, Wen and Wang (1979) refocused the traditional Chinese concept of Shen-k'uei—vital (kidney) deficiency syndrome for Koro. The First Koro case (Chakrabarty, 1982) and the first Koro epidemic were reported from India (Chakraborty et al., 1982; Dutta, 1983).

Koro reporting with new associations and the diagnostic label continued: Drug (Ludimol) induced Koro from Canada (Waldenberg, 1981); Koro as a hypochondriacal stress response by Rosenthal and Rosenthal (1982) who challenged the concept of depersonalization and favored the construct of hypochondriasis in their Koro case; Koro in reactive depression from the UK by Weller and Ameen (1982)—who also challenged the concept of culture-boundness in Koro as was suggested by Yap; Koro-like symptom at the background of cultural belief about *djinni* from Dares-Salaam, Tanzania (Lucieer,). A landmark report came from Berrios and Morley (1984), who turned the tide and gave Koro a new direction of universality. They published a series of 16 cases—15 were from non-Chinese ethnicity from diverse geographical areas like Britain,

France, South Africa, Canada, Greece, Israel, Nigeria, and India. Interestingly, all these fifteen cases suffered from primary psychiatric illnesses. They also hypothesize that Koro-like symptoms in non-Chinese subjects may constitute behavioral phenotypes (overvalued ideas, often to the delusional extent; related to concurrent psychiatric conditions) without any underlying cultural link. They also reported a case with 20 years' belief that his penis is recurrently shrinking and disappeared into the abdomen. This is one of the earliest reports indicating the association of hypochondriacal genital concern or a possibility of "Chronic Koro" diagnosis. Ang and Weller (1984) reported two Koro cases, one a West-Indian and a Greek Cypriot immigrant, in association with psychiatric illnesses. They suggested that Koro here manifests "hyperacute anxiety coupled with a delusional belief occurring in a psychotic setting." It is to be noted that Yap (1965a) also reported Koro's presentation with paranoid thinking and auditory hallucinations but was uncertain about this psychotic spectrum. That is why in his 1969 paper on culture-bound reactive syndrome, he incorporated both neurotic and psychotic dimensions. Considering the worldwide occurrences of Koro and its accompanying nosological diversity and confusion, Edwards (1984) proposed a new terminology for Koro as "Genital Retraction Syndrome," which was widely welcomed in the academic community.

1985: A robust organic boost-up is supported by the Simons and Hughes (1985) publication of a book devoted to the theme of "Culture-bound Illnesses" where Koro is classified under "genital retraction taxon," and the primary role of organic factors in Koro was formulated. They said culture plays a secondary role: the primary being the underlying physiological locus (penile vasoconstriction in response to physical or psychological states). Malinick et al. (1985) reported a Koro case in a black American male from the United States and focused on the link between witchcraft-belief and penis loss. While analyzing different Koro epidemics, Jilek and Jilek-Aall (1985) attempted to re-evaluate the concept of "culture-boundness" in Koro and stressed a sociological perspective, including the broader geopolitical and socio-economic climate of the affected population and the society. Emsley (1985) reported a non-Chinese Koro case in a black male from South Africa and identified the genital symptom as an acute anxiety state with delusional psychotic belief. Moodley (1985) reported Koro after Lorazepam withdrawal in a Scottish man from London. The author believes that this was an example of depersonalization focusing on the genital area due to acute anxiety state and also suggested that because of more reporting of Koro symptoms in association with anxiety-related conditions, Koro may be seen "as an unusual presentation of anxiety."

1986: Some publications of this year stressed the biomedical hypothesis rather than cultural issues in genital retraction pathology's genesis. Joseph (1986) reported two Koro cases associated with abnormal brain electrical activities, implicating epileptic body image distortions involving the genitals. Oyebode et al. (1986) presented an unusual case of Koro in a British man who had a six-year history of recurrent shrinking of the penis. They proposed abnormal physiological penile change and obsessional self-scrutiny as the cause of this Koro-like symptom. Ogunlesi (1986) reported the Koro case from Africa, in a Nigerian Yoruba tribal male, associated with paranoid psychosis.

1987: Several publications highlight Koro's organic or psychological basis and further weaken Koro's cultural theory. Holden (1987) reported Koro in a Zulu immigrant male from Kingston, Canada, at the background of alcoholic hepatitis, avitaminosis, and urinary tract infection. He refuted cultural diagnosis and asserted that Koro might be a reaction to various psychological or physical stressors rather than solely a culture-bound pathology. Mukherjee (1987) found no cultural factor in Koro's report on a white male from Kent, United Kingdom. Kendell and Jenkins (1987) reported Koro in a black American male from Columbia, United States, in association with schizophrenia, which they identified as "delusion of Koro." Money and Annecillo (1987) reported Koro as a body image disturbance from Baltimore, United States.

1988: Reporting of Koro from non-Chinese culture remains unabated. Chowdhury et al. (1988) reported a massive Koro epidemic from North Bengal, India—a region far from any Chinese cultural influence. Ilechukwu (1988) reported two Koro cases from Nigeria. Durst and Rosca-Rebaudengo (1988) described Koro with organic illness from Israel. Mellor (1988) expanded the theory of depersonalization and body image disturbances. The depersonalization in Koro is said to be somatic and localized to the genital area. Fernando (1988) reported Koro in a European male from New Zealand. He designated a non-cultural diagnosis: monosymptomatic hypochondriacal psychosis. Maslowski (1988) reported Koro with schizophrenia from Malta. Perera (1988–1989) reported two Koro cases from Sri Lanka with schizophrenia and the other with OCD-spectrum disorder.

1989: New research findings surfaced from the Indian epidemic: Chowdhury (1989a, 1989c, 1989d, 1991a, 1991b, 1991c, 1991d) from India reported several reports on dysmorphophobic penis-image perception in Koro patients and also found several biomedical factors (Chowdhury, 1989b) as a precipitator of Koro symptoms. Leo et al. (1989) reported Koro from Padua, Italy. The authors suggested that an organic condition (phimosis) affecting genitals may precipitate Koro among Western Europeans.

1990: Turnier and Chouinard (1990) reported Koro with depression from Canada. Anderson (1990) reported a case of Koro after a non-dominant temporoparietal stroke. For conceptual clarity, he preferred the name Genital Retraction Syndrome to Koro. Cortell (1990) reported the first case of Koro from Spain. Bernstein and Gaw (1990, 1991a, 1991b) considered Koro as an "Eastern phenomenon" and proposed Koro's specific category for inclusion into DSM-IV. Given Koro's strong cultural link, they suggested Koro's inclusion as a "culture-specific disorder strongly." The authors also raise the question of whether Koro is a unique cultural syndrome or merely the cultural expression of a universal phenomenon. They try to delineate the difference between Koro and Koro-like syndromes and assert that Koro can occur in the right setting and stimulus even in non-Chinese cultures. They highlighted a possible ground for a primary physiological substratum in Koro. This paper aroused lots of argument and suggestions on the different probability of Koro phenomenologies like increased sympathetic tone and high anxiety (Kennedy & Flick, 1991); body dysmorphic disorder or delusional disorder, somatic type (Stein et al., 1991), or dysmorphophobia or obsessive–compulsive disorder (Lipschitz, 1991). Chowdhury (1990a, 1990b, 1993e) examined the diagnostic status and trait anxiety profile of a cohort of epidemic male Koro cases from India. Amering and Katschnig (1990) compared Koro with a cross-cultural perspective of a panic attack and cited a similarity with the Kayak-Angst phenomena of Greenland and Polar Eskimos.

The Decade of 1991–2000: Biology of Koro

The debate between the culture-non-culture issue in Koro's genesis is continued, as shown in Koro's increased academic interest, exemplified by at least 101 Koro and related publications in this decade. Many of the researchers have stressed the role of biological factors over cultural issues in Koro. Following is the summary of the important contributions of this decade toward Koro phenomenology.

Koro continues to be reported from a vast non-Chinese geographical region like the Middle East (Amman, Riyadh, Jeddah, Qatar); Nepal, New Zealand, Ireland, Russia, Sri Lanka, and South Korea. Increasing contributions from the Urology faculty mark the importance of organic factors in Koro perception (PuraniK & Dunn, 1995). At least six Koro case reports were from urogenital clinical facilities, strengthening our insight about the diverse presentation of Koro in association with organic pathology (where culture has virtually no role). Two Koro reports with forensic presentation—from the United States (Lewis & Ednie, 1997) and New Zealand (Chowdhury & Faulkner, 1997) opened up a new associated pathology with Koro after a gap of 50 years of Palthe's (1937) publication of a forensic Koro case.

The report of an epidemic of "penis-loss" from Nigeria by Illechukwu (1992) is a finding with crucial transcultural significance in this field. It may be regarded as a Koro-variant presentation of a Mass Psychogenic Illness. The author attempts a phenomenological correlation between Koro and the magical penis-loss event. He believes that both are the expression of a common denominator, viz., the genitally focused primordial anxieties.

The discussion paper by Prince (1992) on the cultural cognition of fox-spirit and Koro in Hainan Island (China) gives a new impetus in favor of Koro's culture-boundness. The author provides an excellent anthropological account of the fox-spirit theme in Sino-Japanese folklores and attempts to corroborate its significance with the Koro cognition of Hainan Island epidemic cases. This discussion provides a conceptual bridge between psychiatric morbidity and traditional beliefs. This is a unique theoretical reinforcement to the weaning cultural significance attached to Koro. Three other papers (Chowdhury, 1993c; Tseng et al., 1992; Zeng et al., 1993) also deal with the fox spirit's theme.

Kirmayer's (1992) paper on the castration theme and Koro sheds light on this universal phenomenon's transcultural aspect. This is a comprehensive analysis of the theme of castration anxiety, including its universality, variability, and meaning across cultures. The author attempted to explore the dynamics of castration anxiety and sexual identity in culture-related illnesses of oriental societies like Koro, Dhat syndrome, or magical penis loss and cites an equivalent clinical entity in Western society. He provides a rich discussion on various ethno-physiological influences on the expression of castration anxiety in different cultures, e.g., semen-conservation doctrine, sexual restraining, masturbatory guilt, and interrelation between the expression of psycho-sexual anxieties and folk beliefs, ethno-physiological ideas, and social stresses of the concerned cultural groups.

Few publications enriched our understanding of Koro further—one is of a large cohort of Female Koro presentation in an epidemic setting from India (Chowdhury, 1994), a report of sporadic case from India (Chowdhury & Bera, 1995) and the other on Koro presentation involving tongue from Malaysia (Chin & S'ng, 1995). Chowdhury (1993a, 1993b), in a series of study highlighted the abnormality of penis image among Koro patients.

There are quite a few papers devoted to cultural psychiatry: (a) some are challenging the cultural tag with Koro, and (b) some support the cultural context in Koro.

a. Adeniran and Jones (1994) questioned whether Koro is a culture-bound disorder or a universal symptom. Bartholomew (1994, 1998) strongly refuted the medical postulations in Koro (particularly the epidemic form) and stressed the sociological perspective. Chowdhury (1996a) provided a proposal for new classification as Primary and Secondary Koro and also provided some critical biomedical context of altered physiological penis state in the precipitation of Koro attacks (Chowdhury, 1996b). The year 1995 marked the 100 years of Koro publication. Chowdhury (1998) summarized this long journey focusing on emerging new nosological dimensions of Koro-like monosymptomatic hypochondriacal psychosis, body dysmorphic disorder, or penile dysmorphophobia besides its culture-bound definition.

b. Chowdhury (1991e, 1991f) provided a medico-cultural social construct of the Indian Koro epidemic. Ng and Kua (1996) traced the references of Koro in ancient Chinese history. Ng (1997) reported the history of Koro in Singapore from a Chinese cultural perspective.

Koro symptoms with some unusual associations have been reported and thus widens the purview of Koro as a manifestation of various psychopathologies: Koro with H.I.V. infection (Heyman & Fahy, 1992); Capgras and Koro (Smyth & Dean, 1992); Koro and folie a deux (Menezes, 1992); Capgras, Fregoli and Cotard's syndromes (Wolff & McKenzie, 1994); Koro with infertility (Cohen et al., 1995); and Koro associated with a phobia for AIDS (Chand, 1998). Koro is reported in substance abusers: Heroin (Chowdhury & Bagchi, 1993); Cannabis (Chowdhury & Bera, 1994), and Buprenorphine withdrawal (Chowdhury & Banerjee, 1996).

1992: I.C.D. 10 Included Koro under the category F 48.8—"Other specified Neurotic Disorders" along with Latah and Dhat syndrome—all of which have culture-specific etiologies. It also includes 12 culture-bound syndromes, including Koro under Annexure 2. The suggested diagnostic codes are F48.8 or F45.34 (Somatoform autonomic dysfunction of the genito-urinary system).

1994: DSM-IV, A.P.A. included Koro as one of the entries in the Glossary of Culture-Bound Syndromes in Appendix I.

All these Koro publications across the different disciplines, viz. medicine, neurology, urology, and psychiatry, show its varied presentation and strike at the very root of its sole cultural hypothesis. The controversy between "culture-bound" or "universal" is not new. In fact, it started in the mid-1960s. Several researchers proposed a generalized classification of all mental disorders under a single umbrella. This process began in Kiev (1964), who tried to place different CBSs under common psychiatric categories like Koro and Susto under anxiety states; malojo and voodoo death under phobic disorders, jiwa itchk under depressive disorders, and latah under hysterical disorders. Murphy (1972) traced the history of latah from European colonial times and tried to offer a psychiatric explanation of the disorder. Simons (1985) classified CBSs under different taxons, and they provided seven taxonomical categories—Koro was included under genital retraction taxon. Marsella (1996) provided a catalog of additional nosological terms that were used to define CBSs. In the mid-1990s, a strong opinion was surfaced by the work of many researchers for the need for the inclusion of CBSs under the Western classificatory system (Kirmayer, 1991; Levine & Gaw, 1995; Prince & Tcheng-Laroche, 1987). They felt that all psychiatric disorders are culture-bound in a general sense, as no disease can escape local cultural encoding, shaping, presentation, and communicative style of distress experience (Littlewood, 1991). There were many suggestions, criticisms, and proposals for including CBSs at par with Western psychiatric thoughts (Bhui & Bhugra, 2001; Kapur, 1987), emphasizing culture's role in mental ill-health diagnosis and intervention. This debate was an essential issue in the proposed shift in the current classificatory scheme and groundwork relating to the DSM-IV Task Force working group (Littlewood, 1992, 1996). Despite all these academic noises, the ICD and DSM still kept Koro separately under descriptive annexure of Culture-bound syndromes (Alarcón, 1995).

1995–1999: Koro cases appeared from new geographical territory like Nepal (Chowdhury & Rajbhandari, 1995); Ireland (Phelan & Daly, 1996); Hungary (Kovács & Osváth, 1998); and Amman (AI-Hmoud, 1999)—all are indicative of cultures without Southeast Asian influence. Few case reports from genito-urinary faculties (Puranik & Dunn, 1995; Wilson & Agin, 1997) strongly advocated organic background of Koro.

2000: Few reports strengthen organic background in Koro-like urogenital pathology (Caballero, et al., 2000; Kim et al., 2000) or as a part of post-ictal psychosis (Bayer, 2000). DSM-IV, T. R., APA, listed Koro in the Glossary of Culture-bound Syndromes of Appendix I without any diagnostic code. It contains a descriptive account of 25 Culture-bound syndromes.

The Decade of 2001–2010: Universality of Koro

At least 55 Koro-related publications continued the trend of its diverse associations and new geography. Some researchers questioned its culture-boundness again. The new geographical territory has further expanded to Japan, Pakistan, Oman, Spain, Greece, Turkey, Mexico, and Poland.

A shift in the concept: After P. M. Yap, Prof. Wen-Shing Tseng (2001) of the University of Hawaii, Honolulu is another prominent academician in the field of culture-bound syndromes (CBS). Yap's challenge was to offer psychiatric nosology to a host of CBSs, including Koro, and distinguish and similarities between Eastern and Western psychiatric classifications. On the other hand, Tseng tried to establish Cultural Psychiatry—as a discipline in its own right. He redefined Culture-bound Syndromes to "Culture- related syndromes." He proposed a subdivision of CBSs into six different groups as per the role of culture in causing or shaping the pathology (Tseng, 2006): Pathogenetic (Koro, Dhat); Pathoselective (Amak, family suicide); Pathoplastic (Taijinkyofusho, Brain fag syndrome); Pathoelaborating (Latah); Pathofacilitating (mass hysteria, substance abuse); and Pathoreactive (Hwabyung, Susto). He stressed the changing clinical pattern of many of the CBSs over time. He also provided an example of culture-related syndromes in Western societies as well.

More and more researchers are questioning the cultural tag with Koro, and they provided different explanations and nosology for Koro. Perez et al. (2000) suggested that the CBSs should be conceptualized in the "context of a general dialectic between etic (universality) and emic (cultural specificity) rather than controversy on the need for an annex on CBS in the D.S.M." Altable and Urrutia (2004) questioned the diagnostic use of the term Koro with schizophrenia. They cited an example of "surface grammar" and "deep grammar" in symptom similarity. In the context of their patient, they raised the question of whether the Koro perception is a part of abnormal body experiences of a schizophrenic perceptual abnormality or coexistence of Koro and misidentification syndrome. Garlipp (2008) supports Koro's diagnostic label restriction and recommends its use only in epidemic cases where definite socio-cultural factors play a role. Chowdhury (2008a) provided a clear clinical guideline for secondary Koro presentation (in association with other disorders) as Koro-like symptoms (KLS). Marlowe (2009) challenged Koro's concept as a culture-bound Asian disorder, mainly because of Koro's widespread reporting from diverse regions, ethnicities and secondary to other diseases, ranging from substance abuse to psychosis. The author believes that the term "genital retraction syndrome" is a more useful descriptive term than Koro.

New associations: Association of drug abuse—cannabis, amphetamine, and steroid (Praharaj, 2004) with Koro, further strengthens some organic mechanism behind Koro perception. In some patients, koro-like symptoms are noted with the vasoconstrictive effect of amphetamine (Bloor, 2004; Charlott & Bycroft, 2009).

Koro's reporting from Eastern Indonesian cultural context (Mitchell, 2010) and body heat concept as an explanatory model from India's Koro patients (Chowdhury, 2008b) renewed the cultural flavor in the midst of all these to the construct of Koro.

The Decade of 2011–2020: New Diagnostic Berth for Koro

At least 61 publications appeared during this time. Egypt, Iran, Malaysia, and Australia are the new countries added to Koro geography. Some extraordinary psychiatric associations with Koro have been published like erectile dysfunction (Abdullah & Wahab, 2012); association with another CBS—Dhat syndrome (Kalra et al., 2012), Othello and Capgras syndrome (Marques, 2015), and Alzheimer disease (Tau & Masukar, 2020). There was a massive Koro epidemic in India in 2010 (Ghosh et al., 2013). After many years, two sporadic female Koro cases are reported: India (Srivastava & Pandit, 2013) and the other from England

(Chowdhury & Chawla, 2019). Several Koro epidemic reports appeared from India (Chakraborty & Sanyal, 2011; Dan et al., 2016; Debbarma et al., 2016; Nath et al., 2011; Promodu et al., 2012). A report on Africa's genital shrinkage/vanishing epidemic unfolds a socio-political-cultural dimension (Aikins et al., 2015). Re-focusing on the Singapore Koro epidemic sheds new light on a book (Mendelson, 2011) and a report (Everest-Phillips, 2018). Crozier (2012) did an extensive and scholarly review of Koro's different dimensions as an illness—from its inception by Dutch physicians and its explanation in the ambit of Western psychiatry. He provided a very insightful analysis of Koro phenomena over centuries. He explained appropriate social, anthropological, and global (migration) issues that influence the perception and concept of genital retraction or Koro among professionals.

DSM-5-2013 May: This marks the end of Koro's culture-related nosological status. DSM-5 replaced the term "culture-bound" with the concept of "cultural concept of distress"—that refers to ways that cultural group experiences, understands, and communicates suffering, behavioral problems, or troubling thoughts and emotions. Koro is reclassified in DSM-5 as under ORCD—"Other specified Obsessive–Compulsive and Related Disorders" (300.3). This inclusion takes away the suffix—"culture-bound" from the Koro label but offers a diagnostic code for the first time. This new category also included two other CBSs. This inclusion marks the end of the culture-related journey of Koro after 117 years!

There are seven clinical presentations grouped under the ORCDs:

1. Body dysmorphic like-disorder with actual flaws.
2. Body dysmorphic like-disorder without repetitive behaviors.
3. Body-focused repetitive behavior disorder.
4. Obsessional jealousy.
5. Shubo-kyofu: Similar to BDD with fear of having a bodily deformity
6. Koro: Anxiety that the penis, vulva, or nipples will retract into the body and may lead to death.
7. Jikoshu-kyofu or olfactory reference syndrome: A fear of having body odor.

So the next question comes whether this ORCD inclusion of Koro is how far justified. Let us answer this issue from two standpoints. Firstly what is the reported OCD-link with Koro reporting since 1895? Secondly, how logical is the ORCD inclusion of Koro.

OCD-link with Koro: There are at least 26 publications from different countries where direct OCD-link with Koro has been reported (Table 5.1).

Points in Favor

It is fascinating to note that Koro's second report in 1896 pointed out the OCD dynamics, namely "compulsive sensation" and "compulsive perception!" Indeed, many reported sporadic Koro cases, mainly secondary presentation (in association with other medical or psychiatric disorders), display OCD behavior like obsessive rumination or doubts about penis morphology (size, length, or shortening) and verities of compulsive behavior, and maneuvers of checking and rechecking penis over some time. They usually ran a chronic course (ranged from months to years), usually with other hypochondriacal health concerns and without any dramatic presentation of acute anxiety/panic-like features. They typically have a history of hypochondriacal health concerns and multiple health-seeking behaviors for a cure. These cases definitely may be designated under OCD spectrum. Besides, much recent research on penile dysmorphophobia and Koro or dysmorphophobic concern for the penis points toward definite OCD dynamics in Koro phenomenology. Moreover, Koro's perception (shrinking/retracting penis) spanning over a long period (ranging from weeks to months) generated a concept of "Chronic Koro" which was not apparent during Yap's time. And this chronicity points toward an OCD spectrum definitely.

The present author assumes that some confounding OCD-Koro cases (or hypochondriacal somatization) may be mixed with cases of an epidemic (Chowdhury, 1989e, 1992a, 1992b). Given the inadequate research insights, pressure of time, and flow of patients, this aspect has never been explored in detail in any of the Koro epidemic reports so far.

Table 5.1 Review of World Koro literature regarding Koro with OCD-link

Sl No	Author (year)	Type of report/country	Clinical findings indicative of OCD-link
1	P. C. J van Brero (1897)	Second report from Dutch-Indies (South Celebes)	Postulated Koro as a manifestation of obsessional-compulsive illness
2	P. M. Yap (1965a)	Analysis of 19 cases, Hong Kong	Four patients having compulsive personality
3	J. G. Edwards (1970)	Case report, Koro with Schizophrenia, from the U.S.A	He had traits of immaturity, obsession (perfectionism and compulsive checking). At age 18 years, he was preoccupied with the idea of his small size of penis
4	Arbitman (1975)	Second Koro case report from Canada	Koro in association with depression and marked obsessive–compulsive traits
5	Hes and Nasi (1977)	The first report from Israel	Association of obsessive–compulsive thoughts and sexual conflicts with masturbatory guilt
6	Cremona (1981)	Fourth case report from Britain	At age 21 the patient was admitted to a psychiatric hospital with health-related anxieties, particularly the health of his penis and obsessional thoughts and rituals

(continued)

Table 5.1 (continued)

Sl No	Author (year)	Type of report/country	Clinical findings indicative of OCD-link
7	Keshavan (1983)	Discussion paper, U.S.A	The role of suggestible personality with heightened self-scrutiny and over-concern about genitalia has been suggested
8	Modai and Muniz (1986)	A case report from Israel	A fearful concern of the shrinking penis and the concomitant avoidance behavior, e.g., avoiding pressure on the penis; holding the penis most of the time; inability to bend the body because of fear movement may cause further shrinkage
9	Oyebode et al. (1986)	A case report from the U.K	Six-year history of recurrent shrinkage of penis/ obsessional self-scrutiny of penis size
10	Fernando (1988)	A case report from New Zealand	Hypochondriacal health concern of dysmorphophobic nature (asymmetrical body), improved with Clomipramine
11	Perera (1988, 1989)	A case report from Sri Lanka	The patient was preoccupied with the obsessional doubt that his penis would disappear inside the abdomen, and he repeatedly checks, holds, and observed the organ almost on a half-hourly basis. He responded well with Clomipramine 50 mg twice daily

Sl No	Author (year)	Type of report/country	Clinical findings indicative of OCD-link
12	Hollander et al. (1989)	A case report from the U.S.A	Diagnosis of borderline personality disorder, Tourette's syndrome, obsessive–compulsive disorder, and marijuana abuse developed an obsessive rumination regarding a small and ugly penis at the age of 20. Marked improvement with Clomipramine (60 mg/day). His mother had obsessive–compulsive disorder
13	Heyman and Fahy (1992)	A case report from the U.K	A firm conviction that the penis had gradually been shrinking over the previous three months. He felt that it might disappear altogether, for which he made several visual scrutinies of the penis daily. He responded fairly with Dothiepin (150 mg/day) and cognitive psychotherapy
14	Goetz and Price (1994)	Report from Pennsylvania, U.S.A	Constant ruminations regarding his genitals and responded significantly with Clomipramine (100 mg p.o. qHS)

(continued)

Table 5.1 (continued)

Sl No	Author (year)	Type of report/country	Clinical findings indicative of OCD-link
15	Chowdhury et al. (1994)	Report from West Bengal, India	Mental state examination revealed a strong hypochondriacal bodily preoccupation with obsessive ideas
16	Wilson and Agin (1997)	A case report from New York, U.S.A	The patient had compulsive traits in keeping a detailed daily record of fluctuations of his symptoms. Diagnosed with anxiety disorder with Koro. He responded with Desipramine and by 2 weeks, the genital perception disappeared
17	Nakaya (2002)	A case report from Japan	Have 'continual compulsion to manually pull his penis' to prevent the penis' disappearance during wakening hours, and at night a cloth was tied around the base of the penis. Responded with Fluvoxamine (150 mg/day)
18	Laguna and Napiorkowska-Laguna (2003)	A case report from Poland	The patient responded favorably with Tab Fluvoxamine 100 mg daily for five months
19	Praharaj (2004)	A case report from Delhi, India	Steroid Abuse. He checks and rechecks his genitals several times a day

Sl No	Author (year)	Type of report/country	Clinical findings indicative of OCD-link
20	Kar (2005)	Report from Orissa, India	Fifteen years waxing and waning course. During exacerbations, he spent most of his time measuring the penis by a scale and pulling it to bring it out of the abdomen. He tied a string around it and attached it to a hook above to prevent its shrinkage during the night
21	Stip et al. (2007)	A case report from Quebec, Canada	His anguish took an obsessive form during his hospital stay to check and recheck his genitals frequently in the bathroom
22	Kondan (2008)	A case report from the U.K.	During his typical autonomic arousal episodes, he developed the feeling that his genitals were retracting into the abdomen and then rushed to the toilet to check whether the retraction is occurring. These episodes were frequent for the last ten years
23	Devis et al. (2012)	Discussion paper, U.S.A.	Koro is a culturally-specific form of OCD or related spectrum disorder

(continued)

Table 5.1 (continued)

Sl No	Author (year)	Type of report/country	Clinical findings indicative of OCD-link
24	Silva et al. (2016)	Case report from Portugal	He described these thoughts as repetitive, intrusive, and ridiculous He gradually developed a robust obsessive doubt about his penile condition and forced to verify his penis length several times a day. Responded with Fluvoxamine 200 mg/day and C.B.T.
25	Haghshenas et al. (2017)	A case report from Iran	He is also having a host of anxiety symptoms, along with obsessional thoughts about losing his penis
26	Ghosh and Chowdhury (2020)	A case report from Kolkata, India	The subject also has another culture-bound syndrome Dhat Syndrome and subsequently showed symptoms of obsessive–compulsive disorder

It is hoped that henceforth, researchers will try to explore this OCD-link in epidemic cases as well (Chowdhury, 1992e, 1995).

In order to receive a diagnosis of an OCRD, obsessive–compulsive symptoms must be the key and primary feature that cannot be better explained by something else like a medical condition, drug or alcohol use, or another psychiatric disorder. To complicate things further, people can receive dual diagnoses. For example, when Koro symptoms is a delusional perception in paranoid schizophrenia. Other areas of overlap may be hypochondriacal health concerns relating to sexual organs or functions, drug abuse, or withdrawal, especially cannabis and Koro in depression (functional or organic) where nihilistic delusion of "no penis" is the symptom. Of course, the questions remain whether "No penis" perception or apprehension of "penis loss" (into the abdomen) be considered Koro symptom or nihilistic delusion altogether. A critical area of perceptual transparency of Koro perception is warranted because there are varieties of penis-related perceptions reported as Koro in the literature. From a proper research methodological viewpoint, this area needs careful delineation of the symptom (Chowdhury & Brahma, 2020). In Koro—the perception is sudden, and the penis is retracting/shrinking toward the abdomen (due to inward pull) with fear of death, or sexual disability is the cardinal feature. Even the feeling of "shortness" of a penis without any intra-abdominal pull, is in a real sense, does not qualify for the Koro label. Penis loss or penis theft may be a Koro variant, not Koro in the strict clinical sense. These clinical clarifications are necessary for OCD attribution of Koro.

Points Against

The classical presentation of Koro or Primary Koro sometimes may have some obsessive–compulsive element in their clinical course (checking or rechecking of the penis). Still, the overall presentation mostly does not fit the criteria for OCD spectrum. Virtually, they are more close to an episode of panic attack except that Koro is usually not a recurrent disorder. But like a panic attack, it shows severe anxiety with autonomic arousal, derealization, depersonalization, an ideational component of fear of dying and may be associated with depressive or obsessive symptoms (ICD 10: F 41). In epidemic form, conversion disorder (F 44) and genitally focused hypochondriacal disorder (F 45.2) may be confounded in sporadic cases. OCD is not a one-off phenomenon—it has a long clinical course even if treated. Primary Koro is mostly a one-off phenomenon, with definite socio-cultural dynamics behind it, and very rarely, they are recurrent in nature in epidemic cohorts.

Koro as a "Symptom," not a Diagnostic Entity

This is another recent development where Koro is going to lose its diagnostic entity as a disease category. This is an emerging clinical construct accumulating over the years from the Koro reporting, mainly with secondary psychotic illness and often with extreme hypochondriacal health concerns. Here Koro lacks the classical acute presentation and constitutes one of the symptoms within the primary disorder's varied psychopathological frame.

There is quite a handful of reporting of such Koro-like symptom in association with schizophrenia, paranoid schizophrenia, and psychotic depression, where the shrinking or retracting of penis constitute a part of paranoid ideation (Ang & Weller, 1984; Altable & Urrutia, 2004; Chowdhury, 1992d, 1993b; Devan & Ong, 1987; Ede, 1976; Edwards, 1970; Kendell & Jenkins, 1987; Kranzler & Shah, 1988; Maslowski, 1988; Oyebode et al., 1986; Padi, 1984; Perera, 1988–1989; Yap, 1964b). In some reports, delusion is presenting with Folie a deux or "shared-belief type" of symptomatology where the patient checks the reality of penile indrawing or shortening with wife (Constable, 1979; Menezes, 1992; Ramamourty & Menon, 2014; Westermeyer, 1989) or with a prostitute (Kapugama et al., 2016). Their conviction was shared by the wife or the prostitute and thus added confirmation to the penile pathology. Some authors (Kendell & Jenkins, 1987) called it as "Koro delusion," and some say "Koro pattern of depersonalization" (Edwards, 1970). Some also questioned Koro's separate diagnosis, instead of considering this Koro symptom as part of the cases' broader psychopathology. They suggested the construct of "surface grammar" (similarity in symptom) and "deep grammar" (different psychopathology) (Altable & Urrutia, 2004; Yang et al., 2009) in secondary Koro presentation.

A similar situation is also reported in association with Depression (Anderson, 1990; Ang & Weller, 1984; Arbitman, 1975; Chowdhury 1992f; Hawley & Owens, 1988; Turnier & Chouinard, 1990; Weller & Ameen, 1982). For example, like the self-harming behavior, it may not be a diagnosis in secondary presentation but constitutes a part of the symptomatology. Self-harming behavior may present in various disorders like personality disorder, affective disorder, and schizophrenia. Similarly, Koro may be presented with genitally focused hypochondriasis (Cremona, 1981; Ifabumuyi & Rwegellera, 1979; Kar, 2005; Ntouros et al., 2010; Rosenthal & Rosenthal, 1982) or forerunner of affective disorder (Damodaran & Nizamie, 1993). Garg et al. (2017) termed Koro as a hypochondriacal delusional conviction. Koro is also present in cases with Obsessive–Compulsive rumination of genital scrutiny (Haghshenas et al., 2017; Modai et al., 1986; Nakaya, 2002; Silva et al., 2016; Yap 1965b). In all these secondary presentations, Koro's perception (usually non-acute) may be a symptom of penile ill-health perception and other multiple health concerns or pathology. All these cases were once identified as "Chronic Koro" (Chowdhury & Brahma, 2004), but after careful clinical scrutiny, it sounds more logical to designate them as Koro-like symptoms (Chowdhury, 2008a; Garlipp, 2008)—that is like a *symptom* under the primary diagnosis (like the pressure of speech in mania or mood dysregulation in emotionally unstable personality disorder, or paranoid delusion in schizophrenia), not as a diagnostic entity by its right.

Another challenging area is now coming under clinical debate about whether the perception of "no penis" or "penis loss" (Ogunlesi, 1986) is considered "Koro." Some authors reported Cotard's syndrome, nihilistic delusion with Koro (Alvarez et al., 2012; Bandinelli et al., 2011; El-Tantawy, 2017), or simply "delusion" (Ungvari & Mullen, 1994). Though in classical or primary Koro, the fear ultimately rests with the dissolution of the penis which stays within the body boundary (inside the abdomen) but outside normal viewing, and in that sense, it is not a loss of the penis. But in nihilistic delusion or Cotard's symptom, the penis is lost from the body altogether. So it is a clinical conjecture that this perception or apprehension of penis loss be equated with Koro symptom because there is a fine clinical line of demarcation between these two penis-deprivation states. This situation is further complicated and confounded because penis loss (or vanish) by theft through magic or witchcraft (Risso & Boker, 1968) and sorcery took an epidemic form in Africa, and many authors described these as Koro.

Conclusion

Whatever may be the academic controversy, Koro, after its 117 years of journey as a culture-bound disorder, now will be regarded as "Other specified Obsessive–Compulsive and Related Disorders" (300.3). It seems that there will be no "death" of this cultural tag with Koro in a broader cultural sense. It will remain as culture plays a crucial psychodynamic role in OCD symptom generation (de Silva, 2006; Okasha et al., 1994). Culture is vital, especially concerning the interpretation of stress (Nicoloini et al., 2017; Popa et al., 2014), religiosity (Okasha et al., 1994), and feeling of sex guilt (Inozu et al., 2012, Chowdhury, 1993d, 1996c), many of which are a contributor to Koro symptom formation (Chowdhury, 1992g). Cross-cultural variation in OCD phenomenology (Williams et al., 2017) and the cultural meaning and experience of OCD-related beliefs (Brakoulias & Starcevic, 2011), especially about sexual morphology (Wylie & Eardley, 2007) and functioning (Real et al., 2013) are the emerging areas of research. They may, in some way, refocus the interface between OCD-culture and Koro. The epidemic spread of Koro is visibly a culture-dependent phenomenon (Chowdhury, 1989f, 1992c). World Koro reporting from different cultures, ethnicities, and diverse associated pathologies attests to this trend (Chowdhury, 2015).

References

Abdullah, K. H. A., & Wahab, S. (2012). Koro-like symptoms with associated erectile dysfunction in a Rohingha refugee. *ASEAN Journal of Psychiatry, 13*(2), 221–223.

Adeniran, R. A., & Jones, J. R. (1994). Koro: Culture-bound disorder or universal symptom? *British Journal of Psychiatry, 164*(4), 559–561.

Adriani, N., Kruijt, A. C. (1912). *De Bare'e - Sprekende Toradja's van Midden-Celebes*. Landsdrukkerij.

Aikins, A. de-G., Dzokoto, V. A., & Yevak, E. (2015). Mass media constructions of 'socio-psychological epidemics' in sub-Saharan Africa: The case of genital shrinking in 11 countries. *Public Understanding of Science, 24*(8), 988–1006.

Alarcón, R. D. (1995). Culture and psychiatric diagnosis: Impact on DSM-IV and ICD-10. *Psychiatric Clinics of North America, 18*, 449–466.

Al-Hmoud, N. (1999). Koro-like syndrome in a Jordanian male. *Eastern Mediterranean Health Journal, 5*, 611–613.

Altable, C. R., & Urrutia, A. R. (2004). Koro-misidentification syndrome in schizophrenia? A Plea for Clinical Psychopathology. *Psychopathology, 37*(5), 249–252.

Alvarez, P., Puente, V. M., Blasco, M. J., Salgado, P., Merino, A., & Bulbena, A. (2012). Concurrent Koro and Cotard syndromes in a Spanish male patient with a psychotic depression and cerebrovascular disease. *Psychopathology, 45*(2), 126–129.

Amering, M., & Katschnig, H. (1990). Panic attacks and panic disorder in cross-cultural perspective. *Psychiatric Annals, 20*(9), 511–516.

Anderson, D. N. (1990). Koro: The genital retraction syndrome after stroke. *British Journal of Psychiatry, 157*, 142–144.

Ang, P. C., & Weller, M. P. I. (1984). Koro and psychosis. *British Journal of Psychiatry, 145*, 335.

Anumonye, A., & Adaranijo, H. (1978). Chronic nonspecific urethritis as psychological reaction among Nigerian neurotic patients. *Nigerian Medical Journal, 8*, 3–5.

Arbitman, R. (1975). Koro in a Caucasian. *Modern Medicine of Canada, 30*, 970–971.

Bandinelli, M., Trevisi, M., Kotzalidis, G. D., Manfredi, G., Rapinesi, C., & Ducci, G. (2011). Chronic koro-like syndrome (KLS) in recurrent depressive disorder as a variant of Cotard's delusion in an Italian male patient. A case report and historical review. *Rivista di Psychiatria, 46*(3): 220–226.
Barret, K. (1978). Koro in a Londoner. *Lancet, ii*, 1319.
Bartholomew, R. E. (1994). The social psychology of 'epidemic koro'. *International Journal of Social Psychiatry, 40*(1), 46–60.
Bartholomew, R. E. (1998). The medicalization of exotic deviance: A sociological perspective on epidemic koro. *Transcultural Psychiatry, 35*(1), 5–38.
Bayer, R. S. (2000). Koro-like symptoms and transient post-ictal psychosis. *Qatar Medical Journal, 9*(2), 68–69.
Bergen, L. van, Hesselink, L., & Verhave, J. P. (Eds.). (2017). *The Medical Journals of the Dutch Indies. A platform for medical research.* Indonesian Academy of Sciences.
Berntein, R. L., & Gaw, A. C. (1990). Koro: Proposed classification for DSM-IV. *American Journal of Psychiatry, 147*, 1670–1674.
Berntein, R. L., & Gaw, A. C. (1991a). Classification of Koro. *American Journal of Psychiatry, 148*, 1280.
Berntein, R. L., & Gaw, A. C. (1991b). Classification of Koro. *American Journal of Psychiatry, 148*, 959–960.
Berrios, G. E., & Morley, S. J. (1984). Koro-Like symptom in a non-Chinese subject. *British Journal of Psychiatry, 145*, 331–334.
Bhui, K., & Bhugra, D. (2001). Transcultural psychiatry: Some social and anthropological research issues. *International Journal of Social Psychiatry, 47*(3), 1–9.
Blonk, J. C. (1895). Koro. *Geneeskunding Tijaschrift Voor Nederlandsch-Indie, 35*, 562–563.
Bloor, R. N. (2004). Whizz-dick: Side effect, urban myth or amphetamine-related koro-like syndrome? *International Journal of Clinical Practice, 58*(7), 717–719.
Borrey, F. (1936). A propos du Koro. *La Presse Medicale, 44*(72), 1415.
Brakoulias, V., & Starcevic, V. (2011). The characterization of beliefs in obsessive-compulsive disorder. *Psychiatric Quarterly, 82*, 151–161.
Brero, P. C. J. van. (1896). Naar Aanleiding van het Opstel Over "Koro" van den Heer J. C. Blonk-in de Voring Aflevering van dit Tijdschrift. *Geneeskunding Tijdschrrift Voor Nederlandsch-Indie, 36*, 48–54.
Brero, P. C. J. van. (1897). Koro, eine Eiggentuemliche Zwangsv-Orstellung. *Allegemeine Zeitschrift Fur Psychiatric Und Psychischgerichtliche Medicin, 53*, 569–573.

Caballero, J. M., Avila, A., Cardona, X., Sastre, F., & Bello, M. P. (2000). Genital pain without urogenital pathology: The koro-like syndrome. *Journal of Urology, 163*(1), 243.
Chabot, H. T. (1950). *Verwanschap, Stand en Sex in Zuid-Celebes*. J. B. Wolters.
Chakrabarty, P. K. (1982). Koro: A peculiar anxiety neurosis (A Case Report). *Indian Journal of Psychiatry, 24*, 192–193.
Chakraborty, S., & Sanyal, D. (2011). An outbreak of Koro among 19 workers in a jute mill in South Bengal. *Industrial Psychiatry Journal, 20*(1), 58–60.
Chakraborty, A., Das, S., & Mukherjee, A. (1982, 3–4 December). *Koro makes an epidemic appearance in India. Transcultural Newsletter*, III.
Charlotte, L. F., & Bycroft, J. (2009). Street urology: Beyond the formulary. *BJU International, 104*(5), 722.
Chand, S. P. (1998). Koro associated with phobia for AIDS. *International Journal of Psychiatry in Medicine, 28*(3), 353–356.
Chiang, H. (2015). Translating culture and psychiatry across the Pacific: How koro became culture-bound. *History of Science, 53*(1), 102–119.
Chin, C. N., & S'ng, K. H. (1995). "Koro"–like syndrome affecting the tongue-a case report. *Medical Journal of Malaysia, 50*(2), 175–177.
Chowdhury, A. N. (1989a). Penile perception of Koro patients. *Acta Psychiatrica Scandinavica, 80*, 183–186.
Chowdhury, A. N. (1989b). Biomedical potential for symptom choice in Koro. *International Journal of Social Psychiatry, 35*, 329–332.
Chowdhury, A. N. (1989c). Dysmorphic penis image perception - The root of Koro vulnerability. *Acta Psychiatrica Scandinavica, 80*, 518–520.
Chowdhury, A. N. (1989d). Draw-a-penis test (DAPT). *Journal of Personality & Clinical Studies, 5*, 97–100.
Chowdhury, A. N. (1989e). Neuroticism, extraversion and sex-guilt cognition in the genesis of Koro. *Journal of Indian Psychoanalytical Society, 43*, 57–64.
Chowdhury, A. N. (1989f). Koro among kinships. *Indian Journal of Social Psychiatry, 5*, 24–26.
Chowdhury, A. N. (1990a). Diagnostic nosology of Koro. *Journal of Personality & Clinical Studies, 6*, 207–209.
Chowdhury, A. N. (1990b). Trait anxiety profile of Koro patients. *Indian Journal of Psychiatry, 32*, 330–333.
Chowdhury, A. N. (1991a). Penis root perception of Koro patients. *Acta Psychiatrica Scandinavica, 84*, 12–13.
Chowdhury, A. N. (1991b). Dysmorphic penis perception in Koro. *Indian Journal of Psychiatry, 32*, 330–333.

Chowdhury, A. N. (1991c). Personality profile of Koro patients. *Journal of Personality & Clinical Studies, 7*, 117–118.
Chowdhury, A. N. (1991d). Penis-shaft perception of Koro patients. *Journal of Indian Academy of Applied Psychology, 17*, 41–44.
Chowdhury, A. N. (1991e). Medico-cultural cognition of Koro epidemic: An ethnographic study. *Journal of Indian Anthropological Society, 26*, 155–170.
Chowdhury, A. N. (1991f). Role of medical cognition in psychiatric outbreaks: Study from North Bengal Koro epidemic. *Indian Journal of Behavioral Sciences, 1*, 64–67.
Chowdhury, A. N. (1992a). Ego and the body image. *Journal of Indian Psychoanalytical Society, 46*, 51–60.
Chowdhury, A. N. (1992b). Koro social response (*urban*): A longitudinal study of North Bengal Koro epidemic. *Indian Journal of Psychiatry, 34*, 46–52.
Chowdhury, A. N. (1992c). Psychic infectivity: The role of positive illness cognition in psychiatric epidemic. *Journal of Personality & Clinical Studies, 8*, 125–128.
Chowdhury, A. N. (1992d). Koro in schizophrenia with a case report from industrial set up. *Industrial Psychiatry Journal, 5*(1), 47–59.
Chowdhury, A. N. (1992e). Clinical analysis of 101 Koro cases. *Indian Journal of Social Psychiatry, 7*, 67–70.
Chowdhury, A. N. (1992f). Koro in affective disorder with a case report from industrial setup. *Industrial Psychiatry Journal, 5*(2), 71–83.
Chowdhury, A. N. (1992g). Psychopatho-sexuality in Koro patients. *Journal of Indian Academy of Applied Psychology, 5*, 71–83.
Chowdhury, A. N. (1993a). Glans penis perception of Koro patients. *Acta Psychiatrica Scandinavica, 87*, 355–357.
Chowdhury, A. N. (1993b). Variations in the perception of penis. *Journal of Sexual Health, 3*, 156–160.
Chowdhury, A. N. (1993c). Psychiatric morbidity and the fox connection. *Transcultural Psychiatric Research Review, 30*(4): 399–401.
Chowdhury, A. N. (1993d). Art in Koro. *Journal of Sexual Health, 3*(7), 181.
Chowdhury, A. N. (1993e). Age specific trait anxiety in Koro patients. *Journal of Personality & Clinical Studies, 9*, 15–18.
Chowdhury, A. N. (1994). Koro in females: An analysis of 48 cases. *Transcultural Psychiatric Research Review, 31*, 369–380.
Chowdhury, A. N. (1995). Koro and the Indian psychiatrists. *Indian Journal of Social Psychiatry, 11*, 78–80.
Chowdhury, A. N. (1996a). Definition and classification of Koro. *Culture, Medicine & Psychiatry, 20*, 41–65.

Chowdhury, A. N. (1996b). Koro: A state of sexual panic or altered physiology? *Sexual & Marital Therapy, 11*, 39–46.

Chowdhury, A. N. (1996c). Sex guilt cognition in the genesis of Koro. *Archives of Indian Psychiatry, 3*, 52–59.

Chowdhury, A. N. (1998). Hundred years of Koro. *International Journal of Social Psychiatry, 44*, 182–189.

Chowdhury, A. N. (2008a). Cultural Koro and Koro-like symptom (KLS). *German Journal of Psychiatry, 11*, 81–82.

Chowdhury, A. N. (2008b). Ethnomedical concept of heat and cold in Koro: Study from Indian patients. *World Cultural Psychiatry Research Review, 3*, 146–158.

Chowdhury, A. N. (2015). Koro. In R. L. Cautin & O.S. Lilienfeld (Eds.), *The encyclopedia of clinical psychology* (1st ed., pp. 1626–1629). Wiley.

Chowdhury, A. N., & Bagchi, D. (1993). Koro in heroin withdrawal. *Journal of Psychoactive Drugs, 25*, 257–258.

Chowdhury, A. N., & Banerjee, G. (1996). Recurrent Koro in repeated IV buprenorphine withdrawal. *Addiction, 91*, 145–146.

Chowdhury, A. N., Banerjee, G., Sen, K. D., Bera, N. K., & Sharma, N. K. (1994). Koro in West Bengal again: Report of nine cases. *Indian Journal of Social Psychiatry, 10*, 27–30.

Chowdhury, A. N., & Bera, N. K. (1994). Koro following cannabis smoking. *Addiction, 89*, 1017–1020.

Chowdhury, A. N., & Bera, N. K. (1995). Koro in North Bengal anew: An unusual case. *Journal of Personality & Clinical Studies, 11*, 48–51.

Chowdhury, A. N., & Brahma, A. (2004). Chronic Koro. *Eastern Journal of Psychiatry, 8*, 57–59.

Chowdhury, A. N., & Brahma, A. (2020). Update on Koro research methodology. *Indian Journal of Psychiatry, 62*(1), 102–104.

Chowdhury, A. N., & Chawla, M. (2019). Koro in female. A case report and a mini review. *European Journal of Psychiatry, 33*(4), 182–185.

Chowdhury, A. N., & Faulkner, R. (1997). Koro and offending behaviour: A report from New Zealand. *Transcultural Psychiatry, 34*, 545–546.

Chowdhury, A. N., & Rajbhandari, K. C. (1995). Koro with depression from Nepal. *Transcultural Psychiatric Research Review, 32*, 87–90.

Chowdhury, A. N., Pal, P., Chatterjee, A., Roy, M., & Das Chowdhury, B. B. (1988). Analysis of North Bengal Koro epidemic with three years follow-up. *Indian Journal of Psychiatry, 30*, 60–72.

Cohen, S., Tennenbaum, S. Y., Teitelbaum, A., & Durst, R. (1995). The koro (genital retraction) syndrome and its association with infertility: A case report. *Journal of Urology, 153*(2), 427–428.

Constable, P. L. (1979). Koro in Hertfordshire. *Lancet, 1*, 163.

Cortell, A. M. (1990). Apropos the first case of koro syndrome in Spain. *Medicina Clinica (barcilona), 95*(9), 358–359.

Cremona, A. (1981). Another case of Koro in a Briton. *British Journal of Psychiatry, 138*, 180–181.

Crozier, I. (2012). Making up koro: Multiplicity, psychiatry, culture, and penis-shrinking anxieties. *Journal of History of Medicine & Allied Sciences, 67*(1), 36–70.

Damodaran, S. S., & Nizamie, S. H. (1993). "Incomplete Koro" – A fore-runner for mood disorders: Two case reports. *Indian Journal of Psychiatry, 35*, 60–62.

Dan, A., Mondal, T., Chakraborty, K., Chaudhuri, A., & Biswas, A. (2016). Clinical profile and outcome of Koro: A follow up study from a Koro epidemic in West Bengal India. *Indian Journal of Psychiatry, 58*(suppl 1), 571.

Debbarma, S., Das, S. K., Kumar, A., Debbarma, S., Das, A., & Reang, T. (2016). Koro epidemic: A descriptive study. *Journal of Evolution of Medical & Dental Sciences, 5*(76), 5634–5638.

de Silva, P. (2006). Culture and obsessive-compulsive disorder. *Psychiatry, 5*(11), 402–404.

Devan, G. S., & Ong, H. S. (1987). Koro and schizophrenia in Singapore. *British Journal of Psychiatry, 150*, 106–107.

Devis, D. M., Stever, A. M., Terwilliger, J. M., Williams, M. T. (2012). The relationship between the culture-bound syndrome Koro and obsessive-compulsive disorder. In G. R. Hayes & M. H. Bryant (Eds.), *Psychology of culture* (pp. 213–221). Nova Science Publisher Inc.

Diagnostic and Statistical Manual of Mental Disorders. (1982). 3rd ed. American Psychiatric Association.

Diagnostic and Statistical Manual of Mental Disorders. (1987). 3rd ed. Rev. American Psychiatric Association. American Psychiatric Press Inc.

Diagnostic Criteria from DSM-IV. (1994). *American Psychiatric Association.* American Psychiatric Press Inc.

Diagnostic and Statistical Manual of Mental Disorders. (2000). *DSM-IV-TR* (4th ed). American Psychiatric Association.

Diagnostic and Statistical Manual of Mental Disorder. (2013). 5th ed. American Psychiatric Association.

Dow, T. W., & Silver, D. A. (1973). Drug induced Koro syndrome. *Journal of Florida Medical Association, 60*, 32.

Durst, R., & Rosca-Rabaudengo, P. (1988). Koro secondary to a tumour of the corpus callosum. *British Journal of Psychiatry, 153*, 251–254.

Dutta, D. (1983). Koro epidemic in Assam. *British Journal of Psychiatry, 143*, 309–310.

Ede, A. (1976). Koro in an Anglo Saxon Canadian. *Canadian Psychiatric Association Journal, 21*, 389–391.

Edwards, J. G. (1970). The Koro pattern of depersonalization in an American schizophrenic patient. *American Journal of Psychiatry, 126*, 1171–1173.

Edwards, J. W. (1984). Indigenous Koro: A genital retraction Syndrome of insular South East Asia: A critical review. *Culture, Medicine & Psychiatry, 8*, 1–24.

El-Tantawy, A. M. M. A. (2017). Chronic Koro-Like Syndrome co-morbid with schizophrenia and history of cannabis abuse in an Egyptian patient: Case report. *Arab Journal of Psychiatry, 28*(1), 92–96.

Emsley, R. A. (1985). Koro in non-Chinese subjects. *British Journal of Psychiatry, 146*(1), 102.

Everest-Phillips, M. (2018). Anxiety politics in Singapore: The "Koro Crisis" of 1967. *Asian Journal of Public Affairs, 10*(2), 53–66.

Fernando, N. (1988). Monosymptomatic hypochondriasis treated with a tricyclic antidepressant. *British Journal of Psychiatry, 152*, 851–852.

Garg, K., Kumar, C. N., & Sharadhi, C. (2017). Koro: Much more than just a culture bound syndrome. *Asian Journal of Psychiatry, 29*, 146–147.

Garlipp, P. (2008). Koro-A culture-bound phenomenon: Intercultural psychiatric implications. *German Journal of Psychiatry, 11*(1), 21–28.

Ghosh, S., Nath, S., Brahma, A., & Chowdhury, A. N. (2013). Fifth Koro epidemic in India: A review report. *World Cultural Psychiatry Research Review, 8*(1), 8–20.

Ghosh, S., & Chowdhury, A. N. (2020). A case of two culture-bound syndromes (Koro and Dhat syndrome) coexisting with obsessive-compulsive disorder. *Indian Journal of Psychiatry, 62*(2), 221–222.

Goetz, K. L., & Price, T. R. (1994). A case of koro: Treatment response and implications for diagnostic classification. *Journal of Nervous & Mental Disease, 182*(10), 590–591.

Gwee, A. L. (1963). Koro - A cultural disease. *Singapore Medical Journal, 4*, 119–122.

Gwee, A. L. (1968). Koro - Its origin and nature as a disease entity. *Singapore Medical Journal, 9*, 3–6.

Haghshenas, M., Malekpour, F., Yousefi, E., Shalbafan, M., Behtash, N., & Shirazi, E. (2017). Koro-like syndrome in an Iranian 50 years old man; is it a variant caused by cultural issues? *Journal of Neurology & Psychology, 5*(1), 3.

Haslam, M. T. (1980, December). Medicine and the orient: Shen-K'uei syndrome. *British Journal of Sexual Medicine*, 31–36.

Hawley, R. M., & Owens, J. H. (1988). Koro: Its presentation in an elderly male. *International Journal of Geriatric Psychiatry, 3*, 69–72.

Hess, J. P., & Nassi, G. (1977). Koro in a Yemenite and a Georgian Jewish immigrant. *Confinia Psychiatrica, 20*, 180–184.

Heyman, I., & Fahy, T. A. (1992). Koro-like Symptoms in a man infected with human immunodeficiency virus. *British Journal of Psychiatry, 160*, 119–121.

Holden, T. J. (1987). Koro syndrome associated with alcohol-induced systemic disease in a Zulu. *British Journal of Psychiatry, 151*(5), 695–697.

Hollander, E., Liebowitz, M. R., Winchel, R., Klumker, A., & Dlein, D. F. (1989). Treatment of body-dysmorphic disorder with serotonin reuptake blockers. *American Journal of Psychiatry, 146*, 768–770.

ICD-6. (1949). *Manual of the international statistical classification of diseases, injuries, and causes of death* (6th Rev.). World Health Organization.

ICD-9. (1978). Mental disorders: Glossary and guide to their classification in accordance with the ninth revision of the international classification of diseases. World Health Organization.

ICD-10. (1992). *Classification of Mental and Behavioural Disorders. Clinical description and diagnostic guidelines*. World Health Organization and Oxford University Press.

Ifabumuyi, O. I., & Rwegellera, G. G. C. (1979). Koro in a Nigerian male patient: A case report. *African Journal of Psychiatry, 5*, 103–105.

Illechukwu, S. T. C. (1988). Koro-like syndrome in Nigeria. *Transcultural Psychiatry Research Review, 25*, 310–314.

Illechukwu, S. T. C. (1992). Magical penis loss in Nigeria: Report of a recent epidemic. *Transcultural Psychiatric Research Review, 29*, 91–108.

Inozu, M., Karanci, A. N., & Clark, D. A. (2012). Why are religious individuals more obsessional? The role of mental control beliefs and guilt in Muslims and Christians. *Journal of Behavior Therapy & Experimental Psychiatry, 43*(3), 959–966.

Jilek, W. G. (1982). Culture – "Pathoplastic" or "Pathogenic"? A key question of comparative psychiatry. *Curare, 5*, 57–68.

Jilek, W., & Jilek-Aall, L. (1977a). A Koro epidemic in Thailand. *Transcultural Psychiatric Research Review, 14*, 57–59.

Jilek, W., & Jilek-Aall, L. (1977b). Mass hysteria with Koro symptom in Thailand. *Schweizer Archieve Neurologic Neurochirurgie Und Psychiatrie, 120*, 257–259.

Jilek, W., & Jilek-Aall, L. (1985). The metamorphosis of "Culture-bound" syndromes. *Social Science & Medicine, 21*, 205–210.

Joseph, A. B. (1986). Koro: Computed tomography and brain electrical activity mapping in two patients. *Journal of Clinical Psychiatry, 47*, 430–432.

Kalra, G. S., Bansod, A., & Shah, N. B. (2012). A case report of dhat and koro: A double jeopardy. *ASEAN Journal of Psychiatry, 13*(1), 91–95.

Kapugama, K. G. C. L., Obadaarchchi, L. N., Ruwanpriya, B. V. S., & Kuruppuarachchi, K. A. L. A. (2016). Depression presenting with genital symptoms - a series of unusual case histories. *Sri Lanka Journal of Psychiatry, 7*(2), 23–25.

Kapur, R. L. (1987). Commentary on culture-bound syndromes and international disease classification. *Culture, Medicine & Psychiatry, 11*, 43–48.

Kar, N. (2005, October 12). *Chronic koro-like symptoms - two case reports. BMC Psychiatry, 5*, 34.

Kendell, E. M., & Jenkins, P. L. (1987). Koro in an American man. *American Journal of Psychiatry, 144*(12), 1621.

Kennedy, B., & Flick, G. R. (1991). Classification of Koro. *American. Journal of Psychiatry, 148*, 1278–1279.

Keshavan, M. S. (1983). Epidemic psychosis or epidemic Koro? *British Journal of Psychiatry, 142*, 100–101.

Kim, J., Kim, M., Lee, N., & Park, Y. (2000). A case of urethrocutaneous fistula with koro syndrome. *Journal of Urology, 164*(1), 123.

Kiev, A. (1964). *Magic, faith, and healing*. Free Press.

Kirmayer, L. J. (1991). The place of culture in psychiatric nosology: Taijin Kyofusho and DSM-IIIR. *Journal of Nervous & Mental Disorder, 179*, 19–28.

Kirmayer, L. J. (1992). From the Witche's hammer to the Oedipus complex: Castration anxiety in Western society. *Transcultural Psychiatric Research Review, 29*, 133–138.

Kobler, F. (1948). Description of an acute castration fear, based on superstition. *Psychoanalytic Review, 35*, 285–289.

Kondan, V. R. J. (2008). A case of koro in a Caucasian man. *Progress in Neurology & Psychiatry, 12*(4), 25–27.

Koro Study Team (Chairman: AL Gwee). (1969). The Koro epidemic in Singapore. *Singapore Medical Journal, 10*, 234–242.

Kovács, A., & Osváth, P. (1998). Genital retraction syndrome in a Korean women. A case of koro in Hungary. *Psychopathology, 31*, 220–224.
Kranzler, H. R., & Shah, P. (1988). Atypical Koro. *British Journal of Psychiatry, 152*, 579–580.
Laguna, D., & Napiorkowska-Laguna, D. (2003). Koro - culture-bound or universal syndrome? Review of the literature and case report. *Advances in Psychiatry & Neurology, 12*(4), 457–468.
Lappierre, Y. D. (1972). Koro in a French Canadian. *Canadian Psychiatric Association Journal, 17*, 333–334.
Legendre, J. (1908). Une curieuse epidemic. *Annales De Medicine Coloniale, 11*(2), 280–281.
Leo, D. D., Mauro, P., & Pellegrini, C. (1989). An organic triggering factor in koro syndrome? A Case Report. *European Journal of Psychiatry, 3*(2), 77–81.
Levine, R. E., & Gaw, A. C. (1995). Culture-bound syndromes. *Psychiatric Clinics North America, 18*(3), 523–536.
Lewis, C. F., & Ednie, K. (1997). Koro and homicidal behavior. *American Journal of Psychiatry, 154*(8), 1169.
Lipschitz, A. (1991). Mechanism and classification of Koro. *American Journal of Psychiatry, 148*, 959.
Littlewood, R. (1991). Against pathology: The new psychiatry and its critics. *British Journal of Psychiatry, 159*, 696–702.
Littlewood, R. (1992). DSM-IV and culture: Is the classification internationally valid? *Psychiatric Bulletin, 16*, 257–261.
Littlewood, R. (1996). Psychiatry's culture. *International Journal Social Psychiatry, 42*(4), 245–268.
Lucieer, W. M. (1984–1985). The bitter taste of liberty. *Psychopathologic Africaine, 20*, 17–40.
Malinick, C., Flaherty, J. A., & Jobe, T. (1985). Koro: How culturally specific? *International Journal of Social Psychiatry, 31*, 67–63.
Marlowe, K. (2009). The cultural myth of Koro conceptualization: Time for a rethink. *Transcultural Psychiatry, 46*(2), 375–376.
Marsella, A. J. (1996). Culture-bound syndromes. In R. Corsini & A. Auerbach (Eds.), *Concise encyclopedia of psychology* (2nd ed., pp 223–224) Wiley.
Maslowski, J. (1988). Koro-like syndrome in Maltese subject on the basis of chronic schizophrenia. *Bulletin of Maritime & Tropical Medicine in Gdynia, 39*(1–2), 108–110.
Matthes, B. F. (1874). *Over de Bissoe's of Heidensche Priesters en Priesteressen de Boeginezen* (p. 31). C. G. Vander Post.

Marques, J. G. (2015). Koro, Othello and Capgras syndromes in one patient with drug induced psychosis. *Psychiatrica Danubina, 27*(4), 429–430.
Mellor, C. S. (1988). Depersonalization and self-perception. *British Journal of Psychiatry, 153*(Suppl. 2), 15–19.
Mendelson, S. D. (2011). The Great Singapore penis panic and the future of american mass hysteria. *Create Space Independent Publishing Platform.*
Menezes, S. B. (1992). A case of Koro and folie a deux in a Shona family. *South African Medical Journal, 82*(6), 483.
Mitchell, D. (2010). Koro in Eastern Indonesia 1999 to 2010. *Asia-Pacific Psychiatry, 2*(3), A7.
Modai, I., Munitz, H., & Aizenberg, D. (1986). Koro in an Israeli male. *British Journal of Psychiatry, 149*, 503–506.
Moekti, S., & Denin, S. K. (1978, July). *A non-rational dissemination of castration anxiety in Palembang, 1975*. Paper presented at the First Asian Teaching Workshop on Mental Health and Culture, Jakarta (Personal Communication).
Money, J., & Annecillo, C. (1987). Body-image pathology: Koro, the shrinking-penis syndrome in transcultural sexology. *Sexual & Marital Therapy, 2*(1), 91–99.
Moodley, P. (1985). Koro in non-Chinese subjects. *British Journal of Psychiatry, 146*, 102–103.
Mukherjee, T. (1987). Koro-like states. *British Journal of Psychiatry, 150*(6), 881.
Mulder, J. G. A. (1935). Over Koro. *Geneeskundig Tijdschrift Voor Nederlandsch-Indie, 75*, 837–838.
Mun, C. T. (1968). Epidemic Koro in Singapore. *British Medical Journal, i*, 640–641.
Murphy, H. B. M. (1972, March). *Notes for a theory on Latah* (32 pp.). Paper presented at the Conference on Culture and Mental Health in Asia and the Pacific. Hawai.
Nakaya, M. (2002). Fluvoxamine treatment of a Japanese patient with koro. *Journal of Clinical Psychiatry, 63*(12), 1182–1183.
Nath, A. K., Bhowmik, B. K., & Ghosh, M. (2011). *A socio-cultural study of 'Koro" epidemic in certain villages in Tripura* (pp. 29–30). Brochure of Conference of Indian Psychiatric Society, East Zone.
Nicolini, H., Salin-Pascual, R., Cabera, B., & Lanzagorta, N. (2017). Influence of culture in obsessive-compulsive disorder and its treatment. *Current Psychiatry Reviews, 13*(4), 285–292.

Ng, B. Y. (1997). History of Koro in Singapore. *Singapore Medical Journal, 38*(8), 356–357.
Ng, B. Y., & Kua, E. E. H. (1996). Koro in ancient Chinese history. *History of Psychiatry, 7*, 563–570.
Ngui, P. W. (1969). The Koro epidemic in Singapore. *Australian & New Zealand Journal of Psychiatry, 3*, 263–266.
Ntouros, E., Ntoumanis, A., Bozikas, V. P., Donias, S., Giouzepas, I., Garyfalos, G. (2010, March 15). Koro-like symptoms in two Greek men. *BMJ Case Report.* https://doi.org/10.1136/bcr.08.2008.0679
Ogunlesi, A. O. (1986). Koro symptomatology associated with paranoid psychosis in a Nigerian patient: A case report. *West African Journal of Medicine, 5*(4), 305–307.
Okasha, A., Saad, A., Khalil, A., Dawia, A. S., & Yehia, N. (1994). Phenomenology of obsessive-compulsive disorder: A transcultural study. *Comparative Psychiatry, 35*(3), 191–197.
Oyebode, F., Jamieson, R., Mullaney, J., & Davison, K. (1986). Koro - A psychophysiological dysfunction? *British Journal of Psychiatry, 148*, 212–214.
Padi, M. H. (1984). Koro. *British Journal of Psychiatry, 145*(5), 558–559.
Palthe, P. M. van W. (1934). Koro-Een Eigenaardige Angstneurose. *Geneeskundig Tijdschrift Voor Nederlandsch-Indie, 74*, 1713–1720.
Palthe, P. M. van W. (1935a). Koro-Eine Merkwurdige Angsthysterie. *Internationale Zeitschrift Fur Psychoanalyse, 21*, 249–257.
Palthe, P. M. van W. (1935b). Anauvulling op Het Artikel "Koro", een Eigenaardige Angstneurose. *Geneeskundig Tijdschrift Voor Nederlandsch-Indie, 75*, 836–837.
Palthe P. M. van W. (1936a). "Koro". Une Maladie Imaginaire et Une Phobie Orientale. *La Presse Medicale, 44*(67), 1331–1332.
Palthe, P. M. van W. (1936b). Psychiatry and neurology in the tropics. In C. D. de Langen & A. Lichtenstein (Eds.), *A clinical textbook of tropical medicine* (pp. 525–547). G. Kolff and Company.
Palthe, P. M. van W. (1937). It Significanto Forense del 'Koro.' *Archivio Di Anthropological Criminale, Psychiatry Medicina Legale, 57*, 173–182.
Perera, H. V. (1988–1989). Two cases of koro-like states occurring in Sri Lanka. *Journal of Ceylon College of Physicians, 21–22*, 33–35.
Perez, S., Junod, A., & Pilard, M. (2000). Culture-bound syndromes: Pertinence as a diagnostic category. *Medicine Tropicale, 60*(1), 75–82.
Phelan, D., & Daly, R. J. (1996). Koro-like syndrome associated with brief reactive psychosis in an Irish male. *Irish Medical Journal, 89*(2), 75–76.

Popa, B., Guillet, L., & Mullet, E. (2014). Cultural differences in the appraisal of stress. *Psicológica, 35*, 745–760.

Praharaj, S. K. (2004). Koro and psychosis following steroid abuse. *German Journal of Psychiatry, 7*(3), 49–50.

Prince, R. H. (1992). Koro and the fox spirit on Hainan Island (China). *Transcultural Psychiatric Research Review, 29*, 119–132.

Prince, R. H., & Tcheng-Laroche, F. (1987). Culture-bound syndromes and international disease classification. *Culture, Medicine & Psychiatry, 11*, 3–19.

Promodu, K., Nair, K. R., & Pushparajan, S. (2012). Koro syndrome: Mass epidemic in Kerala, India. *Indian Journal of Clinical Psychology, 39*, 152–156.

Puranik, A., & Dunn, J. (1995). Koro presenting after prostatectomy in an elderly man. *British Journal of Urology, 75*(1), 108–109.

Ramamourty, P., & Menon, V. (2014). Koro presenting as acute and transient psychosis: Implications for classification. *Asian Journal of Psychiatry, 10*, 116–117.

Real, E., Montejo, A., Alonso, P., & Menchon, J. M. (2013). Sexuality and obsessive-compulsive disorder: The hidden affair. *Neuropsychiatry, 3*(1), 23–31.

Rin, H. (1963). Koro: A consideration on Chinese concepts of illness and case illustrations. *Transcultural Psychiatric Research Review, 15*, 23–30.

Rin, H. (1965). A study of the aetiology of Koro in respect to the Chinese concept of illness. *International Journal of Social Psychiatry, 11*, 7–13.

Rin, H. (1966). Two forms of vital deficiency syndrome among Chinese male mental patients. *Transcultural Psychiatric Research Review, 3*, 19–21.

Risso, M., & Boker, W. (1968). Delusions of witchcraft: A cross-cultural study. *British Journal of Psychiatry, 114*, 963–972.

Rosenthal, S., & Rosenthal, P. A. (1982). Koro in an adolescent: Hypochondriasis as a stress response. *Adolescent Psychiatry, 10*, 523–531.

Sachdev, P. S., & Shukla, A. (1982). Epidemic Koro syndrome in India. *Lancet, ii*, 1161.

Sakar, S. L. (1943). A study of the psychology of sexual abstinence from the dreams of an ascetic. *International Journal of Psychoanalysis, 24*, 170–175.

Silva, L., Rapso-Lima, C., Soares, C., Cerqueira, J. J., & Morgado, P. (2016). Koro syndrome in an obsessive compulsive disorder. *European Psychiatry, 33*(Suppl), S618.

Simons, R. C. (1985). Introduction: The genital retraction taxon. In R. C. Simons & C. C. Hughes (Eds.), *The culture-bound syndromes: Folk illnesses of psychiatric and anthropological interests* (pp. 151–153). D. Reidel.

Simons, R. C., & Hughes, C. (1985). *The culture-bound syndromes: Folk illnesses of psychiatric and anthropological interests* (R. C. Simons & C. Hughes, Eds.). Dordrecht.

Slot, J. A. (1935). Koro in Central Celebes. *Geneeskundig Tijdschrift Voor Nederlandsch-Indie, 75*, 811–820.

Smith, M. G., & Dean, C. (1992). Capgras and Koro. *British Journal of Psychiatry, 161*, 121–123.

Srivastava, M., & Pandit, B. (2013). Koro- a case report and review. *International Journal of Physiology, 1*(1), 37–40.

Stein, D. J., Frenkel, M., & Hollander, E. (1991). Classification of Koro. *American Journal of Psychiatry, 148*, 959.

Stip, E., Bergeron, T., Lavigueur, C., Fabian, J. L., & Bentaleb, A. (2007). Koro Syndrome. *Medico Psychological Annals, 165*(3), 147–153.

Strong, R. P. (1945). *Sitt's diagnosis, prevention and treatment of tropical diseases* (7th ed., p. 1145). K. H. Lewis and Company.

Suwanlert, S. (1983, July 11–16). *The second Koro epidemic in North East Thailand*. Poster presentation at the 7th World Congress of Psychiatry, Vienna.

Suwanlert, S., & Coates, D. (1979). Epidemic Koro in Thailand: Clinical and Social Aspects. *Transcultural Psychiatric Research Review, 16*, 64–66.

Tau, M., & Masukar, A. V. (2020). Koro delusion in mild cognitive impairment due to Alzheimer's disease. *Journal of Neuropsychiatry & Clinical Neuroscience, 32*(2), 204–206.

Tseng, W. S. (2001). *Handbook of cultural psychiatry*. Academic Press.

Tseng, W. S. (2006). From peculiar psychiatric disorders through culture-bound syndromes to culture-related specific syndromes. *Transcultural Psychiatry, 43*(4), 554–576.

Tseng, W. S., Mo, M. K., Hsu, J., Li, L. S., Ou, L. W., Chen, G. Q., & Jiang, D. W. (1988). A socio-cultural study of Koro Epidemic in Guangdong, China. *American Journal of Psychiatry, 145*, 1538–1543.

Tseng, W. S., Mo, K. M., Li, L. S., Chen, G. O., Ou, L. W., Zheng, H. B. (1992). Koro epidemic in Guangdong, China. A questionnaire survey. *Journal Nervous & Mental Disease, 180*(2), 117–123.

Turnier, L., & Chouinard, G. (1990). Effect anti-koro d'un antidepresseur tricyclque. *Revue Cannadienne De Psychiatrie, 35*, 331–333.

Ungvari, G. S., & Mullen, R. S. (1994). Koro: The delusion of penile retraction. *Urology, 43*(6), 883–885.

Vorstman, A. H. (1897). "Koro" in de Westerafdeeling van Borneo. *Geneeskundig Tijdschrift Voor Nederlandsch-Indie, 37*, 499–505.

Walendberg, S. S. A. (1981). Koro. *Canadian Journal of Psychiatry, 26*, 104–141.
Weller, M. P. I., & Ameen, N. (1982). Elvis Presley, reactive hypomania and Koro. *American Journal of Psychiatry, 139*(7), 970.
Wen, J. K., & Wang, C. L. (1979). Shen-K'uei syndrome: A culture specific sexual neurosis in Taiwan. In A. Kleinman & T. Y. Lin (Eds.), *Normal and abnormal behaviour in Chinese Culture* (pp. 357–369). D. Reidel Publishing Company.
Westermeyer, J. (1989). A case of koro in a refugee family: Association with depression and folie a deux. *Journal of Clinical Psychiatry, 50*, 181–183.
Wilson, S., & Agin, C. (1997). Genital pain associated with genital retraction: A case of Koro syndrome. *Journal of Pain & Symptom Management, 13*(3), 176–178.
Williams, M. T., Chapman, L. K., Simms, J. V., Tellawi, G. (2017). Cross-cultural phenomenology of obsessive-compulsive disorder. In J. S. Abramowitz, D. McKay, & E. A. Storch (Eds), *The Wiley handbook of obsessive compulsive disorders* (Vol. I, 1st ed., pp. 56–74). Wiley.
WittKower, E. D., & Rin, H. (1965). Transcultural psychiatry. *Archives of General Psychiatry, 13*, 387–394.
Wolff, G., & McKenzie, K. (1994). Capgras, Fregoli and Cotard's syndromes and Koro in folie à deux. *British Journal of Psychiatry, 165*(6), 842.
Wong, K. C. (1918). An inquiry into some Chinese sexual diseases. *National Medical Journal of China, 4*, 26–31.
Wylie, K. R., & Eardley, I. (2007). Penile size and the 'small penis syndrome.' *BJU International, 99*(6), 1449–1455.
Yang, H., Tranulis, C., & Freudenreich, O. (2009). Keeping culture-bound syndromes in cultural context: The case of Koro. *International Journal of Culture & Mental Health, 2*(2), 86–91.
Yap, P. M. (1951). Mental disorders peculiar to certain culture: A survey of comparative psychiatry. *Journal of Mental Science, 97*, 313–327.
Yap, P. M. (1962). Words and things in comparative psychiatry with special reference to the exotic psychoses. *Acta Psychiatrica Scandinavica, 38*, 163–169.
Yap, P. M. (1964a). Suk-yeong or Koro: A culture-bound depersonalization syndrome. *Bulletin of the Hong Kong Chinese Medical Association, 16*, 31–47.
Yap, P. M. (1964b). Koro or Suk-yeong: An atypical culture-bound psychiatric disorder found in Southern Chinese. *Transcultural Psychiatric Research Review, 1*, 36–38.

Yap, P. M. (1965a). Koro - A culture-bound depersonalization syndrome. *British Journal of Psychiatry, 111*, 43–50.
Yap, P. M. (1965b). Koro in a Briton. *British Journal of Psychiatry, 111*, 774–775.
Yap, P. M. (1967). Classification of the culture-bound reactive syndrome. *Australian & New Zealand Journal of Psychiatry, 1*, 172–179.
Yap, P. M. (1969). The culture-bound Reactive Syndrome. In W. Caudill & T. Y. Lin (Eds.), *Mental health research in Asia and the Pacific* (pp. 33–53). East-West Centre Press.
Yap, P. M. (1974). *Comparative psychiatry: A theoretical framework*. University of Toronto Press.
Zeng, W., Mo, G., Chen, G., Li, L., Wen, R., & Liu, T. (1993). Social psychiatry and epidemic koro. Comparison of folk belief among young men in Taiwan, Jilin, and Guandong Provinces. *Chinese Mental Health Journal, 7*(1), 38–40.

Part III

Literature Review

6

Western Publications: Part One—From 1874 to 1970

Preamble: *Western Publications*: From 1874 to 2020. A year-wise search with the term Koro, Genital Retraction Syndrome, Koro-like Symptom, and Koro Delusion is done through databases like PsychINFO, CINAHL, Medline, EMCARE, and EMBASE for English language journals. Some non-English publications were also available (like Dutch, Chinese, French, Polish, Finish, Spanish, German, Turkish, and Arabic) with English abstracts. Some Koro-related topics were also included to better understand the Koro psychopathology, like body image and depersonalization, coital death, psychiatric epidemics, penis theft epidemic, and Mass Psychogenic Illness in Africa. The publication of some related books is also mentioned (not review). The non-English literature search is not at all exhaustive. The publications are divided into three Chapters—from 1874 to 1970 (up to the Singapore epidemic); later parts of the twentieth century—from 1971 to 2000; and the third part—first two decades of the twenty-first century—2001–2020. This division is a bit arbitrary. Singapore Koro epidemic is a landmark event since the Koro publication in 1895. A total of 294 published Koro (and

A. N. Chowdhury, *Koro*,
https://doi.org/10.1007/978-3-030-87962-4_6

related) reports are critically reviewed and evaluated in these chapters. These are presented according to the year of publication and are usually grouped as per decades. The publications that appeared as a letter to the Editor are marked with (L) signs. Some available contemporary newspaper reports on Koro are also documented. Depending on the available information, the "Koro Epidemic" is boxed as per the year reported.

Nineteenth-Century Publications on Genital Retraction or Koro

Preamble: Genital retraction by the name *Suo Yang* is reported in Traditional Chinese medical classics from 476–221 BC. This review is addressing the reporting of genital retraction by the name *Koro* mainly in the Western press. The earliest reference of the term Koro is in 1874, and Dr. J. C. Blonk first used this clinical description from Dutch-India (Indonesia) in 1895. Jilek (1986) reported a genital shrinkage epidemic from Guangdong province, China, in 1865. This is probably the first world reference of recorded clinical material on genital shrinkage illness.

Interestingly, the examples of genital shrinkage symptoms are found in at least three publications in the late part of the nineteenth century, albeit without using the term Koro for obvious reasons, from three geographically wide-apart regions viz. USA (Hammond, 1883), Russia (Ivanov, 1885), and England (Raven, 1886). This section reviewed ten available publications relating to genital retraction or Koro during 1874–1897.

1865: Suo-Yang Epidemic in Hainan Island, China

This is probably the earliest reference of a *Suo-yang* or genital retraction case in recent history and that too of an epidemic form. There is no published report of this epidemic. Dr. Kan-Ming Mo, Honorary

Director, Guangdong Psychiatric Hospital, communicated this information to Dr. Wolfgang Jilek (Jilek, 1986) from the Tang District archives in North-Western Hainan Island of Guangdong Province, China, who reported it in 1986.

1874

[1]. B. F. Matthes
Over de Bissoe's of Heidensche Priesters en Priesteressen de Boeginezen. C.G. Vender Post, Amsterdam, 1874.

This is the first known reference of the term "Koro" in B. F. Matthe's Dictionary of the Buginese Language of South Sulawesi.

Koro = "to shrink"
Lasa Koro = "a shrinking of the penis, a sort of disease that is not unusual amongst the natives and must be very dangerous". (p. 31)

Dr. Benjamin Fredrik Matthes (16 January 1818–9 October 1918), was a Dutch Bible translator and linguist. His *Buginese-Hollandsch* is still considered a standard work in the study of the Buginese language.

1883

[2]. W. A. Hammond: *Sexual Impotence in the Male, New York.*

It contains a hypochondriacal case report with complaints of genital shrinkage (Hes & Nassi, 1977). William Alexander Hammond (28 August 1828–5 January 1900) was an American military physician named the 11th Surgeon General of the US Army during the American civil war. He was the American Neurological Association founder and known for his academic and research works and was the author of many clinical books and articles.

1885

[3]. A. A. Ivanov: Vetjagivanie Polov Chlena. (Retraction of Sex Organ)
Vrach, 1885, 423.

The original publication is not available. It was a report of a Russian case with genital retraction symptoms. The account of this case of genital shrinkage was quoted by Raven (1886) in Lancet as follows:

> … the penis had bodily disappeared, and was recaptured only after prolonged manipulation. Even then the patient seems to have distrusted its tendency to remain in its natural position, for he had tied a string around it above the glans, in order that it should not again escape him. (p. 250)

1886

250 THE LANCET, HOSPITAL MEDICINE AND SURGERY [AUGUST 7, 1886]

[4]. T. F. Raven: Retraction of the penis.
The Lancet, 1886, August 7, 250.

This is probably the first clinical report of genital retraction published in the British Medical Press. It was a case of penile retraction in a 27-year-old Englishman. This publication is listed under "penis (retraction)" in Index Medicus (1886, 8:682) and is abstracted in the classic study of medical anomalies by Gould and Pyle (1896). A copy of the original text is appended here (Fig. 6.1). Dr. Blonk is credited, though, for the first publication by the name *Koro* in the Western medical press and its South-East Asian heritage. Still, in a true sense, Dr. Ivanov from Russia and Dr. Raven from England should be appropriately credited for reporting genital retraction (the first two cases) from Europe.

1895

[5]. J. C. Blonk: Koro.
Geneeskundig Tijdschrift voor Nederlandsch-Indie, 1895, 35, 562–563.

Dr. Blonk, a Dutch military physician and a second-class officer of health, is credited for introducing the concept and name of Koro illness first in the Western World. He used the term Koro to address the clinical phenomenon of penile retraction. Blonk did not witness an attack

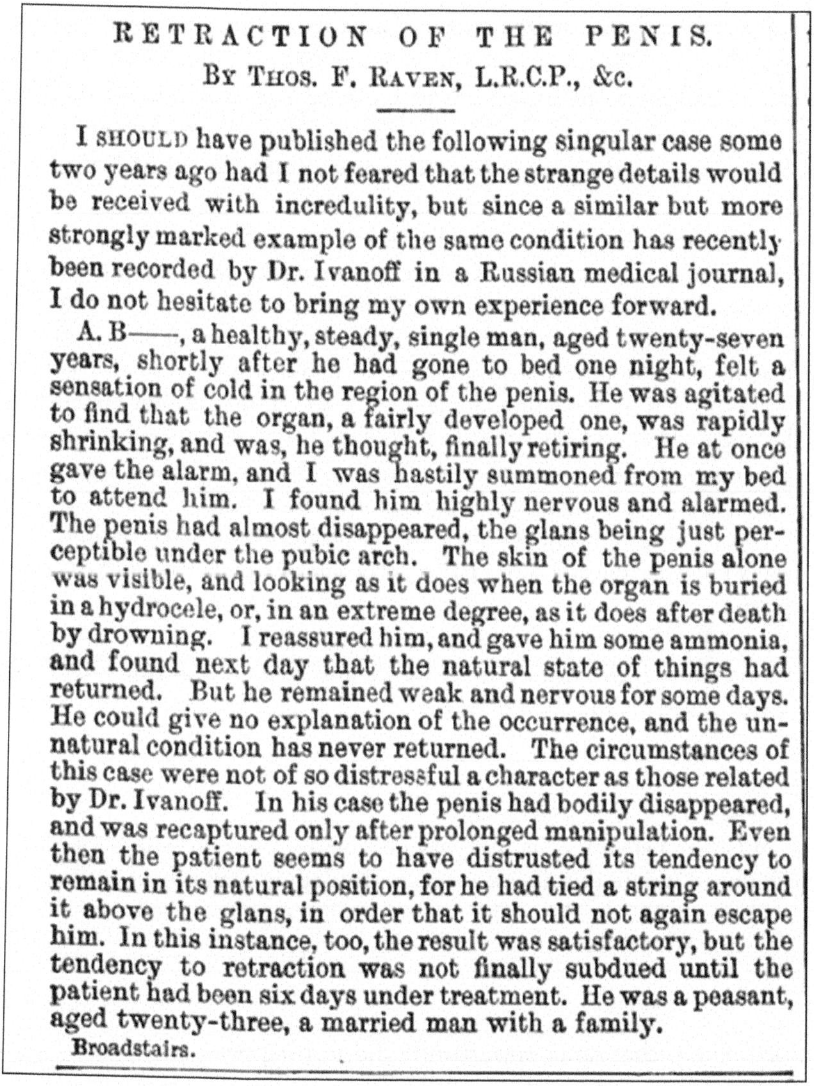

RETRACTION OF THE PENIS.

BY THOS. F. RAVEN, L.R.C.P., &c.

I SHOULD have published the following singular case some two years ago had I not feared that the strange details would be received with incredulity, but since a similar but more strongly marked example of the same condition has recently been recorded by Dr. Ivanoff in a Russian medical journal, I do not hesitate to bring my own experience forward.

A. B——, a healthy, steady, single man, aged twenty-seven years, shortly after he had gone to bed one night, felt a sensation of cold in the region of the penis. He was agitated to find that the organ, a fairly developed one, was rapidly shrinking, and was, he thought, finally retiring. He at once gave the alarm, and I was hastily summoned from my bed to attend him. I found him highly nervous and alarmed. The penis had almost disappeared, the glans being just perceptible under the pubic arch. The skin of the penis alone was visible, and looking as it does when the organ is buried in a hydrocele, or, in an extreme degree, as it does after death by drowning. I reassured him, and gave him some ammonia, and found next day that the natural state of things had returned. But he remained weak and nervous for some days. He could give no explanation of the occurrence, and the unnatural condition has never returned. The circumstances of this case were not of so distressful a character as those related by Dr. Ivanoff. In his case the penis had bodily disappeared, and was recaptured only after prolonged manipulation. Even then the patient seems to have distrusted its tendency to remain in its natural position, for he had tied a string around it above the glans, in order that it should not again escape him. In this instance, too, the result was satisfactory, but the tendency to retraction was not finally subdued until the patient had been six days under treatment. He was a peasant, aged twenty-three, a married man with a family.

Broadstairs.

Fig. 6.1 First report of genital retraction in British Medical Press (Printed with permission: Order License ID 1141766-1, dated 19.8.21)

of Koro. He gathered information about this genital shrinkage malady. He got the term "Koro" from a *djaksa* (native Legal Officer) who was his informant and a Koro sufferer, who reported the maneuver of holding the penis to prevent retraction and described that the attacks might last for hours, leaving the patient too exhausted. Blonk described Koro as:

> At times, sufferers of this disease feel that the penis tends to retract into the abdominal cavity. In cases where timely assistance is not provided, this would actually happen, and the patient would then also succumb. The sufferers are of course very afraid of this. As soon as they notice that the first symptoms are appearing, they take the penis in the hand to prevent it from retracting. Sometimes, however, they cannot maintain this themselves, and this therapy must be taken over by someone else. Sometimes the penis must be held in this manner for hours on end, while in some cases a fairly strong force must be applied.
>
> During these attacks, the patients are plagued by a severe feeling of fear, while after the attack has passed, they are extremely tired and weary. (p. 562)

As Blonk himself did not examine or see any case, he was not sure about the reason for this illness. He stated:

> I could not find out anything about the cause of an attack, not even at what age the first attacks usually occur.
>
> Whether heredity is at play was possible to ascertain with sufficient certainty. Overall, this disease seems to develop on neurasthenic soil.
>
> Questionable is the influence on and connection with sex life. (pp. 562–563)

He was keen to examine a case personally to earn more knowledge, but unfortunately, that same opportunity did not happen:

> Although many patients do not want to know that they are suffering from this disease, a sufferer, a jaksa who was quite intelligent, had promised to notify me when another attack occurred. Since during my stay on Celebes I had to be quite often at the station of that jaksa in charge of the civil medical service, I very much hoped to attend his attack one day, and then be able to check personally see the symptoms. (p. 563)

The copy of the first page of the original text is shown in Fig. 6.2.

[6]. P. C. J. van Brero: Een en ander over de psychosen onder de bevolking van den Indischen Archipel.
Geneeskundig Tijdschrift voor Nederlandsch-Indie, 1895, 35, 23–51, 119–153.

This is a comprehensive review of different exotic disorders and psychopathology reported from the Southeast Asian archipelago. It is a Dutch publication.

1896

[7]. P. C. J. van Brero: Einiges uber die geisteskrankheiten dc bevolkerung des Malaiischen Archipel.
Allgemeine Zeitschrift fur Psychiatrie und Psychisch-gerichtllche Medicin, 1896a, 53, 25–78.

It is the German publication of his earlier 1895 paper.

[8]. P. C. J. van Brero: Naar Aanleiding van het Opstel over "Koro" van den Heer J. C. Blonk in de Vorige Aflevering van dit Tijdschrift.
Geneeskundig Tijdschrift voor Nederlandsch-Indie, 1896b, 36, 48–54.

This paper is practically a commentary and detailed discussion and interpretation of the Koro case, reported by Blonk (1895). Dr. P. C. J. van Brero was the 2nd physician at the mental hospital in Buitenzorg* (now Bogor city), West Java province, and extensively researched "Dementia paralytica." He described Koro as "a strange compulsive idea." This is a Dutch publication.

In referring to Blonk's observation on Koro, he said:

> This interesting observation is important firstly as a contribution to the knowledge of anthropology of the inhabitants in whose midst we live, and secondly as an increase in our knowledge of those peculiar mental disorders known under the name of compulsions (*dwangvoorstellingen*),

First World Medical Reference of 'KORO'

KORO,

DOOR

J. C. BLONK,

Officier van Gezondheid 2e Klasse.

Onder dezen naam is bij de Boegineezen en Makassaren een ziektebeeld bekend, dat, naar ik meen, nog niet is beschreven. Ook is het mij niet mogen gelukken het voorkomen dier ziekte op Java, in de Padang'sche bovenlanden, en te Atjeh te constateeren.

Volgens lijders aan deze ziekte gevoelen zij op onregelmatige tijdstippen dat de penis neiging heeft zich in de buikholte terug te trekken. In de gevallen, waarin niet tijdig hulp wordt verstrekt, zoude dit ook werkelijk geschieden, en de patient dan tevens bezwijken. De lijders zijn daarvoor natuurlijk zeer bevreesd. Zoodra zij dan ook bemerken dat de eerste verschijnselen zich voordoen, nemen zij den penis in de hand om het terugtrekken te beletten. Soms echter kunnen zij dit zelf niet volhouden, en moet deze therapie door een ander worden overgenomen. Uren achtereen moet soms op die wijze de penis worden vastgehouden, terwijl in sommige gevallen een vrij sterke kracht moet worden aangewend.

Gedurende deze aanvallen worden de patiënten geplaagd door een hevig angstgevoel, terwijl zij, nadat de aanval geweken is, uiterst vermoeid en afgemat zijn.

Omtrent de aanleiding tot het optreden van een aanval kon ik niets te weten komen, ook niet op welken leeftijd gewoonlijk de eerste aanvallen zich voordoen.

Fig. 6.2 1895 Publication of J. C. Blonk (first page) (Adopted from Blonk [1895, p. 562])

> precisely because koro in a single, but salient point, deviates from the phenomena of these psychic processes which have hitherto been observed in Europe. (p. 49)

He believed that Koro is a strange obsessional idea and commented as follows:

> For I do not believe it will need to be further argued that we are not dealing here with a disease, but with a complicated disease phenomenon, that the penis will not disappear into the abdominal cavity, and that the patient will not collapse either. Koro belongs to that curious group of mental disorders, which was first given the name of "Zwangsvorstellungen" by von KRAFFT-EBING (1), and which WESTPHAL (2) defines in the following manner, mentioning the properties:
>
> > With obsessional ideas (*Zwangsvorstellungen*) I mean those thoughts which, with an otherwise intact intelligence and without being stipulated by an emotional or affect-like state, come to the fore of consciousness against the will of the pertaining person, do not allow themselves to be chased away, prevent and thwart normal process of thoughts, which the affected person recognises as abnormal, alien to him, and which he confronts with his healthy consciousness. The content of these thoughts/concepts can be varied, is often, or predominantly, absurd in character, and shows no detectable connection with previous contents of thoughts/ideas, but appears incomprehensible even to the sick person himself as if flown to him from the air. (p. 49)
>
> 1. Allg. Zeitschar. F. Psych. Bd. 35. S. 303
> 2. Westphal, Lecture: Medicin. Psych. Society, 5th March 1877, Arch. für Psych., Vol. VIII.

He tried to strengthen his argument in favor of Koro as a manifestation of obsessive–compulsive disorder, more specifically as "compulsive sensation" and "compulsive perception." By referring to Koch's (1891) argument, he stated that:

> KOCH,[3] whose reflections I now follow further, calls these deviations *compulsive thoughts*, whereby using the word *thinking* in its widest sense.

They occur in persons that are psychopathically burdened by birth, and sometimes play such a great role in this that the condition is named after them.

He gives the following definition:

Obsessive-compulsive thoughts are characterized by the fact that they are pathologically conditioned, arise primordially, impose themselves with pathological compulsion and penetrate between the rest of the thinking so that the person affected by them cannot arbitrarily (completely) get rid of them, but that they are alien, obtrusive and / or inapplicable thoughts is recognised.

He states that not everyone is immediately aware of the correctness of the latter, but it never happened that such a person could not be convinced of the incorrectness of his ideas.

He further divides the compulsive thoughts into several types, one of which, it seems to me, must be classified as koro, namely, the compulsive sensation and compulsion perception. (p. 50)

3. Dr. J. L. A. Koch, *Die psychopathischen Minderwertigkeiten*, Ravensburg, 1891. I take this opportunity to recommend the reading of the work of this experienced and human psychiatrist to anyone who heals people. At the end of his book, the writer rightly says: "The field of psychopathic inferiority is a large, but also a very interesting area. Who engages with it, will learn to see many things in life differently from before, to understand people and actions of people that he previously did not understand."

He then tried to clarify Koro perception from illusion and delusion:

These sensations should not be confused with illusions, claims KOCH, precisely because they are immediately regarded as compulsion/coercion, as something strange. This seems less accurate to me because illusions can also be recognized as incorrect. The difference lies, in my view, in that, where the relevant body parts are in contact with objects, such as a pillow or mattress, the boundaries and points of contact are felt beyond any doubt as usual, but in spite of that the compulsion persists.

…

> Meanwhile, it will be noted that there is a fundamental difference between koro and the mentioned "compulsions" in particular, and compulsions in general, namely that the latter does not seem to be recognised as false and the former as such, which is generally considered as a fundamental difference between compulsion and delusion. So, the question arises whether the phenomenon of "koro" is a delusion? (pp. 51–52)

In the last part, he compared Koro "compulsive perception" with paranoid ideas and fanatic beliefs:

> Will this erroneous concept now prove to be correctable in koro? In a sense, correction is already taking place since the sufferer himself sees the phenomenon as something abnormal, which neither the paranoicist nor the fanatic does.
>
> Where there is a fallacy, only the field of action of criticism can be dealt with in general, because the critical faculties are more individually owned. And it is indeed tempting to assume here that the spiritual equipment mentioned above is poorly developed. After all, the treasure of experience and knowledge in a half-civilized people such as that of the Malay is so incomplete that it is not surprising that such views, suffering from inaccuracies in criticism, are generally accepted, much less not as one consider what powerful influence [p. 4] affections of mind generally exert on the course of thought in man, especially among the half-civilized. How prolific is superstition in all its forms! (p. 53)

In the end, he expressed the possibility of cultural, religious, or even mystic influence on this very Koro illness:

> On the other hand, the limited distribution in a particular region gives rise to the idea that the prevailing view there may perhaps be related to religious practices, mysticism, or the like. Then persuasion would prove impossible. I can only suggest a suspicion, being too unfamiliar with the ethnology of our archipelago. Further observations may decide on this. (p. 54)

[* Kraepelin spent three weeks at this Buitenzorg mental hospital in 1904 to investigate differences in incidence and manifestations of mental illness in patients of indigenous, Chinese, and European population groups (Pols, 2006). He concluded that the symptoms of schizophrenia were less severe in indigenous patients and that their prognosis was much better (Kraepelin, 1904).]

1897

[9]. P. C. J. van Brero: Koro, eine eigentuemliche zwangsvorstellung.
Allegemeine Seitschrift fur Psychiatric & Psychischgerichtliche Medicin, 1897, 53, 569–573.

This is a German publication and similar to his earlier Dutch publication in 1896. He cited the typical clinical presentation of Koro as described by Blonk in 1895:

> He was told that in the southern part of Celebes, one of the four larger islands of the East Indian Archipelago, there were sick people whose penis occasionally, for no known cause, tends to withdraw into the abdominal cavity; if it really happens, then it brings about death if the sick themselves or others did not hold onto the penis early on.
>
> These seizures were sometimes lasting for hours, being accompanied by intense anxiety, followed by great exhaustion; they were found in people with a disturbed nervous life who hid their 'illness' forreasons of shame. (p. 569)

He tried to point out some differences between Koro and obsession:

> These compulsive sensations (Zwangsempfindungen) and compulsive perceptions (Zwangswahrnehmungen) are in principle not different from the more generally known obsessional ideas. They only represent varieties. The sensation as such is not disturbed because where the body parts concerned come into contact with other objects, e.g. pillows, the boundaries of which are felt beyond doubt as usual; but regardless of this, the idea of abnormal size and shape persists. However, as has already been noted, there is the fundamental difference between Koro and the 'obsessional perceptions' described in particular, and obsessions in general, namely that the latter is recognized as incorrect and the former, it seems,

> is not recognized as such, which is generally accepted to indicate a fundamental difference between obsessions and delusions. (p. 571)

The author discussed the power of rational thinking, and in that context, he pointed the underdevelopment of thought processes of "semi-civilized people" there very strangely. This assessment carries a Eurocentric bias and accusation:

> ...will the patient be convinced that the penis will not retract into the abdominal cavity and that he will not die? In other words, are you dealing with a mistake in reasoning or a wrong opinion? Wherever there is generally talk of a mistake in thinking, only the 'field of work' can be dealt with, because a person's critical skills are more of an individual property. And it is really tempting to assume here that the mental endowment, which was discussed above, is poorly developed. For the experience and knowledge of a semi-civilized people like the Malay is so incomplete that it is not surprising that such views, suffering from inaccuracies in criticism, are generally (considered) feasible. All the less when you consider the powerful influence that affects [emotions] have on the train of thought, especially in semi-civilised people.
>
> How terribly does superstition thrive there in all its forms. (p. 572)

In conclusion, he stressed the Koro nosology as obsession and reflected a Eurocentric bias again:

> This is the only example of obsession of the local population that I know of. Undoubtedly there are several, but taking into account the sharp boundary between Europeans and natives, the natives' mistrust of the European healing practices, as well as the shame of the patients involved, detection extremely difficult. (p. 573)

[10]. A. H. Vorstman: 'Koro', in de Westerafdeeling van Borneo. *Geneeskundig Tijdschrift voor Nederlandsch-Indie, 1897, 37, 499–505.*

Vorstmann was a medical officer in Palembang (Borneo). This paper contains two Koro case reports from Kalimantan. The first case was a Chinese, a native of the Sintang district of Kalimantan, who had a history of alcohol abuse. Vorstman diagnosed this as delusion as there was no evidence of retraction of the penis. Edwards (1984) provides a detailed account of the first case as follows:

> The patient was found in bed, surrounded by a retinue and with an old man sitting at the foot of the bed. Having on information about the patient's symptoms during the preceding days, Vorstman's examination and questioning failed to yield much insight into the man's problem. Based on prior experience, Vorstman concluded that alcohol abuse, a common native habit, was the background of this case. Upon leaving the house, the Chinese official, who had served as interpreter, remarked that Vorstman was probably unsure of the nature of the patient's illness. He related that for the past eight days the patient's penis had been withdraw into the belly; as a preventive measure the old man at the foot of the bed had been gripping his master's "obstinate limb". Vorstman found this story interesting from the ethnographic standpoint but difficult to believe, especially on anatomical grounds. Subsequently, a different government patrol officer confirmed that the native did believe in such a disease; and the district officer of Nangapinoh informed that in his district there was a corpse of a native who had died of this disease. (p. 6)

The second was an Indonesian patient who was brought in, holding his penis always. Palthe (1935) described this as follows:

> Shortly after his first patient, Vorstman met a second, a Chinese man, who kept holding his penis in the hospital; if the fatigue of his right hand made it impossible for him to hold it any longer, he Vorstman interprets Koro as a compulsory sensation, the content of which relates to ideas and concepts from everyday life. In his opinion there was a superstition in the patient's environment that the penis can retract into the body and thereby cause death. (p. 250)

Koro Literature: From 1901 to 1950

Preamble: At least 21 publications relevant to genital retraction syndrome or Koro are available during this span of 50 years. The 1912 publication of Nicolaüs Adriani and Albert Kruyt points a new light on the origin of the name "Koro." Two reports are of Koro epidemic in mainland China. Few are discussion papers, four papers contain Koro case reports, and three publications include the description of genital shrinkage/retraction symptoms secondary to some psychiatric morbidity. All these three reports were by notable personalities of psychiatry, viz. Prof. Emil W. G. M. Kraepelin (1913), a German psychiatrist, Prof. Paul F. Schilder (1935), an Austrian psychiatrist-psychoanalyst, and Gustav Bychowski (1934), a Polish-American psychiatrist-psychoanalyst. The primary five papers of Palthe in the 30s are valuable documents of early Koro research. The Koro reports by Slot, Mulder, and Chabot are the most useful initial clinical reports on Koro from Dutch-Indonesia.

1908: Koro Epidemic in Szechwan, China

1908

[1]. J. Legendre: Une curieuse epidemie.
Annales de Medicine Coloniale, 1908, 11(2), 280–281. [In French]

It is a report of a Koro epidemic from mainland China in 1908. It is also the first report of a Koro epidemic published in the Western medical press (a French Journal). Dr. J. Legendre was a French military physician, and he personally conducted the investigation. The epidemic affected about 20 male teenage students (age <20 years) of a school in Szechwan, China. The author refers to the condition as *so-in-tchen*, possibly a distorted rendering of *Suo-yang*. He viewed this "genital shrinking" syndrome as an "Asiatic psychosis that can manifest itself collectively and individually," and rumor played a vital role in this epidemic. Victims recovered speedily but had a fear of impotence and the risk, "terrible for a Chinese," of being unable to procreate. The local emergency treatment consisted of applying "methodical traction to the penis."

Edward (1986) described a case seen by Dr. Legendre:

> A young apprentice noticed one evening that his penis was smaller than its norm; self-diagnosing his condition as "so-in-tchen", he began a remedy used in similar cases of imminent death, rhythmic tractions of the penis. This was not an isolated case; the same day and the next a score of others could be found using the same treatment with similar success-many students had recovered. (p. 89)

NB. Simplified Chinese of Szechwan is now Sichuan.

1912

[2]. N. Adriani, A. C. Kruijt: De Baree-sprekende Toradjas van Midden-Celebes.
Landsdrukkerij, 1912, Batavia.

The Dutch ethnographers Nicolaüs Adriani and Albert Kruyt encountered the genital shrinking phenomenon in the Dutch East-Indies in 1912. They said that the name was derived from a tribe in Sulawesi bearing Koro's name. Toraja is an Indonesian ethnic group that speaks the Baree dialect in Sulawesi.

1913

[3]. E. Kraepelin: *Psychiatrie – Ein Lehrbuch fur Studierende und Arzte. 8th edition, Vol. 3, Johann Amborosius Barth, Leipzig.*

It is a treatise on manic-depressive illness. Kraepelin describes the fear of penile shrinkage as one of the hypochondriacal delusions in the depressive state in a German patient. He, however, did not use the term Koro.

Kraepelin made an Asian tour in 1904, and he encountered amok, latah, and Koro (Kraepelin, 1904). He thought amok belongs to the epileptic disorders, latah to hysteria, and Koro to obsessive–compulsive disorder (Jilek, 1995). English version of "Manic Depressive Insanity and Paranoia" was published in Edinburgh in 1921 (Kraepelin, 1921).

1918

[4]. K. C. Wong: An inquiry into some Chinese 'Sexual Diseases'.

National Medical Journal of China, 1918, 4, 26–31.

This is a precious medical record of genital retraction or Koro from China, researched by Edwards (1984). Wong was a well-known scholar of Chinese medical history, and in this article on "Sexual Diseases," he wrote:

> ..... From time immemorial sexual intemperance has been regarded as the primary cause of a host of diseases. Ancient writers dwelt on the disastrous consequences of immoderate indulgence, and this has made such a deep impression on the minds of the people that whenever a newly married couple gets sick, sexual carelessness is at once set down as the cause. (p. 26)

He also noted *Suo-yang* (retraction of penis and/or testes*)* as an acute complication of some sexual disease and locally considered a prodrome of impending death. Wong discussed a condition called "jiase" which Edward believed is similar to Suo-yang. *Jiase*, an acute fever of seven days and ending by a crisis and "is said to be caused by sexual carelessness and by catching a cold or taking cold things, especially melon and ice cream immediately after copulation" (Wong, 1918, p. 27). The usual symptoms are: headache, giddiness, pain in the back and loins, abdominal colic, blurred vision, retraction of the testicles of men and the nipples of women, contracted and cold extremities difficulty breathing. He further added that:

> When the ailment is complicated with retraction of the testicles or penis, it is believed to be very dangerous. A disgusting cure is said to be the woman's pubic hair which is burned to ashes and taken with the water used in washing the private parts. For emergency it is usual to compress the testicles or penis, as the case may be, between the two halves of a wooden box for scales to prevent the disease ascending. (Wong, 1918, p. 28)

1933

[5]. P. M. van Wulfften Palthe (1933): Kranzinnigenverpleging in Ned.-Indie.

Geneeskundig Tijdschrift voor Nederlands Indie¨ [Mental Health Care in the Dutch East Indies], 73, 171–181.

1934

[6]. P. M. van Wulfften Palthe: Koro-Een eigenaardige angstneurose.
Geneeskundig Tijdschrift voor Nederlandsch-Indie, 1934, 74, 1713–1720.

1935

[7]. P. M. van Wulfften Palthe: Koro-eine merkwurdige angsthysterie. [Koro: A peculiar anxiety neurosis]
Internationale Zeitschrift fur Psychoanalyse, 1935a, 21(2), 249–257.

This paper was devoted to an elaborate discussion on the orthography of Koro and its Chinese equivalent syntaxes. The author references Blonk's (1895) and Vortsman's (1897) earlier paper on Koro. This paper contains his impression of local people's ideas and beliefs about Koro as an illness. He very meticulously described his experience of seeing a Koro patient in 1932 as follows:

> A few years ago, we examined a Chinese man who had lived in West Borneo for a long time and who also suffered from Koro. However, after a one-off conversation, he evaded further examination so that almost no evidence could be obtained. At the time, we had the impression that the attack began with a vague feeling of fear, a dark premonition of death, that was secondarily motivated by the fear that the penis may withdraw into the body. According to the statements of our patient, we believed that we were entitled to assume that this 'Koro' was not only associated with fear of death, but also with fear of castration. We also heard of a Koro case of a Malay Radja, whereby it is worth reporting that his whole population lived in fear with their ruler. For many days, it was very restless around the ruler as his people did not go to sleep and spent the nights in prayer until calm returned to the 'Kraton' and the fear of the Koro was again dispelled for some time. This patient was known to me as a typical

> psychasthenic. We also received news from Makassar about cases of Koro among the more educated natives; in other words, only in those groups of the population in which neuroses occur at all. (p. 250)

He also gave a very lovely ethnographic exploration about the orthography and social meaning of the illness from some social inquiry and his experience with another Chinese patient from Canton who also suffered from tuberculosis, seen at State Hospital at Batavia:

> With the help of an interpreter, we were able to learn interesting details from him, notably the name the Chinese give to this 'disease', namely '*Shook Jong*' (Mandarin: *Shoo Jang*), meaning 'shrinking of the penis'.
>
> From further talks with our patient and from information that we received from Dr Kwa, Batavia, supplemented by several details that we received from connoisseurs of Chinese life, we discovered that there are two different aspects that must be strictly distinguished: a (fantasised) disease and a neurosis.
>
> The disease called *Shook Jong* is commonly known to the Chinese. It consists in the shrinking of the penis due to certain causes which we were told include sexual intercourse at very young age or excessive masturbation when the necessary strength is still lacking, or urinating against the wind. (We can compare this with the popular belief in Europe that you get a 'cold' if you urinate against the wind: cold here = gonorrhoea.) If one notices such an abnormal inclination of the penis during coitus, then one should not leave the vagina, but if it happens under other circumstances, then the penis must be held, by helpers, with the hand and with the mouth. If the penis accidentally escapes, death is said to be a certain consequence. (p. 251)

He discussed the traditional use of the instrument *Lie Teng Hok* and penis rod and penis perforation needle used to prevent penile indrawing. Lie Teng Hok is a fine weighing pan used by Chinese goldsmiths and pharmacists. A local traditional Chinese doctor of China Town in Batavia told him that this instrument is dangerous and temporary. For permanent cure, one should follow the principles of Chinese healing:

> The tendency of the penis to withdraw is considered to show that the *yin*-principle, which represents the feminine, is predominant over the *yang*-principle that represents masculinity. (*Yang* and *Ying* stand for heaven and earth, sun and moon, day and night, warm and cold, life and death, positive and negative, strong and weak, male and female.)
>
> Therefore, in order to cure the disease, *yang* medicines must be taken, in other words, medicines which the Chinese in India denote with the qualification '*panas*' (warm) in contrast to the '*dingin*' (cold) medicines which represent the *yin* principle. As an example of good medication in the case of '*Shook Jong*', this venerable medicine man informed me: gunpowder with arak, tin with sulphur and many medicinal herbs. (p. 252)

He explained very eloquently that how cultural beliefs and social custom is active among the indigenous population to offer a "dreadful disease category" to Koro:

> Consequently, we seem to be dealing here with the belief in a disease which is commonly known and feared in a certain region, among a certain people, but whose consequences no one has ever seen. One knows nothing from one's own experience, one knows everything from hearsay, no one has ever seen a person dying from the consequences of a penis retracting into his body, which, however, does not falter one's belief that this is possible. The disease exists because it has a right to it; such seems to be the popular belief: for the penis is the centre, the essentials of life; a dead person has no penis; the penis is drawn inwards. One now turns this line of thought upside down and declares: 'So if the penis shows a tendency to withdraw when we see it shrink, then danger threatens; if it really disappears then one will die'
>
> This collective imagination is typical of primitive thinking. The mystical *pars pro toto* idea, despite all the evidence, supports the belief that a dead person has no penis: he cannot possibly have it. For the same reason, the conclusion drawn from this, that the disappearance of the penis leads to death, is irrefutable, even though no one has seen anyone perish from *Shook Jong* with his own eyes and there are still enough eunuchs in China to this day (which are deprived not only of their testicles but also of their *membrum*), which clearly show the inaccuracy of this opinion. Despite all this, the belief in it is so strong that there are

> Chinese who suck *sub finem vitae* on the genitals of their children or attach a weight in order to prevent (the penis') disappearance. (p. 253)

He also gave an excellent psychodynamic case narrative of how this folk belief facilitated obsessive–compulsive behavior:

> Our above-mentioned patient stated that he was having difficulties with women since his youth; he did not dare to socialise with them and had never engaged in coitus at that time. His sexual need was great, and he therefore masturbated a lot. His parents had warned him about this and told him that if he continued, his penis would shrink and retract inward. In other words, they had threatened him with *Shook Jong*. This had made a great impression on him, and because he still could not stop masturbating, he developed fear and obsessional thoughts which were repeated and which he could only master by firmly anchoring the *membrum*. (p. 253)

He discussed the old Chinese custom of castration as punishment and also to produce eunuchs. He postulated Koro as an example of Freudian "Castration Complex" as follows:

> ... we see here before us a living case of the Freudian castration complex. If the view is correct, that a castration fear manifests itself in Koro, then it is to be expected that Koro also occurs in women. This is actually the case now. A doctor from Borneo told me that Koro often occurred there, even with women who had the feeling that the labia were pulled inwards and that the breasts were shrinking; a woman from Kuala-Kapuas is said to have died from it. Here, too, the idea prevails that the disappearance of one's sexual traits results in death. (p. 253)

The last part of the paper deals with the Koro orthography in Buginese and Macassarian languages. He gathered from an old Chinese man that the original term was *Kuru* or *Kura-* which means turtle in Malay and Chinese. The turtlehead is expressed as a glans penis. In the end, he discussed a favored practice of "penis stick" use—a small 4 cm long rod with a rounded tip (locally called *adia, empalang, oetang*) or large sharp quills (*palang*) to make a perforation in the glans and used predominantly by inhabitants of those under strong Chinese influence in ancient times (Fig. 6.3).

This perforation is suggested to represent some magical practice to wound the genitals "as *psychical technic to neutralize the evil energies at puberty.*" The author speculates that in the past, these were used to prevent retraction of the penis. The concluding paragraph of the paper is quite interesting:

> It is by no means surprising that the tribes in which these penis sticks are used no longer know anything about their original purpose, or at least have not commented on this to the various researchers. For about eight years, I have been asking about the meaning and occurrence of Koro, but no one, neither Chinese nor native, knew anything about it. Only after

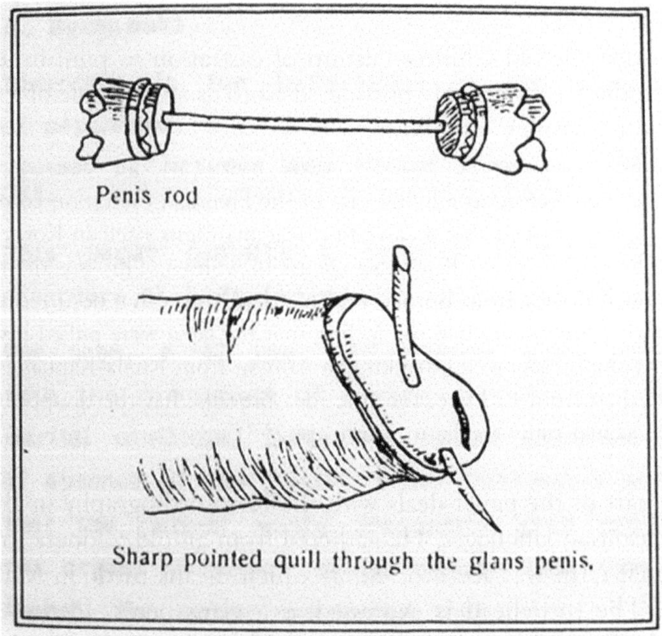

Fig. 6.3 Penis-rod and Sharp quill are probably used to prevent penile retraction (Adopted from Palthe [1934a, p. 1720])

I already knew everything about it, they loosened up when I walked to them; and the same people who previously 'hadn't known anything' now told me all the details with an embarrassed smile, although it was clear that they really were not happy to talk about this because such topics are considered 'magically' dangerous and therefore 'taboo'. (p. 257)

[8]. P. M. van Wulfften Palthe: Anavulling op het Artikel "Koro, een Eigenaardige Angstneurose".
Geneeskundig Tijdschrift voor Nederlandsch-Indie, 1935b, 75, 836–837.

[9]. P. Schilder: *The Image and Appearance of the Human Body.*
Trench Trubner & Co., London, 1935.

It is a well-known and widely referenced book. It contains rich clinical material on different aspects of body image perception and its disorders. According to the author, sui generis, hypochondriacal concerns, or processes crystallize themselves about the experience of altered elements of the body image. In this time-honored monograph on the body image distortion, he cites two cases with genital shrinkage complaints without using the label "Koro." The first patient had varied perceptual deviations, including the shrinking of the penis. The second patient complained of insomnia, nocturnal semen discharge, poor memory, cold extremities, and frequent erections at the sight of the feet of both sex and extreme worry over masturbation. The patient's attention was focused on the penis because of hydrocele, and he was much perturbed by the perception of the shrinking penis.

[10]. J. A Slot: Koro in Zuid-Celebes.
Geneeskundig Tijdschrift voor Nederlandsch-Indie, 1935, 75, 811–820.

It is one of the most valuable and comprehensive clinical documents on Koro by J A Slot, a government doctor in the South Celebes. It provides a detailed report of two native researchers' interviews of a traditional healer in the Macassaran area of Sulawesi. The ethnomedical narratives of Koro were recorded. These were opined as to the affliction of nerves ("nerve contracting disease") or due to physical labor, genital trauma (owing to fall from horseback), and immoderate sexual practices.

The clinical description included an initial stage of cold extremities, palpitation, sweating, paraesthesia of limbs followed by faintness, stiffening of the body, bulging of eye-balls, and retraction of the penis with unconsciousness in fatal cases. The association of fever was viewed as a bad prognostic sign. Indigenous therapies advocated were manual traction of the penis, either self-induced or by others with vigorous limbs massage. Assistance from opposite sex is prohibited because of the belief that even a touch from the opposite sex may yield a fatal outcome. After recovery, a medicinal drink made up of "masculine" ingredients is given to the male patients. The ingredients were a powdered mixture of deer horn, bamboo chips, lasomammelong (lasso = penis), the flowering shoots of the male palmyra (Borassus flabelliformis), and stalk of the arenga palm (Arenga sacchariera). The prognosis was viewed with a bad outcome, especially in chronic cases that might culminate in death. Impotence and sterility in males were said to be the usual sequel.

Prophylaxis included few restrictions like moderate alcohol use and total avoidance of legume like Kentjoes (kaempferia galangal), which also means "retract" or melon because of its springy tendrils and giant scallops and meat, which significantly shrinks when cooked. Stepping over a horse or tortoise stool was forbidden. One has to avoid walking in front of a tortoise because if the animal retracts its head one way, it is a negative sign, but if the head is retracted in the opposite direction away from the person, it is a positive sign as far as the chance for future Koro attack of the viewer is concerned. In Macassares dialect, *Koero* means tortoise. He also mentioned the native use of positive occult influences to prevent this sickness and advises avoiding mysterious negative causes that may precipitate Koro.

The author asserts that there may be a tremendous psychodynamic significance attached to the Macassarese sexual, cultural pattern, viz. transvestite priests/healers, homosexual practice among both sexes' pseudo-hermaphrodites, which play a role in the Koro symptom choice in vulnerable individuals. He mentioned that Koro might occur in several people at the same time and thus resemble mass hysteria. He observed Koro in ordinary farmers who get treatment by occult healing from indigenous healers. Slot stated that Koro is a form of sexual neurosis. He believed that Koro might result from excessive use of alcohol or general exhaustion.

[11]. J. G. A. Mulder: Over Koro.
Geneeskundig Tijdschrift voor Nederlandsch-Indie, 1935, 75, 837–838.

It is a brief note on the ethnomedical aspect of cultural and religious cognition related to Koro among the Sulawesi natives. It is reported that the name Koro locally signifies "shriveling" as meant by Macassars or the Buginese people of South Celebes. He discussed the etiology from Yin-Yang principle among Chinese culture and believed that it acted as a strong primitive folk belief among the Celebes region. He also mentioned some physical conditions like edema of the lower abdomen, hernia, hydrocele, or elephantiasis of the scrotum—which may precipitate fear. He also mentioned Koro in women. He stated the diagnosis of the condition is anxiety neurosis.

[12]. M. Hirschfeld: Men and Women. The World Journey of a Sexologist.
Putnam's Sons, 1935, New York

Magnus Hirschfeld (14 May 1868–14 May 1935) was a German physician and sexologist who was a sexual-rights activist and widely known for his international fame as a sex specialist. He visited many countries and researched on matters related to sex. Edwards (1986) reported that Hirschfeld met Dr. Otto, a German physician who was practicing in Guangzhou, and described this colorful account of a Suo-yang case that he saw on an emergency call in the middle of the night:

> .....There, on the edge of the bed, sits a young man of about twenty-six, his face disfigured by fear, and before him kneels his grandmother, with his wives, his nurse and many servants. With an instrument otherwise used as a gold measure, which can be opened and shut like a pair of jaws, the grandmother has seized the penis of the patient and will not release it even for examination.... The patient has such jong, which means the

> disappearance of the male parts; he has noticed before going to sleep that his member was becoming smaller and smaller. He then called for help, and his grandmother, experienced old woman that she is, has just saved him from death, which would certainly have overtaken him had the member become still smaller and slipped completely back into the body.
>
> In this instance, and in a great many others, Dr. Otto succeeded in setting this fear aside by means of through-going instruction. In other cases he failed, and these men continue to carry their gold measures on their penises day and night, so as never again to fall into so perilous a situation. (Hirschfeld, 1935: 67–68)

1936

[13]. P. M. van Wulfften Palthe: "Koro". Une Maladie Imaginaire et Une Phobie Orientale.
La Presse Medicale, 1936a, 44(67), 1331–1332.

A short article in a French journal.

[14]. P. M. van Wulfften Palthe: Psychiatry and Neurology in the Tropics, in "A Clinical Textbook of Tropical Medicine ," Eds. C. D. de Langen & A. Lichtenstein. G. Kolff & Co., Batavia, 1936b, pp. 525–547.

It is a book chapter in which Koro is discussed in the light of Freud's theory of castration complex. He also noted the Chinese ethnographic explanation of penile retraction in terms of *yin* (feminine) and *yang* (masculine) principles.

[15]. F. Borrey: A Propos du Koro.
La Presse Medicale, 1936, 44(72), 1415. (L)

After reading Wulfften Palthe's (1936a) French-language article on Koro in Indonesia, the author sent this "letter to the Editor" to this French colonial medical journal as a case report, which he saw in November 1935 at the Paul-Doumer Hospital, a French-run facility in Guangzhou.

Edwards (1986) provided a detailed clinical description from Borrey's account as follows:

> A 17 year-old Chinese male presented with "shook-yong". After consulting a number of therapists without relief, the patient's mother took the boy to the hospital. The illness began six months after the boy's marriage at age 12. He confided to the mother that, after every act of coitus, the shaft of the penis diminished in length; he feared that continued sexual relations with his wife would cause total retraction into the abdomen. On the night he first confided the illness, he was sure the penis had diminished by three-fourths its normal size; to prevent further reduction the penis was tied to his right thigh. Over the years, a Chinese doctor prescribed yang remedies, which did not work; nor this prayers and offerings to spirits have any positive effects. The family was particularly concerned since the boy had not yet fathered a son to carry on the family line.
>
> ....The boy asserted his first coitus was normal and he never had a venereal disease. According to the patient, the disorder first began after a voyage on the Xi (West) river: he experienced a slight sensation of penile retraction. (pp. 99–100)

He responded partially with yohimbine-strychnine after five days of hospitalization and was discharged.

Observation: Few essential clinical observations are important in this case: (1) Not presented as classical Koro; (2) The chronicity of the pathology; (3) Post-intercourse correlation (Physiological/ morphological change); (4) Onset after cold exposure; (5) Psychological Impotence and (6) non-response to multiple health-seeking.

[16]. J. Legendre: Une Curieuse Epidemie.
La Presse Medicale, 1936, 44(79), 1534. (L)

After reading Wulfften Palthe's (1936a) French-language article on Koro in Indonesia, the author sent this "letter to the Editor" to this French colonial medical journal, stating the fact of similarity of "so-in-tchen" which he observed and reported thirty years ago (1908). He also added that the illness was also known in Mandarin speech as "koan hoa."

1937

[17]. P. M. van Wulfften Palthe: Il Significanto Forense del 'Koro'. *Archivio Di Anthropologica Criminale, Psichiatria Medicina Legale, 1937, 57, 173–182.*

P. M. van Wulfften Palthe, a Dutch physician, was the hospital psychiatrist for mental diseases at Bongor and Professor of Neurology and Psychiatry in the Medical Academy. He was a well-known name in the area of early Koro research. He was an academician and published quite a few research papers on neuropsychiatric issues from colonial Dutch-Indies. From 1927–1941 he published about 40 research papers in GTNI, mostly on neurological studies but also on the situations of mental health care in Dutch-Indies, including the use of the newly introduced ECTs and studies on Koro.

His 1933 paper summarizes the mental health situation in colonial Indonesia in the early nineteenth century. His four papers (1934, 1935a, 1935b, 1937) and a chapter in a textbook (1936b) are the most valuable early Koro documents. These provide rich and elaborate information on the clinical, epidemic, and endemic aspects, linguistic genesis of the term "Koro," and ethnomedical perspective of genital retraction syndrome in the local cultural context.

He regarded Koro as an unusual form of anxiety neurosis (1934). He believed that Koro in Indonesia appeared to have been imported mainly by the Buginese from Sulawesi to Kalimantan. He referred to the female expression of Koro—the genital and breast retraction. He analyzed the genesis of the illness in terms of folk beliefs and orthography of Koro's word in Macassaran dialects.

The 1935b paper contains a case report, sent to the author as a letter by a practicing physician of Kualakapuas town in southeast Kalimantan. The report states: A farmer of about 35 years of age, probably of Nagadju ethnic group (Edwards, 1984), presented with Koro at the Kualakapuas polyclinic. The patient was a "typical neurotic." He had episodic feelings that the penis shrank into the belly, causing a great apprehension and fear of imminent death. There was a premonitory symptom of a strange sensation in the arms and trunks with radiation to the legs. The experience of penile shrinkage lasted for about an hour. Therapy consisted of penile pull with vigorous massage of the extremities. In females, the chief complaint being that the labia "shoot within." He reported the death of a woman in Mandomai village (central Kalimantan province) from Koro. The local law forbade men to help female illnesses relating to genitalia.

The 1936 publication detailed various psychiatric and neurological morbidities prevalent in the then Dutch-occupied Indonesia or Nederlandish-Indie. This paper's psychiatry section is the English version of the author's earlier Dutch publication (1935b). The author discusses the tropics' ecological influence ("the constant warmth, the loneliness, the eternal green and the absence of any change of the seasons") and the European immigrants' psychic adaptability. The author fails to note any pathological influence of tropical climate. Many Europeans believed in "Tropical Madness" ("an insanity supposed to be caused by the solitude, by the occult influences of the mystic East") and "Jungle Psychosis" (characterized by persistent unsystematized delusions of reference and persecution). It was believed to be the result of magical influence (*dibikin guna-guna*—in the native lexicon) of the tropics.

The author provides a comprehensive discussion of the different "psychopathic disturbances among the natives," viz. Amuek or Amok, Latah, and Koro. Palthe regards Koro as a "sort of anxiety state," which may, in some cases, last for several days. The traditional belief of the Chinese in yin (female) and yang (male) principles have been implicated in Koro, and thus the medicines of yang ("*Panas*" or warm) principles are ruled for its cure. The author believes that this illness represents the collective phantasy of castration fear.

The author traces the historical background of castration (e.g., amputation of the penis) as a means that prevailed in Chinese society as punishment or for creating eunuchs. Moreover, there was a widespread belief in the East-Indies that the destruction of the genital organ implied life's destruction. The author advocates all these socio-cultural customs enhanced the faith in penile retraction or shook yong in the population.

Palthe's 1937 case report was of forensic and legal importance because the Koro attack precipitated Amok's onset, leading to murder. The case was a 40-year-old fisherman of Badjavanese ethnicity, a resident of the northwest coast of Flores, arrested for murdering his wife during a fit of Amok. A court-ordered psychiatric examination disclosed that he was a Koro sufferer. Three years earlier, the first attack was precipitated by cold water during bathing when the patient felt a sudden cold shock run all over his body with eventual penile retraction. Medicines from a native healer offered him a gradual cure. In 1933, after his trip to Mecca (he belonged to the Islamic faith) he had no Koro sensation until the night of his attack or running amok. On that night of the murder, he woke up suddenly, felt cold chills and retraction of the penis, which turned him "furious" with fear and perplexed and clouded his consciousness. He had total amnesia regarding the event of the murder. He had neither marital maladjustment nor any sexual conflicts. He had no abnormality in any organ systems, nor did he have any somatic anomalies of the body and genital organs. He was of good nutritional status, was of normal behavior, and was mentally lucid.

1943

[18]. G. Bychowski: Disorders in the body-image in the clinical pictures of psychoses.

Journal of Nervous & Mental Diseases, 1943, 97, 310–335.

Gustav Bychowski was a Polish-American psychiatrist-psychoanalyst and was a prolific writer. This paper contains a detailed academic and clinical discussion on body image disorders, varied psychopathological manifestations, and rich case notes.

One case showed how depression was instrumental in causing the genitally focused symptom. The subject was a 46-year-old Hebrew male. He had several bereavements (father and then-wife), conflicts in new love relation (whether to marry or not), forbidden sexual impulses, religious ethos—all culminated into depression with intense sexual battle relating to a new heterosexual relationship. The author states:

> The most striking phenomena associated with this depression was the peculiar feeling that his sexual organs were somehow foreign to his body

> and that at times he could not even feel that they were there. The impression was so strong that the patient would frequently grab himself by his sex organs in order to be certain that they were there. (p. 321)

More interesting to observe, he gradually felt the same was happening to other organs, though to a minor degree. Despite all therapeutic interventions, the patient committed suicide. The author concluded that:

> The complex nature of body image which gradually develops from early childhood on and undergoes various changes throughout whole life is responsible for its variations under different physiological and pathological conditions. (p. 333)

1945

[19]. R. P. Strong: Stitt's Diagnosis, Prevention and Treatment of Tropical Diseases.
K.H. Lewis & Co., London, 7th Ed., 1945, p. 1145.

It is a short note on Koro in a book on tropical diseases. Koro was identified as a particular form of anxiety neurosis with a high prevalence among the Buginese and Macassarians in the Celebes and North Borneo. The condition was known as "shook yang" among the Chinese.

1948

[20]. F. Kobler: Description of an acute castration fear, based on superstition.
Psychoanalytic Review, 1948, 35, 285–289.

The author saw one case in 1941 at a hospital in Foshan (Fatshan), a small town north of Canton in the province of Kwangtung, South China. Fritz Kobler was acting head of the Neuropsychiatry department at Medical College of the National Central University of Nanking. The subject developed acute anxiety of penile retraction during his inpatient stay. His family discharged him from the hospital shortly after the onset of these symptoms. It is a psychoanalytical discussion paper on

Koro, based on the finding of this Chinese case. The author viewed the genital retraction symptomatology as the expression of acute castration fear intermingled with cultural beliefs and superstitions. He also noted grasping the penis in hand or clamping it in a mechanical device to prevent retraction. Kobler commented that:

> The attitude of the family is one of believing the anxiety of the patient to be justified, sharing his fear to be danger of death in the very near future and not at all one of considering the patient to be mentally ill. The common local population considers this condition not as a disease but is equally convinced that the related symptoms are facts....The condition disappears after one or two days. (p. 285)

The author also tried to explain this genital retraction concerning masturbatory guilt, anxiety, and often as a chronic course. The author described a typical child play with a penis:

> I was even informed by other doctors that some patients utter the fear that the penis might gradually become smaller and smaller and in this way disappear. Possibly there is a relationship existing between this symptom of anxiety and certain masturbatory habit of children to play with the penis by alternatively pushing in behind preputium and skin until the penis disappears and then letting it appear again. In this case, the anxiety of the disappearing penis would mean an anxiety over masturbation. (p. 289)

1950

[21]. H. T. Chabot: Verwantschap, Stand en Sexe in Zuid-Celebes; Perhubungan-Kerabat, Tingkat-Bangsa Dan djenis-kelamin Di Sulawesi-Selatan.

J. B. Wolters' Uitgeversmaatschappij, 1950.

Hendrik Theodorus Chabot, was a sociology professor at the University of Indonesia at Makassar and had extensive fieldwork among the local population at Makassar. It is a book entirely devoted to discussing Koro psychodynamics' conceptual frame concerning the socio-cultural and sexual construct and codes of the Makassarese community. He stressed the impacts of rapid social changes and implicated sociopsychological factors for the development of Koro symptomatology. The elements he identified were: keen competitiveness of Macassarese people to attain social stability and material wealth, sexual conquests among them, and failure or feelings of anxiety and powerlessness in this process of social competition.

There is an excellent case vignette gathered from a Macassaran informant as follows:

> A man about 45, with wife and children, took a second wife. Afraid of the first wife's jealousy, he tried to keep the new relationship secret but in time the second marriage became known. One evening, he came home tired and fatigued. He got the shivers, broke out in a cold sweat, and felt that his penis was shrinking. At his cry for help, the neighbors came running. Only men helped him. One man tightly held the patient's penis while another went for a *sanro*, a native healer. The *sanro* performed one ritual and after a while the anxiety disappeared, ending the day's attack. (p. 165)

Note

The Medical Journal of the Dutch-Indies 1852–1942 [Bergen L. van, Hesselink, L, Verhave, J. P. (Eds.), 2017].

This is a valuable compilation of Dutch-Indies' medical history, published by the Indonesian Academy of Sciences in November 2017. It mentions all the valuable publications in G*eneeskundig Tijdschrift voor Nederlandsch-Indie (GTNI)*—from 1852–1942. It contains a photograph of 1937—of Dr. V. W. Palthe arranging for electric shock therapy to a patient.

There is a detailed description of Mental illness specific to the Dutch-Indies in a sub-chapter, "*Psychiatric care of the mentally ill*" (pp. 330–347). It is commented that: "Physicians working in the Dutch Indies have focused on three specific forms of mental illness unknown outside the colonies: *amok, latah, and koro.* These conditions are common in Southeast Asia, in particular in the Dutch Indies and Malaysia. European psychiatrists working in the Dutch Indies have made several early and original observations on these conditions." It also contains a brief discussion on each of these illnesses.

Some historical reference of Koro from this section is worth noting here:

> Koro is the fear that one's penis will retract into the pelvis and is generally observed among Chinese men. These men often went to great lengths to prevent this from happening because they believed it would ultimately result in death.... Koro was recorded in the medical literature for the first time in 1895 by J.C.Blonk, who described it as an irresistible compulsion or an acute anxiety neurosis exacerbated by alcoholism....In 1934, P.M.van Wulfften Palthe, professor at the Medical Academy, provided an extensive analysis of koro. He elaborated on how affected men attempted to prevent their penis from retracting by holding it, often assisted by their wife and children, or by using contraptions or penile piercings. ...He explained it using psychoanalytic ideas as an anxiety neuroses related to the castration complex. J.A.Slot observed that, in South Kalimantan, the condition could affect several individuals at the same time and therefore constituted a form of mass hysteria. He observed the condition in common farmers and noted the general use of occult healing methods by indigenous healers.... According to him, the condition followed excessive use of alcohol or general exhaustion. (pp. 339–340)

Observation: Considering the historical analysis of Koro's publications, it is evident that the three Dutch medical personalities brought Koro's medical entity from the colonial landscape of the Netherland Indies (Indonesia) to a broader Western medical press. J. C. Blonk (1895) first introduced the topic to Dutch medical literature, and PCJ van Brero, a leading Dutch psychiatrist, further expanded the concept clinically and published it in Dutch (1895) and German (1896a) journals (Section one). After almost 30 years gap, Wulfften Palthe's, Professor of Psychiatry, different publications brought the Koro as a medical entity in the Western academic world anew: his Dutch magazine (1934); German psychoanalytic literature (1935b); French medical literature (1936a); and Italian Journal of Psychiatric Anthropology (1937) and his work in a Dutch textbook of tropical medicine which was translated into English (1936b) opened the topic to British, German, and American academia.

It is fascinating to note that local "Koro" from the Indonesian landscape entered into the wider Western medical press and psychiatric academia.

Koro Literature: From 1951 to 1960

Preamble: In this decade, six publications are relevant in the context of Koro as an emerging diagnostic entity in the mental health field. Professor P. M. Yap's pioneering article advocates for the first time a nosological position for Koro as a culturally linked psychological abnormality. A short scholarly book on "Culture and Mental Disorders" came from the USA, written by Ralph Linton, Professor of Anthropology at Yale University. Silvano Arieti and Johannes M Meth's credit is that they incorporate Koro in their textbook "American Handbook of Psychiatry." There is no separate publication on the 1955 Guangdong (China) Koro epidemic, but it is mentioned in a review article by Jilek (1986).

1951

[1]. P. M. Yap: Mental diseases peculiar to certain cultures: A survey of comparative psychiatry.
Journal of Mental Science, 1951, 97, 313–327.

This is one of the pioneering scholarly papers on transcultural psychiatry. By elegant analysis of Western psychiatric nosology and Oriental psychiatric manifestations, he attempts to bridge the universal cultural influence on a mental illness over place and time. It also describes the concept of normality as envisioned in Western psychiatric perspectives. Citing different unusual behaviors from different cultures, he concluded that "The idea of the abnormal varies with the time." In the category of culture-specific mental disorders, the author follows two broad divisions. Firstly, autopathological—those conditions regarded as abnormal in cultures in which they are found but regarded as normal in another cultural setting. Secondly, autonormal—behaviors are perceived as normal in their own culture but regarded as a disease condition in

Euro-American civilization. The author briefly references psychic contagions with many examples from medieval Europe in the former category. He includes the criteria of Koro, Latah, Amok, and Witigo psychosis under this heading with a brief account of each. For Koro he states:

> That it is psychogenic illness resting on superstition there can be no doubt. There is a wealth of folk-lore in connection with this disease, but it is probable that actual hysterical anaesthesia of the penis, or some disturbance of the "body-image" occurs… Nosologically Koro is, I believe, an acute anxiety state (penis) in persons with sexual conflicts and preoccupations. (p. 318)

In the category of "Autonormal and heteropathological forms of behavior," the author includes the following varieties: homosexuality, possession, the potlatch of British Columbia, the touch taboos of the Dobuan islanders, thanatomania, and yogism. There is an excellent analytical overview of cultural factors as a contributor to mental symptoms viz. richness of psychiatric symptomatology and patient's intellectual and cultural resources; the cultural basis of delusion, obsession, and compulsion, and repressive social mechanisms and the analogy between schizophrenic and primitive ways of thought, etc. The author also highlights socio-cultural cues to the proneness of mental conflict in different social groups.

This paper showed Yap's deep understanding of the cultural influence on the expression of mental symptoms or illness and an academic warning not to examine an odd behavior from other cultural lenses. This is one of Koro's first academic discourses. This analytical paper is a must-read for all cultural psychiatrists and Koro researchers.

1954

[2]. G. Devereux: Primitive genital mutilations in a neurotic's dream.

Journal of American Psychoanalytical Association, 1954, 2, 484–492.

George Devereux, was an anthropologist, student, and colleague of Prof Linton, who researched culture and personality and cultural issues in psychoanalytic therapy and dream. This paper provides an excellent analytical discussion on a young nurse's dream content and its symbolic relation (anthropological interest) with manifold phallic mutations. The author notes penile encrustations with small precious stones (in Indonesia), Koro, and ampallang in the context of castration fear and fantasy. He also provides a case history of a Jewish adolescent who maneuvered his circumcised penis in a way that approximated the imaginary Koro situation. With rich cross-cultural examples, the author tries to highlight the fact that "a fantasy, thought or wish which is culturally implemented in one society may appear in another society in the guise of an idiosyncratic, unconscious or partially conscious, fantasy."

[3]. H. Teirich: Koro complcx: Casc rcport.
Psyche (Stuttgart), 1954, 7(10), 633–636. [Article in German]

[4]. Sri P. H. Manson-Bahr: Kuru, Latah, Running Amok and Koro.
In, Tropical Diseases—A Manual of the Diseases of the Warm Climate. Cassell and Company, Ltd., London, 1954.

It is a brief chapter in a book dealing with four types of diseases prevalent in the South-East Asia regions. The author describes each of the disorders with a brief epidemiological background and clinical features. Interestingly, the term "Kuru" is a native name for a central nervous system disorder of the Mount Michael area in the Eastern Highlands of New Guinea.

Koro is defined as a form of anxiety neurosis, where sexual conflicts are identified as the source of anxiety. An analogous state in women is also described as diminishing the labia, and shrinkage of the breasts constitutes the cardinal feature. The author listed different pathological conditions as Koro precipitator, viz. edema of the lower abdomen, hernia, hydrocele, and elephantiasis of the scrotum.

1955: Koro Epidemic in Guangdong, China

1956

[5]. R. Linton: Culture and Mental Disorders.
Charles C. Thomas, Springfield, Illinois, U.S.A., 1956.

It is one of the earlier books devoted to the theme of cultural influence on mental symptoms. The author, Ralph Linton, was the Sterling Professor of Anthropology at Yale University, USA. The author provides the results of a systematic survey on cultural correlation with mental disorders, viz—culture and normality; cultural influence in neurosis and psychosis and Hysteria in cultural perspective. In the second chapter, he described Witigo and Koro (pp. 67–69) and contained a discussion on Koro's psychopathology. He cited van Wulfften Palthe who knew a Chinese from Borneo who had Koro illness. He also mentioned that Palthe also saw a Chinese patient hospitalized for tuberculosis, and from him, he knew the Chinese term *shook yang* (penis shrinks). Palthe highlighted two factors in Koro's phenomenology: an imaginary organic illness and acute anxiety of neurotic origin. Linton believed that it is not neurosis but psychosis. He cited an example of a female Koro patient from Borneo ("feel that their breasts are shriveling up and that their labia are being sucked inward"). He said: "The above examples of culturally and geographically localized psychosis indicate the extent to which cultural beliefs can influence delusion and behavior in mental disorders."

1959

[6]. S. Arieti, J. M. Meth: Rare, unclassifiable, collective and exotic syndromes.
In, American handbook of Psychiatry, vol 1, pp. 546–563, 1959. Basic Books, New York.

This chapter is in a book where Koro was included as a culture-bound mental disorder under the heading of rare, unclassified, collective, and exotic psychotic syndromes. A two-point diagnostic criterion for Koro was postulated: fear from the experience of shrinkage of the penis and the cultural interpretation of this experience. They also described some other culture-related disorders.

Koro Literature: From 1961 to 1970

Preamble: A total of 22 reports on Koro or related topics have been reviewed from this decade, among which seven were new Koro cases, viz. from Taiwan, Singapore, Hong Kong, England, France, and the USA. Three were newspaper reporting of the 1967 Koro epidemic of Singapore. There were no separate published reports of the 1966 Guangdong (China) Koro epidemic cited by Jilek (1986).

Publications of this decade are immensely crucial in Koro research because three remarkable events mark these, viz. (1) the publication of seven academic papers by Dr. Pow Meng Yap of Hong Kong, including his 1965 article, "Koro – A culture-bound depersonalization syndrome"—a superbly masterful report which all Koro researchers have extensively cited till date; (2) Dr. Yap's relentless and untiring effort to establish the nosological status of Koro in the sphere of academic psychiatry; and (3) the occurrence of a massive Koro epidemic in Singapore (first time outside China). The Chinese concept of *Yin-Yang* imbalance and Koro symptomatology is also discussed and focused on with great detail by Dr. Ah Leng Gwee and Dr. P. W. Ngui of Singapore, and Dr. Hsien Rin of Taiwan. This decade has provided plenty of clinical and academic input to the construct of Koro illness, especially from the Chinese cultural perspective. The first case of "Koro-like depersonalization" was reported from the USA, a faraway country from China.

1961

[1]. Van H. R. Gulik: *Sexual Life in Ancient China. Leiden, 1961.*

It is a valuable book that contains a socio-anthropological and cultural history of sexuality in Chinese culture, tracing back some 2000 years of Chinese erotic history. Robert Hans van Gulik (9 August 1910–24 September 1967) was a highly educated orientalist, diplomat, and musician. He wrote many scholarly monographs on Chinese art and culture, music, and animals. In his in-depth study of *Sexual life in Ancient China,* he incorporated various cultural myths and traditional practices related to sexuality, from the Chinese "secret texts" and several old erotic albums. There is a discussion on symbolic connotations of the turtle with Koro's social cognition. It analyses the gradual shift of social values attached to the turtle with references from Ming dynasty documents: The Chinese people used the turtle as an artistic and literary symbol for longevity and life's vital forces until the Ming dynasty. Later, it was symbolically connected with Koro's illness cognition because of the similarity between this long-lived creature's retractable head and the glans penis.

1962

[2]. P. M. Yap: Words and things in comparative psychiatry with special reference to the exotic psychoses.
Acta Psychiatrica Scandinavica, 1962, 38, 163–169.

This paper is an example of Yap's sincere attempt to clarify the term 'exotic psychosis' often used by Western scholars. He argued that there are some culture-bound presentations in every culture. These are to be viewed and labeled as per available psychiatric nosology with comparative psychiatry aims and objectives. The paper is a transcultural analysis of the nosological aspects of "exotic psychoses." The author proposed that the term "exotic psychoses" (to designate the various culture-linked psychological illnesses, including Koro) should be replaced by the term "atypical culture-bound psychogenic psychosis." The paper was quite elaborately written with few subheadings.

Under the heading "The object of Comparative Psychiatry" he stressed the importance of linking clinical experience with the epidemiological data for a balanced and meaningful nosology without bias. Then he discussed the need and "The purpose of Nosology" for research and communication as a common conceptual language to address cross-cultural psychiatry. Then he cited "Practical Consideration," where he stressed the need for a unified definition of symptoms because symptoms are the same, but their cultural conceptualization differs. For example, "echolalia in the Malay might be a symptom of a fright-induced state, whereas it would more likely be a part of the schizophrenic syndrome in the West." Or "Koro is interpreted as a phobia based on castration fear." When applied to Koro, the word "phobia" is not used in a sense commonly accepted by most clinical psychiatrists, namely "ideas against which the patient actively struggles." He cited many examples from the literature supporting his contention to have a consensus on CBS's nosological status acceptable in both the hemisphere.

1963

[3]. H. Rin: Koro: A consideration on Chinese concepts of illness and case illustrations.
Transcultural Psychiatric Research Review, 1963, 15, 23–30.

It is the first Koro report published in Transcultural Psychiatric Research Review (TPRR). It contains a detailed discussion of the Chinese concept (yin-yang disturbances) of genital retraction with two detailed case reports. The first case was with multiple neurotic elements and sexual conflicts, and in the second one, the Koro symptomatology is discussed in the background of the paranoid state. Both the cases were Chinese.

[4]. T. A. Baasher: The influence of culture on psychiatric manifestations.
Transcultural Psychiatric Research, Review 1963, 15, 51–52.

Dr. Taha A. Baasher was a prominent psychiatric leader and academician from Africa and the Middle East. It is a discussion paper devoted to the transcultural analysis of mental illness symptoms in the context of African culture. The author cited examples of the cultural effect on mental illness cognition in different ethnic groups like Uduk and Jumjum of Sudan. Penile shrinkage like Koro is also encountered in some Sudanese youths, which resembles that found in Chinese cultures. The author states:

> The condition is seen in patients with immature personality, and is associated with false concepts regarding the harmful effects of masturbation, which is believed to maim the penis, paralyse the hand, and rot the brain. It is interesting to note that in Southeast Asian there is the parallel belief that masturbation would bring about *suo-yang* or *Koro*. In the Sudanese

> who complained of shrinking of the penis, there was no belief that the penis would disappear into the abdomen. The latter symptom seems to be rooted in the cultural soil; hence it is reasonable to suggest that psychiatric conditions like Koro are anxiety states and that the different patterns which have been observed are culturally determined. (p. 52)

[5]. A. L. Gwee: Koro: A cultural disease.
Singapore Medical Journal, 1963, 4, 119–122.

Dr. Gwee was a neurologist and founding editor of the Singapore Medical Journal. He is regarded as one of the leading authorities on Koro at his time. This is one of the pioneering reports on Koro's cultural aspect of Chinese socio-cultural beliefs and traditional practices. Citations and illustrations of various old Chinese medical texts regarding penile shrinkage are essential in this paper. The author discusses the psychodynamics of penile retraction in terms of fear of castration and presented three Chinese cases with a follow-up of seven years.

Case 1: A Chinese schoolboy of 8 years had an insect bite on the penis. A couple living in the house first identified the retraction of the penis and, after applying balm and holding of the penis, resolved the situation. Subsequently, he had three such penile retraction attacks and was attended to and treated by doctors. In each episode, the penis was tied with a loop of string to prevent retraction. One important point to note is that initial observation was made not by the boy himself but by an apprehended couple. The boy and the parents were subjected to long hours of persuasion as a part of therapy.

Case 2: A single Chinese male of 34 years old developed acute retraction while urinating during a cinema show at night: "he felt a loss of feeling in the genital region suddenly, and straightaway, the thought occurred to him that he was going to get a penile retraction." He had spermatorrhoea symptoms during defaecation (Dhat syndrome—my addition), a prostitute visit, and gonorrheal infection. He is also aware of "shook yong." Reassurance and psycho-sexual education cured his symptoms.

Case 3: A married Chinese male of 38 years old had his first penile retraction attack at age 18 when he took purgative. For the last two years, he was physically weak and noticed each time he defecates, and he had feelings of penile retraction. Ultimately, he developed the same perception during intercourse, which was so much fear and anxiety arousing, he abstains from intercourse. Reassurance and psycho-sexual education cured his symptoms.

The author described some popular Chinese folklore and medical texts relating to the penis' retraction and death. Considering the cultural belief, he advocates Koro's nosological state as follows: ".... this condition is one of acute hysterical panic reaction brought on by auto- or hetero -suggestion and conditioning by the cultural background."

1964

[6]. P. M. Yap: Suk-yeong or Koro: A culture-bound depersonalization syndrome.
Bulletin of the Hong Kong Chinese Medical Association, 1964a, 16, 31–47.

This is the lecture's transcript delivered before the Hong Kong Psychiatry Association on 22 May 1964. This is one of the detailed clinical accounts of 19 Koro cases seen by the author, with an extensive literature survey available at this time. The author described the detailed demography, symptomatology, and treatment and followed up his case series in an orderly fashion. The etiology section expanded the traditional Chinese concept of yin-yang imbalances, patients' sexual and personality history and traits, family dynamics, and situational stresses. There is a lengthy discussion on the idea of depersonalization, body image, and psychoanalytical explanation in Koro perception. The last part is dedicated to nosology and diagnosis. He concluded with a compelling clinical reason that Koro is an example of depersonalization syndrome.

[7]. P. M. Yap: Koro or Suk-yeong: An atypical culture-bound psychiatric disorder found in Southern Chinese.
Transcultural Psychiatric Research Review, 1964b, 1, 36–38.

This is an abstract of Yap's paper at the Joint meeting of the Japanese Society of Neurology and Psychiatry and the American Psychiatric Association, held in Tokyo in May 1963.

A brief account of 19 Koro or *Suo-yang* cases is described, along with their clinical manifestations. The detailed clinical description is reported earlier (Yap, 1964a). It is noted that only a feeling of numbness or coldness in the penis might be the sole complaint in some cases. Koro's association with clouding consciousness and paranoid thinking, and auditory hallucinations of depression is also recorded.

The author regards Koro as a form of localized depersonalization of the penis. He asserts that the portion of the body image corresponding to the penis is very weak since the penis is a toneless organ and is not under voluntary muscular movement or control. Its proprioceptive perception is dependent on episodic emotional arousal. The cultural belief in *Suo-yang* has a dual role in Koro's symptom manifestation, viz. pathoplastic and pathogenic. *Suo-yang* may be classified as an anxiety state, keeping in mind its difference from the normal anxiety state in that its culture-dependent relationship in both form and content. Thus, the author places *Suo-yang* as one of the culture-bound psychogenic disorders.

1965

[8]. P. M. Yap: Koro: A culture-bound depersonalization syndrome.

British Journal of Psychiatry, 1965a, 111, 43–50.

This is the first clinical report on Koro published in the British Journal of Psychiatry. It is a time-honored, most extensively cited paper. It contains a detailed clinical description, historical background, etiology, and nosological clarification of 19 Koro cases, that he collected over 15 years in Hong Kong. This is for the first time; after 1895, Koro was discussed with such an elaborate nosological analysis and identified as a "culture-bound depersonalization syndrome." He gave the standard definition of Koro as:

> The term "koro" refers to an unfamiliar state of acute anxiety with partial depersonalization leading to the conviction of penile shrinkage and to fears of dissolution.

This paper first reported Koro's association with drug abuse (heroin withdrawal phase), schizophrenia, general paresis, and manic-depressive disorder. It also said the different personality types of Koro cases as per DSM criteria for the first time. The detailed sexual history of the patients was another essential feature of this account. He mentioned quite a few significant clinical issues in his case series which are still crucial for any Koro researchers to examine among their cohorts: sexual conflict and maladjustment; feeling of sexual inadequacy, cold as a physiological precipitator of Koro; paraesthesia in the genital area; hypochondriacal concern, compulsive personality and associated other mental disorder like depression and paranoid delusion. All these associations have been reported time and again in subsequent Koro research over the years.

The hypothesis of Koro-depersonalization as its phenomenological dynamics was presented as:

> This is a unique example of a depersonalization syndrome whose form and content, and indeed occurrence and distribution, are determined by a combination of social and cultural factors acting on predisposed personalities. The depersonalization is seen as a dissociative mechanism affecting the integrity of the body-image. Unlike ordinary states of depersonalization, the Koro patient has insight into his own condition only in a restricted sense, and moreover does not suffer a general disturbance of affective responsiveness. (p. 49)

Observation: One significant issue was missing in this research. Yap excluded 8 cases of Koro from his study sample: 6 had schizophrenic background; 1 patient was of general paresis due to syphilitic infection; and 1 case presented with the sub-delirious state due to heroin withdrawal. These were virtually Secondary Koro (Koro in association with other disorders). This particular concept was not matured enough at that time, so Yap probably finds no interest in studying them in detail.

[9]. A. R. K. Mitchell: Koro—A culture-bound depersonalization syndrome.
British Journal of Psychiatry, 1965, 111, 553–554. (L)

This letter supports P. M. Yap's above publication with a Koro case report, who attended a British Military Hospital in Singapore in 1964. The patient was a 28 years old married Chinese male who "presented himself to the unit medical officer with a friend firmly grasping his penis, stating that the organ was visibly shrinking into his abdomen and that if it disappeared completely, he would die." The case was managed symptomatically without any result. The attending psychiatrist did not know Koro at that time. The author made a precious comment: "The failure to manage this case adequately arose not only out of ignorance of the basic condition but also by approaching it through a Western-orientated psychiatric formulation of the psychopathology." In this context, he cited Yap's cautionary note regarding the errors in classifying disorders in a foreign culture.

[10]. F. Bodman: Koro.
British Journal of Psychiatry, 1965, 111, 369. (L)

In response to Yap's above paper (1965a), the author cited one Koro description in a Westerner, "a clinical description in non-technical language of Koro occurring in a middle-aged man of good education and mature personality, to be found in Victor Gollancz's *More for Timothy* (pp. 91–92)."*

[* This book was published by Orion Publishing Company, London in 1957, Imprint Gollancz, ISBN 100575009780].

[11]. P. M. Yap: Koro in a Briton.
British Journal of Psychiatry, 1965b, 111, 774–775.

This is a Koro case report in a Briton and the second report in the Koro literature on Koro association with drug abuse (amphetamine). A 43-year-old married man of three children, of a worrying and nervous disposition, whose one of the testicles was forced into the inguinal canal after a fall at a younger age. He was worried about his small penile size compared to "unduly long testes," for which he avoided undressing in front of others. Since the age of 22, he has had three episodes of depression with pain in the neck, back, and testicles. "One unusually cold morning, he felt his penis shrinking to about half an inch" but "elongated on urination," and this feeling lasted for 24 hours. The author discussed the role of penile self-observation and self-scrutiny in developing localized depersonalization in the development of Koro perception. He also mentioned physical factors in penile depersonalization like cold, anxiety, or potential of adrenergic vasoconstriction of erectile tissue. He also said of an Englishman who experienced penile diminution after taking large quantities of amphetamine.

[12]. H. Rin: A study of the aetiology of Koro in respect to the Chinese concept of illness.
International Journal of Social Psychiatry, 1965, 11, 7–13.

It contains a detailed clinical description of two Koro cases reported earlier (Rin, 1963). This is the first Koro report published in the International Journal of Social Psychiatry.

The author cited Koro's multiple diagnostic terms in the literature, like an imaginary organic illness; actual anxiety states—a culture-bound variant of hysteria and psychosis. He postulated that: "The panic state of *suo-yang* can be explained as an extreme form of fear of total castration resulting in death, but beyond this, it is a symbolic manifestation of fear of losing vitality, of becoming sick and weak, and it is deeply related to the fundamental Chinese concepts of sexuality."

The author presented clinical details of two male cases of Suo-yang, which were also reported earlier in his 1963 publication.

Case 1. A 32-year-old single Chinese male migrated from Hankow, Central China, complaining of panic attacks and multiple somatic symptoms. He noticed his penis was shrinking and withdrawing into the abdomen after intercourse with a prostitute for the last month. He consulted various herb doctors, who diagnosed him with *shenn-kuei* or deficient vitality and prescribed traditional medicine (drinking boy's urine and eating human placenta to supply *chih*—energy or vital essence). The detailed psycho-sexual history showed the presence of irresistible sexual drive, gambling, panic attacks with multiple hypochondriacal symptoms (often to a psychotic extent). A significant oral demand was evident in replenishing vital energy with various herbal medicines and huge rice meals.

Case 2. A 39-year-old married Chinese man migrated from the Kiangsy province of Central China and was admitted with a paranoid state. He has marked delusional symptoms like ideas of reference, ideas of being poisoned, and multiple hypochondriacal complaints. He was quite anxious and felt a sharp pain in the perineum and a cold (leng) sensation in the penis at night. Subsequently, he developed several strange feelings like a retraction of the penis, loosening of the scrotal skin, the possibility of his testicles dropping off, and pain in the left testicle. Subsequently, he developed a wide range of paranoid ideas with many strange somatic delusions, including the feeling that because of his loose scrotal skin *jing* (semen) was leaking out. Psychosexual and past history showed passive, dependent character with insecurity in early life, marital conflict, the pressure of work, alcohol consumption, and domestic and legal difficulties. All these cumulatively stressed him. The author believes these caused decompensations and regression with the development of a panic state of *Suo-yang* (loss of vitality), which was incorporated within his delusional system. The author discussed the Koro phenomenology in the light of oral dependence and deprivation in upbringing and the concept of *yin-yang* philosophy in sexuality in Chinese culture.

1966

1966: Koro Epidemic in Guangdong, China

[13]. H. Rin: Two forms of vital deficiency syndrome among Chinese male mental patients.
Transcultural Psychiatric Research Review, 1966, 3, 19–21.

This paper presents two forms of culture-bound psychiatric syndromes in Chinese subjects. They are *Suo-yang* or Koro and *pa-leng* or Frigophobia (morbid fear of cold). The author describes three cases of Koro and three instances of Frigophobia. Both are related to the Chinese concept of vitality and believe that its deficiency will have serious consequences.

Reviewing his cases, the author drew a comparison between these two clinical states. It revealed a set of characteristics of each in so far as the similarities and dissimilarities were concerned. Four similarities between Koro and Frigophobia were enumerated as follows: (1) a core symptom of extreme fear of loss of bodily energy or vitality; (2) imagined loss or deficiency in vital strength attributed to disharmony between yin and yang elements. According to the Chinese traditional belief, these are two complementary forces that have to be in harmony to ensure health. In Koro, the yang elements (semen and blood) are involved, and in Frigophobia the yin elements, i.e., the cold and wind; (3) association of the core symptom with various other psychiatric symptoms; and (4) self-administration of multiple remedies intended to counteract the loss of vitality.

1967

[14]. P. M. Yap: Classification of the culture-bound reactive syndromes.

Australian & New Zealand Journal of Psychiatry, 1967, 1, 172–179.

This is a discussion paper, based on the author's lecture at the Annual Scientific Meeting of the Australian and New Zealand College of Psychiatrists in Perth, in 1967, where he attempted to classify culture-bound reactive syndromes. He started with the emphasis of Comparative Psychiatry that: "The final aim of nosological endeavor in psychiatry, as with any other branches of medicine, must be to classify illness in terms of their causes." The author discussed some unusual forms of mental illnesses like Amok, Latah, and Koro. They have different presentations in different cultures. The author opined that "it is essential to apply the concept of clinical psychopathology to the study of these disorders, and attempt to integrate them into a recognized classification of disease." He also discussed the limitations of the existing classification with a detailed analysis of the concept of "psychogenic" or "reactive" psychosis.

He tried to put the available CBS under four broad classes: Primary fear reaction (Latah, Susto, Thanatophobia); Hypereridic (morbid rage) reaction (Amok); Specific, Culturally imposed noso-phobia (Koro), and Trance Dissociation (Possession syndrome). He tried to put Koro in this classification as follows:

> Koro is a partial and localized depersonalization state confined to the penis, occurring against a background of acute anxiety and arising from fears of sexual exhaustion. It is found among young men in Hong Kong and S.E. Asia who are exposed to a folk-belief in the existence of a mortal illness due to penile shrinkage. (p. 177)

The paper contains many supportive arguments favoring the need to define and classify culture-bound disorders in the background of ongoing psychiatric research. He hoped that: "Many more research remains to be done into the social and ethnological factors that combine to produce the culture-bound syndromes" (p. 178).

1967: Koro Epidemic in Singapore

* * *

Box 6.1 Media Coverage of Singapore Koro Epidemic

❖ 5 November 1967: this article appeared in *The Sunday Times*, Singapore:

'A STRANGE MALADY HITS SINGAPORE MEN AND THE SMA STEPS IN'
The Sunday Times, 5 November 1967.
The 'malady' in question was a mass psychologically-induced panic – called Koro – where hundreds of Singaporean men found that their genitals were shrinking into their abdomens. At the peak of the 'epidemic', the Singapore General Hospital was seeing 70 to 80 cases a week.

Rumour has it that it had to do with inoculated pigs.

Weeks earlier, rumours began spreading in Singapore that eating pork that had been inoculated against the swine flu would cause your genitals to shrink – a condition known as *Koro*, *suo yang* (缩阳), or *shook yong*.

[https://mothership.sg/2016/11/sporean-men-panicked-in-1967-over-strange-case-of-shrinking-genitals-known-as-koro/]

❖ **From The Straits Times: 7.11.67**

"DO NOT FEAR KORO"

"Do not fear Koro", read the headline of the S.T. article on Nov 7, 1967.

.... Rumours had first spread on Oct 28, 1967, that eating pork caused koro - a retraction of the male sexual organ.

Panic ensued as an average of 80 people called daily at the outdoor dispensaries of government hospitals claiming to be suffering from the disease, said a Straits Times report on Nov 7.

A Health Ministry press conference was subsequently called to dispel the rumours and clarify that koro was not connected to consuming pork. A panel of medical experts' pinpoined psychological fear as the main cause of the epidemic.

The epidemic was apparently so severe it "led to almost a standstill in the sale of pork both in markets, eating stalls and restaurants", the report said.

[https://www.straitstimes.com/singapore/from-the-straits-times-archives-past-mass-hysteria-cases-in-singapore]

* * *

❖ **HEADLINE from the Canberra Times**

November, 2, 1967, Page 6 [http://nla.gov.au/nla.news-article10698133]

KORO 'NOT THREAT TO MANHOOD'

* * *

1968

[15]. A. L. Gwee: Koro—Its origin and nature as a disease entity. *Singapore Medical Journal, 1968, 9, 3–6.*

It is a discussion paper on Koro with rich information about Chinese cultural beliefs and traditional Chinese medical references on genital retraction pathology. It contains an elegant analysis of Koro, its definition, an orthography of the term Koro with a citation from ancient

Chinese medical texts (five sources—both in Chinese script and in English translation), and one acupuncture meridian diagram used for the treatment of genital retraction in Traditional Chinese Medicine (TCM). Appendix I–V described different Chinese medical texts from various dynasties that explained *Yin-Yang* concepts about sexual diseases, including the "retraction of penis."

A few crucial orthographic information is provided, e.g., previously referred to as shook yin, but it was changed to shook yang for the last hundred years. From the etiological point of view in TCM, the disease is related to the middle female meridian, governed by the liver, prone to anxiety, worry, and fear. This explains the acute anxiety reaction associated with the retraction symptom. He stated that social and cultural belief in shook yin or shook yang is still very prevalent among Singapore's Chinese population. He suggested that Koro is an acute panic reaction with the delusion of penile retraction (maybe hysterical delusion affected by cultural suggestion). He explained the Singapore Koro epidemic as "mass hysterical delusion with the panic reaction." He elaborated on how rumor, social belief, and suggestibility worked hand in hand to generate and spread the Koro epidemic among the susceptible population. Very interestingly, he mentioned how some social phenomena trigger the population's vulnerability. The examples are the role of estrogen hormone pellets injection to chicken and its relation with reported gynecomastia in some males. This news adds extreme fear and anxiety after the announcement of the swine-fever immunization of pigs. This is a precious paper in the context of the Singapore Koro epidemic.

[16]. M. Bourgeois: A Koro syndrome in a patient from Charenton: An ethno psychiatric transposition.
Annales Medico-Psychologiques, 1968, 1, 749–751. (Article in French)

This paper emphasizes the importance of intercultural psychiatric contributions to psychopathology. He described some symptoms (fear of castration and death, reactional hypochondria, focalized depersonalization, etc.) in a 37-year-old male. The symptomatology was related to the Koro or suk-yeong syndrome (penis retraction) native to the Far East.

[17]. C. T. Mun: Epidemic Koro in Singapore.
British Medical Journal, 1968, i, 640–641. (L)

It is the first brief report of the Singapore Koro epidemic in the British medical press. Mun provides a valuable description of the issue of psycho-social precipitant of the epidemic. The author also provided two case illustrations: a 16-year-old schoolboy and a 4-month-old male baby whose mother complained that the baby was suffering from penile retraction. Interesting to note that the author pointed out a significant physiological penile state for the onset of the Koro symptom: "The onset usually followed a normal physiological cause of retraction and shrinking of the organ -for example, after a bath, after passing urine, after illnesses, etc." He also mentioned that though the epidemic was mainly confined to Chinese subjects, other ethnic groups were also affected.

[18]. B. K. Garg: Koro in Britain.
British Medical Journal, 1968, June 15, 700. (L)

It is a case report of Koro in an 18-year-old Chinese male who presented at midnight at the hospital casualty in Durham, UK. He developed this acute feeling of penile retraction during the passing of urine. He had the same symptom after two weeks at midnight. The author stressed the importance of considering this symptom among the immigrant population in the UK.

1969

[19]. P. W. Ngui: The Koro epidemic in Singapore.
Australian & New Zealand Journal of Psychiatry, 1969, 3, 263–266.

It is a detailed report of the Koro epidemic of Singapore. In the first portion of the paper, the author discusses Koro illness's historical background with the traditional Chinese medical concept and the South-East Asian socio-cultural background.

The second part contains a detailed reporting of the Koro epidemic on 29 October 1967, just after the outbreak of swine fever in July 1967. A total of 536 cases (521 males and 15 females) were seen in OPDs

(Out-Patient Department) of the two General Hospitals, viz. Outram Road and Thomson Road Hospitals. Six patients were below the age of 6, with one only 7-month old. The apprehensive parents brought them to the clinic.

A detailed demographic and clinical analysis of 226 cases (220 males and six females) was provided as follows: Ethnicity—96% Chinese; 1.4% Malays; 1.8% Indians; and 0.4% Eurasians. Age—96.6% were between 11 and 40 years age group, a majority (48.6%) between 21 and 40 years; 30.5% between 16 and 20 years; and 15.5% between 11 and 15 years of age. Marital status—76.8% of males were single, and 5 out of 6 females were single. Education in the males, 54% had a primary level education, 39.5% secondary level, and 0.9% higher education. In the females, 2 were uneducated, 3 had primary, and one had secondary level education.

Symptomatology: 72.3% of males presented with the classical picture of Koro. The three most common symptoms were—fear in the form of acute anxiety in 90.5%, genital shrinkage in 74.5%, and genital retraction in 60.9% cases. Other complaints were: palpitation (41.4%), breathlessness (10.9%), collapse (9.5%); body pain (6.8%), visual blurring (6.8%); fainting (6.4%); vomiting or nausea (5.9%); paraesthesia (5%); genital pain (3.6%); and bodily spasm (2.7%). Five females had complaints of retraction of the nipples of the breast, and one female had a sensation of retraction and shrinkage of her vulva. In the males, 24.5% had past knowledge of Koro, and 76.4% believed that eating pork was related to the Koro attack. 43.6% of males attributed their Koro attack to pork, 4.6% to venereal disease, and 3.2% to sexual activity.

The precipitating factors noted were: 2 cases with sexual activities (one after masturbation, one following sexual intercourse), 25.9% had the attack during micturition, 1.2% after defecation; 17.3% after exposure to chill, cold weather, or air-conditioning, and in 15.9% cases the attack came on during or soon after the bath. In total, in about 61% of cases, their attacks were precipitated by activity or conditions focused on their genital organs.

In two cases of subnormality, both siblings were recorded. They showed the features of Laurence-Moon-Biedl syndrome. Attack frequencies showed that 81.4% of males had a single attack, 8.2% had two episodes, and 10.5% had more than two attacks.

Previous knowledge of Koro: Among the males—24.5% had past knowledge of Koro illness. Among all the cases, 76.4% had either direct or indirect knowledge of Koro concerning eating pork.

Treatment: 74.5% of respondents were admitted and treated with psychotherapy (as reassurance); 11.5% were treated with tablets; and 2.3% were given injections. However, the nature of medicine was not reported.

Prognosis: 81.4% had a solitary Koro attack, 8.2% had two episodes, and 10.5% had more than two attacks. Almost all cases recovered well. Only 7.7% complained that their sexual vigor was affected, and 18.6% reported an impact on their general well-being.

The author commented that Koro should be regarded as a culture-bound psychogenic illness because cultural beliefs play a significant role in its genesis. In favor of this contention, he cited the example of this Koro epidemic, which was initiated only after rumors that Koro could be caused by eating infected pork. A photograph of "li teng hok" or jeweler's instrument, grasping the retracting penis of a Koro patient, is an extra credit of the paper.

[20]. Koro Study Team (Chairman: A. L. Gwee): The Koro "epidemic" in Singapore.
Singapore Medical Journal, 1969, 10, 234–242.

The third survey report of the Singapore Koro epidemic has some detailed discussion on the epidemic pattern according to postal areas, ethnic distributions, and incidence frequencies of cases at hospital OPDs. The survey covered 235 patients (227 males and eight females) called by letters for the interview. The paper provides an excellent account of basic demography, ethnic profile, details of clinical presentations with two photographs of "li teng hok," the device (jeweler's instrument) that was used for clasping the retracting penis. The clinical material is almost the same as that of Ngui's (1969) report. Some important epidemiological features are:

1. Under-five cases: 6 male (projected fear of others)
2. Peak age was between 16 and 20 years for males and 11 and 15 years for females.
3. They tried to plot the incidence among the 28 postal zones of Singapore: Postal areas 3 and 13 had the highest incidences (5.1 and 5.7 per 10,000 populations, respectively).
4. The epidemic has an abrupt and steep rise and falls with a short incubation period.
5. The authors described the penile symptom as "delusion of genital shrinkage (74.5%)" and "delusion of penile retraction (60.9%)"—not elaborating any detail or further about their differences.

   The report mentioned some complications resulted from a remedial measure like manual (72%) or mechanical traction of the penis, but no detailed account was given.
6. The role of media was stressed in both its acceleration as well as in mitigation of the epidemic:

   > The present epidemic shows also how easily public fears can be caused by injudicious propaganda and statements, and how easily too they can be assuaged. The newspapers, television and radio would seem to be powerful tools in such circumstances. It also seems apparent that the best way to deal with a rumour –initiated condition is prompt and effective counter propaganda which can take effect practically instantaneously. (p. 240)

There is an excellent description of the preventive strategy developed to mitigate Koro's epidemic spread by the Singapore Medical Association's public announcement on 4.11.67 and by the Ministry of Health on 6.11.67 with sufficient media coverage. The message was "koro as a result of fear, and not a physical disease with fatalities, and it has no relation with pork from pigs inoculated with swine fever vaccine." Astonishingly then the incidences dropped significantly. The letters to general practitioners, study proforma, and letters to participants are included in appendix I–III.

Observation: One issue of controversy may arise from the descriptions and distribution of symptoms. They described three sets of cardinal manifestations of the Koro illness: firstly, a delusion of penile retraction and impending death; secondly, a panic syndrome with fear, feeling of collapse, palpitation, sweating, nausea, breathlessness, visual blurring, and bodily spasm, pain, or paraesthesia and thirdly, complications resulted from remedial measures. The question one may ask about the justification for the use of the term "delusion" and secondly the "impending death" is the ideational component of the physical nature of the illness. It is not delusion per se rather reactive anxiety to the perceived danger from the penile retraction. In conclusion, they said Koro is a panic syndrome linked with cultural indoctrination.

In the symptom distribution, it was reported as follows: fear (90.5%), delusional of genital shrinkage (74.5%), a delusion of penile retraction (60.9%), and palpitation (41.4%). No clarification was given regarding the difference between shrinkage and retraction and invited some conceptual confusion. By genital, whether they mean both penis and scrotum is not clear. No detail of female presentation is given.

[21]. P. M. Yap: The culture-bound reactive syndromes.
In, Mental Health Research in Asia and the Pacific. Eds. W. Gaudill and T. Y . Lin. East–West Center Press, Honolulu, 1969, pp. 33–53.

A chapter in a book contains the nosological proposition for the "culture-bound reactive syndromes," which was an attempt to balance between the German and Scandinavian scientific taxonomies for reactive psychoses to exotic terms (Jilek, 1982). Yap proposed that "reactive syndromes" often present with a mixture of psychotic and neurotic symptoms. He proposed that reactive syndromes can be divided into four main groups: primary fear reactions, hyperidic rage reactions, culturally imparted nosophobia, and trance dissociations. The author also provides the following schematic categorization for culture-bound syndromes, where Koro was included within the category of the emotional syndrome:

1. Paranoid Syndromes
2. Emotional Syndromes
    - Depersonalization states: Koro
    - Fear-induced depressive states: Susto
3. Syndromes of disordered consciousness:
    - Impaired consciousness: Latah reaction
    - Turbid states: malignant anxiety, amok, neginegi
    - Dissociated consciousness: certain types of possession syndrome, hsich-ping, windigo psychosis.

This article reflects the academic discourse and the author's relentless attempt to provide an acceptable (at least to the Western world) nosological berth for Koro and other culture-bound psychiatric entities.

[Note: This paper was presented at the Conference on mental health in Asia and the Pacific at the East–West Center, Honolulu, Hawaii, March 28–1 April 1966, which was abstracted in the *Transcultural Psychiatry*, 1966, 3, 101–103.]

1970

[22]. J. G. Edwards: The Koro pattern of depersonalization in an American Schizophrenic patient.
American Journal of Psychiatry, 1970, 126, 1171–1173.

The author distinguishes the "Koro pattern of depersonalization" from "Koro," the folk illness. The former is probably universal in its distribution and more common than generally supposed—an example in an American schizophrenic is described. He was born in Greece but brought up in the USA. He had traits of immaturity, obsession (perfectionism and compulsive checking), and had impotence. At age 18 years, he was preoccupied with the idea of his small size of the penis. His schizophrenic illness started at age 22 years with all the cardinal symptoms of psychosis. He said he wanted to forget his past and wished to be called "Nameless." When one ward staff called him by his real name, he suddenly experienced acute anxiety with a sensation of penile shrinkage, which lasted for about an hour. He had no prior knowledge of Koro or similar genital symptom. The author discussed this clinical episode in the light of "subjective ideas of genital change" or "Koro pattern of depersonalization." The interpretation of the sensation of penile shrinkage varies from culture to culture and era to era. In certain Eastern countries, folk belief allows for the occurrence of "Koro." In contrast, it may be seen as genital delusion or delusion-like or may be related to the medieval concept of witchcraft in Western societies.

References

Adriani, N., Kruijt, A. C. (1912). *De Bare'e - Sprekende Toradja's van Midden-Celebes*. Landsdrukkerij.

Blonk, J. C. (1895). Koro. *Geneeskunding Tijaschrift voor Nederlandsch-Indie, 35*, 562–563.

Edwards, J. W. (1984). Indigenous Koro: A genital retraction Syndrome of insular South East Asia: A critical review. *Culture, Medicine & Psychiatry, 8*, 1–24.

Edwards, J. W. (1986). *Preliminary draft of thesis: Genital retraction Syndrome in cross-cultural and biomedical perspective. A Preliminary view* (181 p.).

Gould, G. M., & Pyle, W. L. (1896). *Anomalies and curiosities of medicine*. W.B. Saunders.

Hess, J. P., & Nassi, G. (1977). Koro in a Yemenite and a Georgian Jewish immigrant. *Confinia Psychiatrica, 20*, 180–184.

Jilek, W. G. (1982). Culture—"Pathoplastic" or "Pathogenic"? A key question of comparative psychiatry. *Curare, 5*, 57–68.

Jilek, W. G. (1986). Epidemic of "Genital Shrinking" (Koro): Historical review and report of a recent outbreak in South China. *Curare, 9*, 269–282.

Jilek, W. G. (1995). Emil Kraepelin and comparative sociocultural psychiatry. *European Achieve of Psychiatry & Clinical Neuroscience, 245*, 231–238.

Kraepelin, E. (1904). Psychiatrisches aus Java. *Centralblad Fur Nervenheilkunde Und Psychiatrie, 27*, 468–469.

Kraepelin, E. (1921). *Manic Depressive Insanity and Paranoia* (R. M. Barclay, Trans. & G. M. Robertson, Ed., p. 92). E & S Livingstone.

Pols, H. (2006). The development of psychiatry in Indonesia: From colonial to modern times. *International Review of Psychiatry, 18*(4), 363–370.

van Bergen, L., Hesselink, L., & Verhave, J. P. (Eds.). (2017). *The medical journals of the Dutch Indies: A platform for medical research*. Indonesian Academy of Sciences.

van Palthe, P. M. W. (1935). Koro- Eine Merkwurdige Angsthysterie. *Internationale Zeitschrift fur Psychoanalyse, 21*, 249–257.

Vorstman, A. H. (1897). 'Koro' in de Westerafdeeling van Borneo. *Geneeskundig Tijdschrift Voor Nederlandsch-Indie, 37*, 499–505.

7

Western Publications: Part Two—From 1971 to 2000

Koro Literature: From 1971 to 1980

Preamble: A total of 20 publications of this decade are reviewed. There are some discussion papers: eight reports are on the Koro epidemic in Thailand and Indonesia; nine are reports of Koro cases. Among the new topics are the first reporting of two cases from non-Chinese or non-Southeast Asian countries—one from Canada and the other from the African continent (Nigeria). There is no officially published report of the 1974 Koro epidemic of Guangdong, China. It is mentioned by Jilek (1986). The description of a mini Koro epidemic in Palembang, Indonesia, in 1975 is personal communication to the author from Dr. Sofyan Moekti, MD, M.Sc., Head of Palembang Municipal Health Service and Lecturer, Department of Medical Faculty, Sriwijaya University, Sumatra, Indonesia.

In 1979 "Penis-Disappearing" epidemic in Lagos, Nigeria, has no separate published report. In his book "Comparative Psychiatry," Professor H. B. M. Murphy (1982) mentions this Koro-like phenomenon as personal communication (page 275) from Dr. Femi Morakinyo of Ilelfe,

A. N. Chowdhury, *Koro*,
https://doi.org/10.1007/978-3-030-87962-4_7

who described a minor outbreak of such cases in 1979 in Lagos, Nigeria. Afterward, this topic was elaborately discussed by Ilechukwu (1988) in the Transcultural Psychiatry Research Review. Because of Nigeria's increasing importance in the non-Chinese Koro world geography, the report regarding the perceptual deviation of penis-image by Anumonye and Adaranijo (1978) is included here. Ilechukwu reported a massive "penis-loss" epidemic of 1990 in Nigeria in the Transcultural Psychiatric Research Review in 1992.

1971

[1]. Editor, TPRR
Transcultural Psychiatric Research Review, 1971, 8, 32–34.

This is an abstracted Editorial report in "Research and Observations: Southeast Asia of TPRR." This report is based on two earlier published accounts of the 1967 Koro epidemic of Singapore by Gwee (1968) and Ngui (1969) and another paper on Koro by A. L. Gwee, presented at the World Federation of Mental Health Workshop—"Mental Trends in a Developing Society," held in Singapore in April 1970. The concept of the syndrome in traditional Chinese medicine as "transposition of the symptoms of Yin and Yan" was discussed by Gwee and Ngui, and some salient demographic and clinical data of the epidemic. The presence of anxiety in three-quarters of the patients interviewed was a significant clinical observation. Both the authors questioned Yap's proposition of Koro as a depersonalization syndrome. They asserted that in Koro, the traditional social concepts and individual psychic vulnerability were also significant contributors.

The Editor commented that although there was some difference between Koro in Makassarese (and other Indonesian people) and the Chinese syndrome of Shook Yang, the term "Koro" had earned wider acceptance, even in the designation of the Chinese shook Yang cases also, in the Western literature.

1972

[2]. Y. D. Lapierre: Koro in a French Canadian.
Canadian Psychiatric Association Journal, 1972, 17, 333–334.

This is the first Koro case report from Canada and Koro's first report in association with an organic illness. The author described a 55-year old French Canadian with organic depression (3 days after lobectomy operation for bronchial carcinoma). He had a history of solitary attacks of depression with auditory hallucinations in the past. For a few months before lobectomy, he also had impotence. After a few weeks of his Koro attack, he was diagnosed with a cerebral tumor in the left fronto-temporal region. Three days after his lobectomy operation:

> while having a bath he developed the definite impression that his penis twisted upon itself and curved back into his abdomen. As this made him very tense he pulled on it and this relieved his anxiety temporarily, though the impression recurred intermittently throughout his hospital stay. (p. 333)

Interesting to note the shifting of perception and anxiety in this case. The author stated that:

> When calm, he believed that these symptoms originated in his imagination. However, when the symptoms and his anxiety recurred he was convinced of the veracity of his impression of penile withdrawal and that if it were in fact to occur, he feared for his survival. (p. 333)

Subsequently, he developed some confusion and inappropriate behavior. Organic cerebral involvement was suspected and was confirmed by EEG—a tumor in the left fronto-temporal region. Radiation was given, and he died after five months. The author suggests that this is an example of psychogenic localized depersonalization due to post-operative stress, which generated distorted penile perception and, subsequently, the development of Koro syndrome. This case is an important and one of the earliest examples of Koro in association with organic illness.

1973

[3]. I. Marks, M. Lader: Anxiety states (anxiety neurosis): A review.
Journal of Nervous & Mental Diseases, 1973, 156, 3–18.

It is a review article on anxiety states. In the section on epidemics of acute anxiety, the authors discuss Koro (the 1967 Singapore epidemic) and designate it as reminiscent of other forms of acute anxiety with cultural specificity and showed the Western similarity in the feeling of homosexual and panic attack, which is seen in solitary episodes and not in epidemic form.

[4]. T. W. Dow, D. A. Silver: Drug-induced Koro syndrome.
Journal of the Florida Medical Association, 1973, 60, 32.

Koro's third case report is associated with drug abuse (amphetamine, methadone, cannabis, and L.S.D.) from Montreal, Canada. It describes a case of 20-year-old Canadian youth presented with complaints of vague aches, feelings of depersonalization, and panic over a feeling that his penis was shrinking. He took six amphetamine tablets (Benzedrine) and one methadone tablet 24 hours preceding the Koro attack. He had a 5-years history of intermittent L.S.D., cannabis, and amphetamine abuse. He responded well with a high dose of oral diazepam and remains symptom-free at two months' follow-up.

1974

1974: Koro Epidemic in Guangdong, China

[5]. F. Sirois: Epidemic Hysteria.
Acta Psychiatria Scandinavica, 1974, suppl. 252, 1–45.

It is an elegant masterpiece of a global review of 72 psychiatric epidemics of the last 98 years (1876–1972) with a historical survey of contagious pathology and different factors contributing to the epidemics. It lists three epidemics with genital symptomatology: two were of Koro epidemics—the 1908 China epidemic and the 1967 Singapore epidemic. The third was a "phantom epidemic of Gonorrhea" reported from the USA. It is a valuable document for those working on the mass psychogenic aspect of mental illnesses.

1975

1975: Koro Epidemic in Palembang, Indonesia

[6]. R. Arbitman: Koro in a Caucasian.
Modern Medicine of Canada, 1975, 30, 970–971.

It is a case report of a 44-year-old Caucasian, the second Koro report from Canada. Koro here was associated with depression, marked obsessive–compulsive traits, and a habit of heavy alcohol drinking. This is the first research where the author explores Koro patients' body perception using the human figure's drawing test, which revealed an incomplete sketch with no genitals. The author concludes that the patient had a poor self-image reflected in the deviation of body image, predominantly in the genital area.

1976

1976: Koro Epidemic in Thailand

[7]. A. Ede: Koro in an Anglo Saxon Canadian.
Canadian Psychiatry Association Journal, 1976, 21, 389–391.

It is the third Koro case report from Canada. It presents the case of a 21-year-old unmarried man, Canadian of Anglo-Saxon origin, of Newfoundland, who suffered from delusions of persecution and from the belief that his penis was shrinking into his abdomen. A year before his psychiatric hospitalization, he had an operation for a coccygeal cyst. He reported that he "never felt right" after this operation and felt that his penis was shrinking for the first time. Four days after his hospital admission, he had a panic-like experience and felt that his penis was shrinking into his abdomen (second attack). He responded favorably with intravenous diazepam injection. This patient's genital delusion is like the Koro syndrome seen in south China, Indonesia, and Malaya, except that (a) in those places, the patients were neurotic, whereas this patient was psychotic, and (b) the Southeast Asian patients believed they would die after full retraction of the penis. But this man had no such thoughts; instead, his worry was being "a man without a penis."

[8]. K. Keophanukrangsii: Shrinking sex organs.
Journal of Psychiatric Association of Thailand, 1976, 21, 477–488. [In Thai]

This is a report with case vignettes and epidemiological data of the 1976 Koro epidemic of Thailand.

[9]. J. W. Edwards: The concern for health in sexual matters in the "Old Society" and "New Society" in China.
The Journal of Sex Research, 1976, 12(2), 88–103.

This is a significant scholarly research paper focused on the Chinese concept of sexuality, sexual disease, sexual behavior (contraception, sex, health, coition and health, masturbation) in a comparative context of China's traditional and modern medical philosophy. Interesting to note that the author discussed at length the concept of *Chia Se* (sexual disease) and its relation (acute form) with *Su Yang* (Shrinking Penis disease) and suggested that "…Koro represent the atypical Chia Se- Su Yang syndrome" (p. 93).

The author gave a detailed description of *Chia Se-Su Yang* as follows:

> … the disease is caused by cold drafts on the body, during intercourse or by "taking cold things, especially melons and ice cream immediately after copulation" (Wong, 1918). Alternatively described as an acute fever (Wong, 1918) and Cold (Read, 1926), Chia Se is characterized by violent headache, back pains, distortion of vision, cold extremities, which contract and turn purplish black in color, retraction of the man's testicles or the woman's nipples, and general debility; weakness in the kidneys and lungs…. (p. 92)

The author further stated that:

> Though both sexes are susceptible to the ailment, occurrence in the male is more widely recognized, no doubt because in traditional Chinese belief the acute form of Chia Se, characterized by deterioration of the testicles and shrinking (retraction) of the penis, is a dreaded and lethal disease. In contemporary Chinese societies, the belief in the reality of this disease complex still persists. (p. 93)

It is a must-read paper for any Koro researcher to develop a practical insight into Chinese medical concepts about sexual diseases, including Koro. The author is a serious Koro researcher who minutely traced and unfolded many important historical details on *Su Yang*.

1977

[10]. W. Jilin, L. Jilek-Aall: Mass hysteria with Koro symptoms in Thailand.
Schweizer Archiv fur Neurologie, Neurochirurgie & Psychiatrie, 1977, 120(2), 257–259. [In German]

This is the report of the 1976 Koro epidemic of north-eastern Thailand. Within a few days, at least 200 patients, most of them Thai and 66% of males were treated at local hospitals. The symptom patterns are pretty impressive: the main presenting symptoms included acute anxiety, subjective feeling of shrinking of the penis and impotence in men, shrinking and/or itching of the external genitals, and frigidity in women; further complaints included nausea, dizziness, abdominal pains, headaches, and facial numbness. All patients recovered after a brief symptomatic intervention. The news media also expressed the popular paranoid opinion that the epidemic was caused by Vietnamese people who poisoned food and tobacco to destroy the sexual vitality and general health of the Thai people. This ideology has a unique appeal in the context of a specific sociocultural and politico-historical Southeast Asia situation. It is suggested that an adequate interpretation of Koro and analogous hysterical symptom formation would have to consider in the local context. Koro is regarded as a pathogenic anxiety syndrome interfering with genital body image and sexual functioning.

[11]. W. Jilek, L. Jilek-Aall: A Koro epidemic in Thailand.
Transcultural Psychiatric Research Review, 1977, 14, 57–59.

Report of the 1976 Koro epidemic of Thailand, published in the "Southeast Asia" section of TPRR. It contains the epidemic report collected from different Thai news dailies like *Thai Rath; Dao Siam; Daily News; Bangkok World; Bangkok Post, and Nation Review*. The following are the few vital epidemic data that were reported in the newspapers.

1. The north-western border areas of Udon Thani, Sakhon Nakhon, Nong Khai, and Maha Sarakham were mainly affected.
2. Reported admission data: 171 persons in Nong Khai and Maha Sarkaham; in Nong Khai—20–30 new cases every day; in Maha Sarakham, 37 male and 22 female in one day.
3. One Buddhist monk was also affected.
4. Main presenting symptoms: shrinking of the penis and sexual impotence in men; shrinkage and /or itching of the external genitals; and frigidity in women.
5. Fear of imminent death was present in all cases; some lost consciousness.
6. The widespread belief among the local Thai population was that: Vietnamese shopkeepers and restaurant owners had mixed some poisonous powder into noodles, rice, flour, meatballs, salted pork, iced coffee, soft drinks, and tobacco.

7. Despite the Government's announcement of no such foul play, some media reporting strengthened this community's popular paranoid belief.

The authors ask many people on the streets of Bangkok and Chieng Mai. They responded positively with this alleged conspiracy plot by Vietnamese immigrants, aiming to destroy the sexual vitality and general health of the Thai population. The authors stressed the importance of local socio-political and historical factors in developing the Thai Koro epidemic rather than the psychodynamic theories.

[12]. J. P. Hes, G. Nassi: Koro in a Yemenite and a Georgian Jewish immigrant.
Confinia Psychiatrica, 1977, 20, 180–184.

Koro, observed among inhabitants of Southeast Asia, seems to be extremely rare outside that geographical region. This Koro case report is the first one from Israel. It describes two Koro cases—a 29-year-old Yemenite Jewish immigrant and a 44-year-old Georgian Jewish immigrant. Critical clinical findings noted are: association of obsessive–compulsive thoughts and sexual conflicts with masturbatory guilt, an association of agitated depression (second case), and role of strict Jewish social sexual norms and customs in the genesis of Koro symptom. Two important references cited in this paper need special mention: (1) an earlier (1883) record of a penile-shrinking sign with hypochondriasis, and (2) the statue of Pietro Barbino by Valerio Cicolide Settignano (1560) in Florence, France, concerning the archetype of turtlehead symbolism and penis.

1978

[13]. S. Moekti, S. K. Denin: A non-rational dissemination of castration anxiety in Palembang, 1975.
Paper presented at the First Asian Teaching Workshop on Mental Health and Culture, Jakarta, July, 1978.

It is a report of a mini Koro epidemic of Bangka island situated north-east of Palembang, Sumatra. It involved 13 persons (11 males and two females). Eight cases, including the females, were of Chinese ethnicity. Nine patients were in the 10–14 year age group. Consumption of sea fish was attributed as the cause of the illness, owing to which sale of that particular fish temporarily declined in the market badly.

The main symptoms were a feeling of retraction of the penis or scrotum into the abdomen in males (100%) and the feeling of breast "withdrawal" into the thoracic cavity and chest pain in females (100%). Other symptoms include paraesthesia of the anogenital region (53.3%), abdominal pain (27.2%), cold sweat (25%), and fever (15.4%). The duration of the sickness varied from less than one hour to more than five hours. Affected persons showed a treatment preference of *Shinshe* (Chinese traditional healer)—3 cases to *Dukun* (Indigenous witch doctor)—2 patients and self-treatment with "ginger drink"—6 cases. No treatment was sought by two. The epidemic was checked by rapid information dissipation and community assurance through T.V., radio, and press conferences about the illness's nonrationality. The authors suggested this Koro epidemic to be due to the nonrational dissemination of castration anxiety.

[14]. K. Barrett: Koro in a Londoner.
Lancet, 1978, ii, 1319.

This is the second Koro case report from Britain. An unusual presentation of penile shrinkage is reported in a 33-year-old British engineer. One early morning at 3 a.m., he experienced a feeling of impending doom with the shrinking of the penis. He rapidly developed palpitation, sweating, nausea, and other panic attack symptoms for 20 min. He responded favorably with diazepam but over the following year, beginning at the same time of the day, he experienced 12–15 similar attacks, albeit decreasing intensity and duration. He subsequently married and had no more such complaints except some mild, non-specific anxiety attacks.

[15]. A. Anumonye, H. Adaranijo: Chronic non-specific urethritis as psychological reaction among Nigerian neurotic patients.
Nigerian Medical Journal, 1978, 8, 3–5.

It is an exciting paper where 54 male referred cases were seen at the Psychiatry OPD of Lagos University Teaching Hospital from 1971 to 1975, who had primary complaints relating to genitalia and were diagnosed with chronic non-specific urethritis. Four cases had symptoms of the shrinking penis—2 University students (the penis is getting smaller) and two clerks (with a venereal disease). The authors reported this as an example of a very uncommon presentation in Nigerian culture and compared these with South-Asian Koro symptoms. One important finding is the symptom of crawling, pinching, burning, and irritation at the penis' tip. The authors described the crawling sensation in the urethra, genitalia, or even the whole body, which is also a feature of depressive illness in Nigerian culture. They provided a diagnostic grouping of the cases: anxiety reaction (11 patients), depressive symptom (23 patients), psychophysiological/ somatization reaction (14 patients), and hysterical conversion (6 cases).

[16]. S. Suwanlert: Thai cultural concepts related to Koro syndrome.
Journal of Psychiatric Association of Thailand, 1978, 23(3), 261–275.

It is a very concise analysis of cultural beliefs and practices in Thai society about the etiology of Koro epidemic of 1976. The author suggested some probable conceptual framework in the background of Koro illness in North-East Thailand. He traced the penis-image concept from Chinese culture, as many Thai people have a history of Chinese ancestry. In the North-East region, there were significant Hindu Brahmin groups who worship phallic symbols. Many local men wear amulets, which are short of penis image around their waist to provide protection and potency powers for their sexual organs. There are many native shrines of Mother Spirit (*Chow mae*) in the villages where people observe phallic worship with offerings and vows. The author believed that these imageries and the importance of penis images in the community facilitated Koro in these communities. It is interesting to note that he cited one ubiquitous daily conversational gesture among men: "Oh, you must be so afraid that it makes your penis shrunk."

He mentioned some sociocultural events that influenced sexual identity in Thai society. This is the modern contribution of free sex, the availability of great sexual outlets, and the liberalization of sexual morality through large numbers of prostitutes, night's clubs, pornographic materials, paid wives, and sexual tourism. The third issue he proposed is the folk healers' judgment of penis shrinkage and death, strengthening and reinforcing the already existing cultural fear from penile shrinkage. Lastly, he explained the rumor's role that triggered the sexual panic of loss of penis and masculine power from Koro. It may be recalled that there were rumors in circulation (from political refugees from Laos) in the 1976 Koro epidemic. It was believed that chemical adulteration of food, concomitant loss of potency among males, and increased sexual appetite among females reinforced the unconscious mass fear of death, sexual power loss, and Koro symptom formation. It is an essential paper with ethnographic quality and highlighted the Thai social-cultural background of the 1976 Koro epidemic.

1979

1979: Koro–like Epidemic in Lagos, Nigeria*

*H. B. M. Murphy (1982), in Comparative Psychiatry, page 275, mentioned this Koro-like phenomenon. Dr. Femi Morakinyo of Ile-Ife had described a minor outbreak of such cases in 1979 in Lagos, Nigeria.

[17]. O. I. Ifabumuyi, G. G. C. Rwegellera: Koro in a Nigerian male patient: A case report.
African Journal of Psychiatry, 1979, 5, 103–105.

It is the first Koro case reported from Africa. It describes Koro in a 36-year-old Nigerian married man having four children. A psychiatric referral was done for his recurrent acute anxiety with multiple hypochondriacal concerns. The onset history, a year before, is very interesting:

> ...feeling of pain in both shoulders and the waist and heat at the centre of the head. This was followed usually by extreme fear and panic reaction during which the patient feared desperately that his penis was shrinking into his abdomen. At the height of his anxiety he would run into the bush only to be pursued and brought back by relatives and friends.
> Prior to his referral, he had consulted several indigenous healers, who prescribed various herbs which he had to apply to his penis. It was at the height of the second attack that the patient was referred for psychiatric treatment. (p. 104)

Sexual invalidism and losing his wife was a significant concern. The frequency of sexual intercourse has diminished. Interesting to note the complaint of heat on the head as a symptom. The authors suggest that the lack of psychiatric facilities and the stigma attached to mental disorders are more responsible for Koro symptom formation. Koro here is associated with a secondary diagnosis of recurrent anxiety with multiple hypochondriacal symptoms. As this presentation of Koro occurred in a far-off non-Chinese culture, the authors question the validity of Koro's concept of culture-boundness.

[18]. S. Suwanlert, D. Coates: Epidemic Koro in Thailand—Clinical and Social aspects.
Transcultural Psychiatric Research Review, 1979, 16, 64–66.

It is the report of a week-long field investigation of the 1976 (November) Koro epidemic of Thailand by an official team, of which both the authors were members. The report contains the findings of an interview of 350 Koro patients (338 males and 12 females). A total affectivity number of 2000 is reported.

The 350 cases' demographic data showed the following features: Sex: 96.6% males and 3.5% females. Age range: 6 to 72 years, with most patients between 11 to 20 years. Marital status: 60% single, Education: 62% had attended school for at least four years, Occupation: 40% farmers; 20% students; 16% government employees and business people;

10% porters and traders; 8% Buddhist monk and 6% others. Ethnicity: although the Chinese comprise 10% of the population at risk, not a single Chinese case is reported.

The clinical picture included three phases: (1) Prodromal Phase—characterized by somatic symptoms like vertigo, genital pain or numbness, diarrhea, which occurred after eating the suspected food or smoking the suspected cigarettes. (2) The penile shrinking phase lasted for about 20 minutes. It was marked by a sensation either of penile shrinkage, genital numbness, nipple pain, or discomfort on urination, accompanied by panic. Symptoms in women included complaints of vaginal dilatation. (3) Recovery phase—where the fears of continuing impotence, genital shrinkage, and possible sequel in the form of mental illness were marked.

Of the patients, 95% sought treatment either from folk healers (70%) or from local hospitals (25%). In so far as the cause attributed to the illness is concerned, 94% were convinced that they were poisoned—70% of them felt it was through foods which were processed principally by the local Vietnamese while 24% thought it had occurred through cigarettes.

The authors discuss the salient features of the social responses to the epidemic. They noted that there was no evidence of poison or infection found in elaborate chemical and bacteriological tests of a wide range of foodstuffs. The "indecisive" official reactions only intensified people's fear and prolonged the epidemic. Deleterious repercussions of the outbreak on the fruit industry and other commercial enterprises, affecting the local Vietnamese initially and Thai farmers later, are noted. The social after-effect of the epidemic, which resulted in the ostracism of the Vietnamese, is discussed. Fear of social stability was the critical cause of the epidemic, the authors conclude.

[19]. P. J. Constable: Koro in Hertfordshire.
Lancet, 1979, i, 163.

It is the third Koro case report from Britain. It describes Koro's case in a 50-year-old Briton, who developed acute anxiety one night at about 2.30 a.m. because of his feeling that his "penis was vanishing into the abdomen," a conviction that was also shared by his wife who summoned the doctor that night. He had no previous psychiatric illness except some emotional turmoil and anxiety emanating from his current life situation.

1980

[20]. M. EL. Fakharani: Koro-Ein Syndrom im Kulturwandel? Beobachtungen aufder ost-indonesischen Insel Flores.
Curare, 1980, 3, 241–244. [In German]

It is a Koro report among the Ngada aboriginal tribe from the Flores island of Indonesia's central highlands. Koro is known as "mbaze." A rapid local socio-cultural change has been attributed as a stress factor.

Koro Literature: From 1981 to 1990

Preamble: A total of 59 Koro and related publications of this decade is reviewed, among which some are case reports, some are Koro epidemic reporting, and a few are discussion papers. The case reports are from various parts of the globe and different ethnicities, viz. British; Canadian; Italian, Chinese; American; Tanzanian; emigrant Chinese in Singapore; Jewish; West-Indian and Greek-Cypriot immigrants to Britain; Haitian; Ethiopian; Israeli; Zulu immigrant; Spanish; Homing refugee in the USA; French; Sinhalese (Sri Lanka); Maltese; and Indian. The Koro epidemic reporting was of the 1982 Thailand epidemic, the Guangdong epidemic of China, and a Koro-like epidemic in Nigeria.

This decade's four publications are important landmarks in cultural psychiatry, especially the culture-bound syndromes, including Koro. The first one is the valuable book on the intercultural distribution of mental illness with transcultural comparative perspectives by Professor H. B. M. Murphy (1982). The second is another book, exclusively devoted to studying culture-bound syndromes with anthropological and social analysis by Ronald C. Simons and Charles C. Hughes (eds.) (1985). Both the monographs are examples of scholarly masterwork in cultural psychiatry and are of immense value to all students of transcultural psychiatry.

The other two publications are on Koro itself. The first one is a chapter on Koro by Robert T. Rubin (1982) in a book. The second is the paper by Bernstein and Gaw (1990), arguing in favor of a distinct nosological status of Koro for DSM-IV. This article highlights the phenomenon of Koro as a specific psychiatric diagnosis and invited more professional responses. Sirois's publication on epidemic hysteria is included to complement the epidemic understanding of Koro illness, and the paper on Shen-K'uei Syndrome is reviewed to understand the traditional Chinese medical concept about sexuality.

1981

[1]. A. Cremona: Another case of Koro in a Briton.
British Journal of Psychiatry, 1981, 138, 180–181. (L)

It is the fourth case of Koro reported in an Englishman. A patient is a young man of 24 who had a history of nocturnal enuresis up to age 8, cross-dressing in his sister's clothes, and masturbation at age 12. At age 14, he developed irrational fear, obsessive–compulsive symptoms, hypochondriacal concerns, labile mood, outbursts of violence, heavy drinking, and recurrence of nocturnal enuresis.

At age 18, an unsuccessful attempt at sexual intercourse further increased his health-related anxieties, particularly his penis's health. At age 21, he was admitted to a psychiatric hospital with severe anxiety and obsessional thoughts and rituals. One afternoon, he suddenly felt that his penis was shrinking "about half an inch in length" after discharge from the hospital. The terrifying fear of penile disappearance and eventual death made him too panicky and agitated. Since then, he continued having a "shrinking" sensation all the time, with a few acute episodes occurring every day. Later he began hearing a single threatening male voice and developed depression. He was hospitalized again. Treatment with several drugs failed to improve his overall mental state, and two years later, his Koro-like symptoms remained as distressing as ever.

[2]. S. S. A. Waldenberg: Koro.
Canadian Journal of Psychiatry, 1981, 26, 140–141. (L)

It is a case report of Koro from Canada. A 38-year-old Canadian of British origin developed penile and testicular shrinkage complaints after consuming Ludiomil tablet (100 mg) each for eight preceding nights to treat his depression. Discontinuation of the antidepressant medicine relieved his symptoms spontaneously. This is one of the rare reports of Koro symptoms in association with antidepressant medication.

[3]. J. K. Wen, C. L. Wang: Shen-K'uei Syndrome: A culture-specific sexual neurosis in Taiwan.
In, Normal and Abnormal behavior in Chinese culture. Culture, Illness and Healing (Studies in Comparative Cross-cultural Research). Eds. A Kleinman and T Y Lin. Springer: Dordrecht, 1981, Vol. 2, pp. 357–369.

This book chapter describes the medico-cultural traditional Chinese concept of "vital or kidney deficiency" or Shen-k'uei with typical culture-bound illness behaviors. In classical Chinese medicine *Shen* (Kidney) is the reservoir of vital essence in semen (*ching*), and k'uei denotes deficiency. The authors described this medico-cultural concept in three culture-related illness behaviors as follows:

> For example, Rin (1966) described two rare forms of this syndrome among Chinese male patients in Taiwan: *Koro* and *frigophobia*. Both are recognized as culture-bound psychiatric syndromes among Chinese. In the one fear that the penis is shrinking and that its retraction into the abdomen will lead to death and in the other fear of cold owing to loss of seminal essence, which is believed to reduce the body's *ch'i* (vital essence) and through it the male component (*yang*) which produces an imbalance between hot/ cold bodily constituents, relate to traditional Chinese cultural beliefs and rules concerning male genital sexuality. Although both conditions can be explained in terms of contemporary psychiatric concepts, their symptomatology and illness behavior are meaningful only in the context of Chinese culture. A third form of the *shen-k'uei* syndrome is a psychological condition popularly associated with excessive semen loss owing to frequent intercourse, masturbation, nocturnal emission or

> passing of "white turbid urine," which is believed to contain semen. (p. 357)

Interesting to note that the third condition is similar to an Indian culture-bound syndrome called "Dhat Syndrome." The discussion in this chapter is beneficial for understanding Koro's cultural psychodynamics among the ethnic Chinese subjects.

1982

1982 Koro Epidemic in Thailand

1982 Koro Epidemic in North-East India

[4]. W. G. Jilek: Culture—"Pathoplastic" or "Pathogenic"? A key question of Comparative Psychiatry.
Curare, 1982, 5, 57–68.

It is an elegant analysis of comparative psychiatry aspects, including culture-bound syndromes with historical notes and references. It provides a detailed discussion of mental illness's cultural influence, either pathoplastic or pathogenic, with brief examples of psychiatric clinical entities from various cultures. Different dimensions of cultural changes and the consequent impact on mental health have been analyzed with models from multiple such transitional societies.

Koro is discussed concerning the hysterical quality of culture-bound syndromes with critical analysis of Yap's 1969 Classification Schemes of culture-bound syndromes. It also contains a detailed report of the 1976 Thailand Koro epidemic with a discourse on local socio-cultural and politico-economic perspectives. Koro epidemic was regarded as "a paradigm of collective sociocultural pathogenesis." The author cautioned that the ritualized possession and trance states and religious rituals must be separated from the psychopathological arena "to avoid Eurocentric and positivistic fallacies in psychiatric diagnosis."

[5]. J. A. Harrington: Epidemic Psychosis.

British Journal of Psychiatry, 1982, 141, 98–99. (L)

It is a short report of three distinct mass psychogenic outbreaks occurring in the countryside of Thailand.

The first was an epidemic of "Rok Joo" or genital shrinkage disease (Koro), which affected at least 50 tapioca plantation workers in Nakhon Ratchasima Province. The workers believed that the illness began only after they ate canned sardines from their employer. Some male workers attributed the cause to "Krungthong 85" cigarettes. The disease also spread to other areas like Sarakham village of Sakon Nakhon Province, where people believed that genital shrinkage illness was due to noodles and "Pla Too" (mackerel). A provincial member of parliament (MP) also shared the same belief ("I am fascinated, it did shrink") as that of the terrified people there.

The second account is of a somewhat different type of mass psychogenic illness, reported from Saraburi Province, where almost 100 people in two villages were suffering from a supposed rabies infection after eating a pig that a stray dog bit. The affected men, women, and children became naked and were lying around in their houses and "going wild like mad dogs." There was a local rumor that a pig raiser had sold a pig a few days ago, and it was their firm conviction that a rabies-infected dog had bitten the pig.

The third report is of a state of mass fear from a giant snake that had eaten many cows and chickens before the disease outbreak in Wat Praputtabart of Lop Buri Province. The snake, whose body was said to be as long as a large coconut tree, lived in a cave near the temple. An abbot gave the verdict that the snake was the "guardian of a spirit."

A brief discussion into the Thai traditional belief in spirit or "phi" is undertaken, revealing that *"phi"* may possess people either temporarily or permanently and alter behavior, set people dancing, talk in riddles, or even change their sex. The author suggested that mass psychogenic reactions are an example of epidemic psychosis originating from fear out of false rumor or misinterpretation of events. All these lead to a group or collective panic state.

[6]. R. T. Rubin: Koro (Shook Yang): A culture-bound psychogenic syndrome.
In, Extraordinary Disorders of Human Behaviour. Eds, C. T. H. Friedman & R. A. Faguet. Plenum Press: New York, pp. 155–172, 1982.

This is an excellent and compact review essay on Koro with definitions and historical perspectives, including its genesis, terminology, and Chinese traditional beliefs and practices. It provides three pictures of penile clamps used in penile traction of the penis in Koro cases, one from van Wulfften Palthe's 1934 report and the other two from Gwee's 1969 account of the Singapore Koro epidemic. It draws a comparative analysis between oriental Koro case reports and Koro or Koro-like cases in westerners (with abstracts of six published case reports). It also contains a short review of psychodynamic theories, diagnostic points, and treatment of Koro as evinced in Koro literature. The author suggests that Koro is a "coherent collection of symptoms stemming from diverse etiologies."

[7]. J. B. Cai: Five case reports of Suo-yang zen (Koro).
Chinese Journal of Nervous and Mental Diseases, 1982, 8(4), 206–208. [In Chinese]

It is a report of 5 Koro cases collected by the author over four years in Guangdong, China. All five cases are male—2 single and 3 married, aged between 20 and 30 years. All the married cases gave the cause of their disorder as intercourse with a menstruating woman, and the single case pointed to genital injury. All the cases had a traditional belief about Suo-yang's deadliness. The author described the clinical presentation in each case as follows:

1. Main symptom: mental anguish concerning retraction of the penis
2. In 3 cases, the penis was insensitive
3. In 3 cases, cold air went into the abdomen

4. In 4 cases, abdominal pain
5. 1 case each—sweating, uncontrolled spasms of limbs, hypersensitivity, and dulled awareness

Treatment: Psychological counseling and acupuncture or medicine (glucose acetate and tranquilizers). All cured within 2–7 days.

[8]. S. Rosenthal, P. A. Rosenthal: Koro in an adolescent: Hypochondriasis as a stress response.
Adolescent Psychiatry, 1982, 10, 523–531.

It is a case report of Koro in a 13-year-old male from the USA, who had acute anxiety associated with a feeling of penile shrinkage and eventual death. He was treated successfully with individual and family therapy, and a one-year follow-up evidenced their disappearance. The authors believe that this case illustrates an example of pathological interaction between social beliefs, sexual myths, and family-induced stressors on the one hand and the boy's critical developmental stage on the other. The authors proposed that this Koro-pattern response of the case demonstrates the larval form (an immature mechanism) of hypochondriasis, not depersonalization. They state:

> This adolescent demonstrates many of the elements implicated in current theoretical formulations of the psychodynamics of hypochondriasis. This symptom can be used to deal with anger, unmet dependency needs, and guilt over aggressive and sexual impulses, and to protect against low self-esteem by substituting an image of self as ill or physically defective in place of one as a worthless person.
> … the massive family-induced stressors of rejection, verbal and physical attack, and the absence of maternal support produced surging emotions of fear, anger, and depressive affect. The physiological penile sensations produced by fear (and possibly other dysphoric emotions) triggered the patient's conviction of penile shrinkage, abetted by castration anxiety from the overt violence in the household and his unconscious anticipation of retaliation by the stepfather for this aggressive fantasies. (p. 529)

[9]. H. B. M. Murphy: Neurosis and other minor disorders.
In, Comparative Psychiatry: The International and Intercultural Distribution of Mental Illness. Springer-Verlag, Heidelberg, 1982, pp. 269–277.

It is one of the treatises in cultural psychiatry and contains some valuable findings of cross-cultural variation of various aspects of mental illnesses across the globe.

In Chapter 10, under the heading of "Neurosis and other Minor Disorder," an elegant analysis of Koro and other sexual neurosis is presented. The author discusses the applicability of the Oedipus complex theory, viz. the castration fear in different societies like Makassarese, Chinese and African, which he thinks is an essential contributor to the mass psychogenic reaction in these societies. He interprets the sexual neurosis concerning "Jiryan" and "dhat" in India in the background of the mythical context (Shivaism) of phallic symbolism and castration anxiety. However, according to him, the Koro epidemics in Singapore (1967) and Thailand (1976) were expressions of social stress that challenged ethnic solidarity. He cites the examples of the existing stormy socio-political situation in these countries and the mounting ethnic tension displaced on to castration because the "loss of the means of making a livelihood are more serious matters in Asia millions die of famine than loss of genitals."

[10]. F. Sirois: Perspectives of Epidemic Hysteria.
In, Mass Psychogenic Illness, A Social Psychological Analysis, Eds. M. J. Colligan; J. W. Pennebaker & L. R. Murphy. Lawrence Erlbaum Associates Publisher, Hillsdale, New Jersey, 1982, pp. 217–236.

Koro is discussed under the epidemic typologies as an example of a "large diffuse outbreak." It is a valuable analysis of 88 psychiatric outbreaks focusing on epidemiological variables of outbreaks that occurred in occupational settings. A three-fold stage of psychiatric outbreaks is given: the prodroma, the epidemic moment, and the rebound phenomena. The author opines that the extent of any epidemic is dependent on psychodynamic psychology-related group factors. The most critical social contributors of socially shared psychopathology identified are: religious intolerance, political unrest, economic insecurity, cultural clashes, changing social orders, natural disasters or devastating diseases, and poorly educated, superstition-prone impoverished classes.

[11]. M. P. I. Weller, N. Ameen: Elvis Presley, Reactive hypomania and Koro.
American Journal of Psychiatry, 1982, 139(7), 970. (L)

It is a case report of a Koro-like state at the background of a depressive episode in a 16-year-old Greek Cypriot immigrant in the UK, and it coincided with the death anniversary of Elvis Presley. He had a depressed mood, elective mutism, abdominal pain, and believed that his penis was shrinking inside the abdomen. He responded well with amitryptiline 75 mg daily treatment. Three years later, again, on the death anniversary of Elvis Presley, he developed hypomanic episodes. The patient stated that Elvis is his "hero" and is a big fan of Elvis. He also said that he was Elvis Presley. The author suggested this case from a Western country is an example of Koro in the context of a depressive illness rather than culture-bound, as was initially proposed by Yap.

1983

[12]. M. S. Keshavan: Epidemic Psychosis or Epidemic Koro?
British Journal of Psychiatry, 1983, 142, 100–101. (L)

It is a comment on Harrington's (1982) letter in the British Journal of Psychiatry. The author designated the "Rok Joo" epidemic as Koro and asserted that it was a body image disturbance. Keshavan cites examples of his work with 40 neurotic patients whose complaints were related to the loss of semen, 50% of whom viewed the loss as a threat to their masculine vitality. The role of suggestible personality with heightened self-scrutiny and over-concern about genitalia may lead to the genital shrinkage symptom.

[13]. Suwanlert. S: The second Koro epidemic in North East Thailand.
Poster presentation at the 7th World Congress of Psychiatry, 1983, Vienna, July 11–16.

It is a brief report of the 1982 Koro epidemic (second epidemic) in Thailand.

1984

1984 Koro Epidemic in Guangdong, China

[14]. W. M. Lucieer: The bitter taste of liberty: A study in ethnopsychiatry.
Psychypathologic Africaine, 1984–85, 20, 17–40.

It is a colorful account of a case study from Dares-Salaam, the capital of Tanzania, Africa. It is an excellent account to show how urban socio-political changes impact the young psyche and facilitate cultural beliefs and practices. The author provides a vivid history of how a young man of 25 years met an unknown girl with whom he had several enjoyable intercourses and who stayed together. He did not know the girl's whereabouts; neither was he certain how the girl could dress so brightly and use such expensive perfumes. Then in the third week of the relationship, doubt crept into his mind. He wondered whether she was a real human or *"Djinni"* (a fairy who is "intelligent, imperceptible, and capable of appearing in different forms"). The following intercourse, when she started to clean his penis, developed an intensely cold feeling in the genital area, lower abdomen, and his penis and scrotum shriveled. "He became very afraid, had heart palpitations, and started sweating and trembling. In a panic, he chased the girl away and ran into his brother's room. His brother, after hearing the story, developed the same symptoms." The index case developed a state of depression. "sometimes bordering on stupor and during which he felt himself to be dead and with genitals that were slowly disappearing. He saw and heard people preparing his burial and digging his grave."

He had two further attacks of panic state with other somatic distress. The first attack was after an accidental meeting and a short conversation with this girl, after which he was admitted to a hospital. After his discharge, he was having steady sexual relations with two girls. However, when he met and had intercourse with a third girl, the second attack precipitated. "After intercourse, he saw her becoming bigger and bigger while he felt became very small. He then realized that she was the same female djinni in a different human configuration." The author very nicely discusses this Koro-like symptom in the background of the cultural belief about djinni. He stated: "Although life with her may be deliriously existing, one word or act which displeases her may bring her revenge, she may kill you or send rats that will eat your penis at night." The position of women and attitudes toward them in Tanzanian society has been nicely portrayed by refereeing to popular local verses. The reactivation of traditional folk beliefs in spirits and djinni in the face of rapid cultural transition has been implicated in the background of this symptom formation.

[15]. G. E. Berrios, S. J. Morley: Koro-like symptom in a non-Chinese subject.
British Journal of Psychiatry, 1984, 145, 331–334.

This is the fifth case report of Koro in an Englishmen. It is a very unusual case of Koro-like symptoms. The subject had "a 20-year old belief that his penis recurrently shrank and disappeared into the abdomen." He also had a secondary psychiatric diagnosis of agoraphobia with panic attacks (DSM III-300.22) and social phobias (DSM III-300.23). The origin of penile concern started in childhood when his penis was pulled in a game by his peers. On one occasion, two years before the referral, he was unable to find his penis while attempting to urinate and wet his trousers. He responded well with treatment with phenelzine (30 mg bd) and behavioral psychotherapy for one year.

This paper's real credit is its detailed analysis of 15 non-Chinese Koro cases from diverse geographical areas like Britain, France, South Africa,

Canada, Greece, Israel, Nigeria, and India. Interestingly, all these fifteen cases suffered from primary psychiatric illnesses of which were common: affective disorder-anxiety and depression, and non-affective psychosis-schizophrenia. Analyzing the premorbid psychosexual complaints, the authors suggest that Koro is the expression of a form of sexual pathology. They also hypothesize that Koro-like symptoms in non-Chinese subjects may constitute behavioral phenotypes without any underlying cultural link. This phenotype includes over-valued ideas, often to the delusional extent, related to concurrent psychiatric illnesses. They also provided the treatments in each case and found it interesting to note that the Koro attack was associated with 'fear of death' only in two cases.

[**Note**: This paper was discussed and abstracted by H. B. M. Murphy in Transcultural Psychiatric Research Review, 1986, 23: 159–161. Concerning the penis loss ideation, Dr. Murphy mentioned shame-dominated and guilt-dominated cultures in Chinese and English culture.]

[16]. P. C. Ang, M. P. Weller: Koro and psychosis.
British Journal of Psychiatry, 1984, 145, 335.

This is a report of two Koro cases, one a West-Indian and the other a Greek Cypriot immigrant, in association with psychiatric illnesses. There was a conviction of penile retraction into the abdomen with fear of turning female at the background of schizophrenia in the first. In the second, there was a depression of MDP. The authors suggest Koro here could be considered "hyperacute anxiety coupled with a delusional belief occurring in a psychotic setting."

[17]. J. W. Edwards: Indigenous Koro, A genital retraction syndrome of insular Southeast Asia. A critical review.
Culture, Medicine & Psychiatry, 1984, 8, 1–24.

This paper is the most masterly review on Koro after Yap's 1965 paper in the world Koro literature. It contains the detailed emic construct of Koro with descriptions of early case reports by Dutch physicians.

It cites Raven's (1886) article first in the context of Koro. An orthography of Koro with a geographical note of Celebes has been attempted. It stresses the importance of biomedical factors in the precipitation of genital retraction symptoms. He suggests a tripartite concept in "genital retraction," a term he preferred in place of Koro: (1) valid physiological retraction; (2) panic fear of genital retraction in response to a real or imagined environmental insult; and (3) chronic somatization where the patient exhibits culturally patterned illness.

The author cites a personal communication of one Koro case report from unpublished field research of a medical anthropologist Kenneth Payne, who, between 1974 and 1976, studied the ethnomedical beliefs and practices of the Tagabawa Bagobo people in south-central Mindanao of the Philippines. The Bagobo believe in a shrinking penis disease called *lannuk e laso* (laso = penis; lannuk = to go inside), caused by sorcery and tainted food, used to make one's opponents weak. Although there is no female Koro report, the effect of sorcery on females is a "tongue-tie." A typical case history runs as follows:

> The subject, age 35, was married to a woman aged 33; both had offspring from prior marriage, but the couple had no children together during their ten years of marriage. The husband was very traditional, a good provider for his family, and a hard worker. That his harvests were larger than his neighbors' crops created a suspicion of envy and fear of sorcery. About the time of the subject's attack, his brother, a sufferer of 'lannuk e laso', suddenly died; the death was attributed to sorcery. The subject initially complained of milky urine; later his urine turned deep yellow, a course of events duplicating his brother's final days. He complained of intermittent pain and extreme lower back pain when the penis "went inside". During the crisis the subject's wife massaged lower abdomen and held his penis to prevent its further contraction. The wife attributed her husband's attack to lifting heavy loads. Sometime after the attack, the wife ran off with another man, claiming that her husband was "not good sex". Sexual dissatisfaction was a common complaint of Bagobo women. (p. 8)

Exquisitely, the author provided the different dimensions of Koro, viz. the origin of the term "Koro"; emic constructions and case descriptions from the earlier literature; ethnological descriptions in the context of

Chinese, Indonesian, and Malaysian culture; and biomedical consideration for Koro symptom. Since the inception of the term "Koro" in 1874, this exhaustive review and analysis are valuable documents to all Koro researchers worldwide.

[18]. M. H. Padi: Koro.
British Journal of Psychiatry, 1984, 145(5), 558–559. (L)

This case report very elegantly described how the "penis-shrinking" fear is transmitted by auditory hallucination and forms a delusional content that influences behavior and precipitated acute anxiety and fear of shrinking penis that ultimately required hospital admission (in Hong Kong). It is a Koro case report in a 23-year-old immigrant Chinese single male from England in the background of schizophrenic illness. After returning to the UK, he needed another admission when he blamed his mother and sister for causing his penis to shrink. Afterward, he also believed that his penis would shrink if he ate noodles. His schizophrenic symptoms responded well with the neuroleptic medications but not his Koro symptoms. The author suggested that Koro with diagnoses like schizophrenia may be viewed as "an encapsulated delusional disorder similar to paranoia and paranoid states" and thus non-responder to usual neuroleptic medications.

1985

1985 Koro Epidemic in Guangdong, China

[19]. M. P. I. Weller: Koro.
British Journal of Psychiatry, 1985, 146, 452. (L)

The author here suggested a physiological mechanism of Koro symptom formation. He states: "Under states of high anxiety there will be over-arousal, with vasoconstrictor sympathetic impulses to the arterioles of the penis. In some people, predisposed by cultural or personal experience, the detumescence may become a focus for the pre-existing anxiety, thereby creating a vicious cycle."

[20]. C. Malinick, J. A. Flaherty, T. Jobe: Koro: How culturally specific?
International Journal of Social Psychiatry, 1985, 31, 67–73.

It is an excellent comparative discussion paper on the Western world's witchcraft traditions and African Black culture with a Koro case report of a 51-year-old black American male from Chicago, USA. The subject firmly believed that he developed importance after an oral sex attempt with a prostitute, and his penis began to shrink. He believed that the prostitute had cast a spell on him. He maintained this shrinking penile state almost for three post-hospital admission days, and on the fourth day, the penile morphology became normal. In retrospect, he thought that the prostitute was a witch. He also believed that in the event of the complete disappearance of the penis, he would die. The authors provided an excellent discussion focusing on the link between witchcraft beliefs and penis loss. Though it is reported as a Koro, careful analysis shows that the symptoms may also be explained as an episode of cultural delusion.

[21]. Guangdong Transcultural Psychiatric Research Group: The koro epidemic in Hainan island (A preliminary report).
Paper read at the Regional Conference of the World Psychiatric Association's Transcultural Psychiatry Section, Beijing, August 17–31, 1985.

This is a preliminary report of the 1985 Koro epidemic in Hainan island. It is reported that about 2000 persons (and another 2000 on the mainland) were affected. The outbreak resembles an epidemic hysteria, where acute anxiety is focused on the penis and rarely on a woman's breast, short duration, and recovered completely with reassurance and traditional medicine or devil-repelling measures. They also mentioned the episodic nature of the Koro epidemic in a ten-year cycle. i.e. 1955, 1966, and 1974. The details of this research are published afterward elsewhere.

Note: This paper was discussed and abstracted by H. B. M. Murphy in *Transcultural Psychiatric Research Review*, 1986, 23: 159–161. Concerning the long tradition of penis retraction pathology in Chinese culture and references in traditional medical texts (100 BC–100 AD), Dr. Murphy raised an important issue:

> Regardless of whether we regard the condition as (within China) a syndrome in its own right or merely an expression of an anxiety neurosis, there is definitely a puzzle to be solved in explaining why it should have been so persistent in this society and so little known in all others.

Dr. Murphy also discussed the paper by Berrios and Morley (1984) in this review.

[22]. W. G. Jilek, L. Jilek-Aall: The metamorphosis of 'culture-bound' syndromes.
Social Science & Medicine, 1985, 21(2), 205–210.

This is a very extensively researched and valuable work that challenges the concept of culture-bound syndromes with two specific examples, viz. Koro is a paradigm of transcultural metamorphosis and spirit sickness (of Salish Indian)—as a paradigm of intra-cultural metamorphosis. The authors made a critical analysis of Koro epidemics' geopolitical and diverse cultural backgrounds in Singapore, Thailand,, and India (along with a concurrent example of socio-political stress in each country). They conclude that Koro symptomatology reflects the social dimensions (socio-economic, ethnic, cultural, and biological survival) than the oedipal castration anxiety or any culture-specific pathogenicity. They analyzed Koro's cultural and social demographics and refuted the Oedipus complex theory in Koro symptomatology manifestation. They concluded that:

> … to explain the etiology and epidemiology of *Koro* we can no longer rely on either the model of oedipal castration anxiety, nor on the model of culture-specific pathogenicity. If we look for a common denomination in the affected populations at the time of the *koro* outbreaks we

> shall find it in the experience of a threat to their socioeconomic, ethnic, cultural and biological survival. In these contexts, the individual with *koro* anxiety responds to the collective fear of genocidal extermination by a well-defined enemy who is perceived as threatening the survival of one's ethnic group by attacking its procreative capability. In this perspective an explanation for the pathognomonic symptoms – feelings of shrinking of the organs subserving procreation (male and female genitals, female breast) – is more likely to come from research in comparative primate ethology than from psychoanalytic theorizing. (p. 208)

Similarly, they assert that the prevalence of anomic depression defined as spirit possession by *Salish* ritualists responds to social stresses generated by the despair of powerlessness in the face of threatened ethnic group survival. This research is a significant attempt to re-evaluate the concept of culture-bound syndromes, especially considering the individual psychodynamics and the broader geopolitical and socio-economic climate of society's affected population in real-time.

[23]. R. C. Simons, C. Hughes: The Culture-bound Syndromes: Folk Illnesses of Psychiatric and Anthropological Interests.
Eds. R. C. Simons and C. Hughes, D. Dordrecht, 1985.

It is an extraordinary and invaluable book for psychiatrists, anthropologists, and medical sociologists. In their elegant and in-depth analysis of the cultural influence on mental illness, the authors do an extensive review of the world literature along with a proposal for a novel and new construct of the semantic dimensions of culture-bound diseases.

A comparative study between DSM-III and the patterns of different folk illnesses and the probable neurophysiological evidence of such diseases—are the two important, valuable additions of this work. A proposal for the classification of culture-bound diseases is made by providing a scheme of "taxon"—"to designate the set collectively," to avoid semantic confusion in terminologies across the cultures. Seven such taxons are described: Startle Matching; Sleep Paralysis; Genital Retraction; Sudden Mass Assault; Running; Fright illness and Cannibal Compulsions. The authors suggest that "the taxon name also serves as a rubric for aberrant instances not connected with culturally elaborated beliefs and practices." It contains 39 chapters addressing the different categories of "Taxons."

The Genital Retraction taxon (pp. 151–194) is under the heading of "Folk illnesses of psychiatric interest in which a neurophysiological shaping factor is only suspected" contains six articles wholly devoted to the different aspects of Koro. In addition to introducing the theme of Genital Traction by R. C. Simons and Concluding comments by C. C. Hughes, it contains four published reports. It includes a vibrant discussion on Koro with examples from three different cultural groups, viz. Chinese (Gwee, 1963), American (Edwards, 1970), and African (Ifabumuyi & Rwegellera, 1979), along with Edwards's (1984) masterly review article on Koro or genital retraction syndrome. The authors believe that an underlying physiological state (penile vasoconstriction in response to physical or psychological conditions) is the initiating point upon which cultural elaboration produces Koro symptoms. The individual's cognitive state about his culture is the critical factor in developing anxiety in this context. Anxiety then leads to the sequence of events:

> Since the physiology associated with anxiety includes as one of its manifestations reduction of blood flow to the penis and consequent further penile retraction, perception of this retraction will further increase anxiety, frequency of monitoring and frequency of receiving the Bad News. Frequently receiving The Bad News will even further increase anxiety and its effects. This is an example of a self-incrementing causal loop. (p. 152)

[**Note:** L. J. Kirmayer abstracted this book under Abstract and Reviews in *Transcultural Psychiatric Research Review*, 1987, 24(4), 275–284.

This book is reviewed by Michael R Phillips, Hunan Medical College, Changsha, P.R.C., published in *The Journal of Psychohistory*, 1988, 15(3), 383. He opined that "This edited volume is a must-read for all transcultural psychiatrists and psychologically oriented anthropologists. It provides the background papers and adds a new perspective to the liveliest debated topic at the interface of culture and mental health- the so-called culture-bound syndromes (CBSs)."

K. V. Staiano also reviewed this book in *American Journal of Physical Anthropology*, 1987, 79, 129–130.]

[24]. R. A. Emsley: Koro in non-Chinese subjects.
British Journal of Psychiatry, 1985, 146(1), 102. (L)

It is a case report of a secondary Koro in a 25 year single black male from Cape, South Africa. The onset of penile symptoms was sudden after a failed attempt at coitus. Fear of impotence was there for the last eight months. With clomipramine treatment 75 mg a day, he became mute and catatonic. However, he overcame the symptoms with haloperidol 30 mg daily but remained convinced that his penis was shrinking. The author proposed the diagnosis as an acute anxiety state with delusional psychotic belief, though he stressed the importance of the psychogenic mechanism.

[25]. P. Moodley: Koro in non-Chinese subjects.
British Journal of Psychiatry, 1985, 146, 102–103. (L)

It is a case of Koro-like symptom in a 60-year-old Scotsman from London, at the background of withdrawal state from Lorazepam, which was prescribed for his cardiac dysrhythmia. On the 10th day after discontinuation, he developed agitation, restlessness, whole body shrinking, numbness around the mouth, and the perception that his penis and testicles are disappearing as if he is changing into a woman. There was no fear of death or attempted maneuvers to prevent the alleged penile or testicular "loss." The author believes that this was an example of depersonalization focusing on the genital area due to an acute anxiety state. He also suggested that because of more reporting of Koro symptoms in association with anxiety-related conditions, Koro may be seen "as an unusual presentation of anxiety."

[26]. G. Tollefson: Delusional hypochondriasis, depression, and amoxapine.
American Journal of Psychiatry, 1985, 142(12), 1518–1519.

This is not a Koro paper, but the clinical argument here may sometimes be applicable for Koro symptoms, especially in major depression. The author stated that often major depression might have mood-congruent psychotic symptoms like delusional hypochondriasis. In such cases, the clinical picture may include somatic delusions such as dysmorphophobia or hallucination, like an olfactory reference. The author presents a case of a 33-year-old woman who, after an operation for lower extremity varicosities, developed poor sleep and dysphoria along with the belief that her bones "were crackling and bubbling" and various valves "were bursting." She was diagnosed with major depression with somatic delusion. After a failed trial with phenelzine and alprazolam, she responded well with amoxapine, titrated from 50 to 350 mg over a month. The author commented that delusional depression might react poorly to conventional tricyclics, and thus the addition of a neuroleptic medication may be helpful.

1986

[27]. A. B. Joseph: Koro: Computed tomography and brain activity mapping in two patients.
Journal of Clinical Psychiatry, 1986, 47, 430–432.

It contains two fascinating Koro case reports in association with abnormal brain electrical activities. The first case, a 32-year-old black Haitian man, had multiple stereotyped Koro episodes preceded by an olfactory hallucination of perfume. Brain electrical activity mapping (BEAM) showed abnormal activity in the right temporoparietal region. His clinical diagnosis was atypical psychosis with Koro and psychomotor epilepsy.

The second case, a 32-year-old black Ethiopian, presented with multiple, repetitive stereotypic episodes of Koro in the context of paranoid psychosis. His CT scan revealed mild bilateral frontal lobe atrophy, moderate bilateral temporal and parietal lobe atrophy, and moderate atrophy of the cerebellar vermis. BEAM showed paroxysmal slowing and sharp waves over the right hemisphere, predominantly from frontal and anterior temporal regions, significantly increasing theta activity from temporal lobes and the right frontal lobe. In BEAM, visually evoked potentials were abnormal over the right parietal and temporal areas, while auditorially evoked responses were abnormal over the right temporal lobe only. He has been diagnosed with atypical psychosis, Koro, and psychomotor epilepsy.

The author highlights the dimension of epileptic body image distortions involving the genitals. In his opinion, these cases can be diagnosed as sexual epilepsy, which was mediated by right temporoparietal or bitemporoparietal dysfunctions. This paper is a valuable addition to the probability of biomedical causation of penile retraction/shrinkage pathology.

[28]. F. Oyebode, R. Jamieson, J. Mullaney, K. Davison: Koro—A psychophysiological dysfunction?
British Journal of Psychiatry, 1986, 178, 212–214.

This is a Koro case report of a 56-year-old Englishman who had a six-year history of recurrent shrinking of the penis. At the time of clinical contact, he was also having the features of endogenous depression. The unique feature here is the psychophysiological findings on the penile plethysmographic test. The authors found that the "condition of penile shrinkage corresponds with a true physiological change in penile circumference below a baseline." They offer two possible explanations. The patient had dysfunctional autonomic control of penile size, causing a more frequent diminution in penis size than expected. Or alternatively, the penile changes were within the normal range, but because of his heightened awareness (due to personal factors, obsessional self-scrutiny, or sexual conflicts), the perception became abnormal. This finding is a vital proposition in favor of a biomedical hypothesis of the genital retraction pathology.

[29]. W. G. Jilek: Epidemics of genital shrinking (Koro); Historical review and report of a recent outbreak in south-China.
Curare, 1986, 9, 269–282.

It is an excellent review paper on all the major Koro epidemics with a brief historical account of their genesis. It contains a new piece of information about a 42-year-old Indonesian Koro case of Surabeya. For the first time in the English literature, it also cites a detailed report of the 1908 Szechwan Koro epidemic (China), as reported by Legendre (1908).

A precious bit of information collected by the author from the archives of the Tang district of Guangdong Province was a massive Suo-yang epidemic in the Hainan Islands (China) in 1865. He briefly described three Koro epidemics viz. Szechwan, China (1908), India (1982), and Guangdong, China (1984–1985), and gives a detailed account of each epidemic type, the social rituals involved, and the unique socio-political atmosphere prevalent during the epidemic in each of the countries.

This paper describes four Koro cases of the Guangdong area, one of whom had concomitant temporal lobe epilepsy. Traditional healing rituals for exorcising the victim from this "potentially killing intruder" by severe beating resulted in two victims' death. The last part of the article is devoted to discussing folk beliefs and traditional treatment methods of Koro in Guangdong, which revealed a view in fox-spirit possession as the cause of penile retraction pathology.

There is a valuable description of the fox spirit with cross-cultural references. Zhong Kui's cult, a legendary Chinese physician—hero, and God, is also discussed. The social background analysis of these five large Koro epidemics from five different geo-cultural areas of the globe prompted the author to discard the oedipal theory or cultural specificity construct as the cause. The author stresses the importance of the role of stressful socio-political events to generate collective anxieties. The author considers the "procreative abilities are an important determinant of a person's value."

[30]. I. Modai, H. Muniz, D. Aizenberg: Koro in an Israeli male. *British Journal of Psychiatry, 1986, 149, 503–506.*

It is a report of Koro in a 56-year old Jew from Israel. Psycho-diagnostic tests (RIB, TAT) revealed that he had very low masculine self-esteem and perceived women as big and threatening. The patient also had concomitant depression. The patient identified masturbation as the reason for his illness as it was "weakness the penis and the body, and causes loss of sperm." Jewish laws and traditions' socio-cultural code and ethics are discussed concerning the patient's guilt over masturbation.

Three crucial clinical findings are worthy of mention: (1) acute fear after viewing a black cat at night; (2) a pre-Koro concern with penile pain after intercourse, (which despite a urologist's opinion of being non-pathological), rendered him with the firm conviction of having a fatal disease and (3) intensification of penile shrinkage after his dismissal from the job.

The description of his illness-behaviors, especially the fear about the shrinking penis, concomitant avoidance habits (e.g., avoiding pressure on the penis; holding the penis most of the time; inability to bend the body because of the fear that movement may cause further shrinkage) and detailed accounts of his distress, all indicate the presence of a strong hypochondriacal-obsessive component.

[31]. G. Q. Chu, T. W. Yeh, W. C. Wang: Koro—Analysis of 87 cases.
Xin 1 Xue (New Medicine), 1986, 3, 1–4. [In Chinese]

It reports and analyzes 87 cases of the 1985 Koro epidemic of the Tan County area of Hainan Island, China.

[32]. A. O. Ogunlesi: Koro symptomatology associated with paranoid psychosis in a Nigerian patient: A case report.
West African Journal of Medicine, 1986, 5(4), 305–307.

This is a case report of a 42-year old male of the Nigerian Yoruba tribe who presented Koro symptomatology at the background of paranoid psychosis. It is a compelling case and showed how cultural norms and values generate symptoms even in a psychotic episode. The patient was a married (third time) apprentice of "Babalawo (Ifa oracle diviner)" and a farmer. He had a three-week history of disturbing behavior when he expressed his belief that he will die, and his "penis is about to escape." One confusion remains here that what is the meaning of penis escape? Is that equivalent to the disappearance of penis because there is no mention of "retraction of the penis into abdomen" in the report? Another exciting fact observed at this point was:

> About two weeks prior to his presentation, he pressurized his relatives to invite elders in the neighborhood to come and perform a sacrifice to forestall the escape of his penis. However when the time was ripe for the sacrifice, he ran away claiming that that the elders had come to kill him. (p. 306)

When he was asked about his penis during the mental state examination, he checked his penis by hand and said it was there. Initially, he was treated with amitriptyline and then with neuroleptic medication, and he recovered from his hallucination and belief about "penis escape." The author tried to explain the various socio-cultural and psychological factors in the genesis of this penile symptom. Ifa oracle followers believe in evil forces that can inflict personal harm or disasters, crisis, or illness in the community.

So the probability remains whether this was a case of Koro or of "penis vanishing," a construct that took epidemic form in Africa in later years.

1987

1987 Koro Epidemic in Guangdong, China

[33]. F. Oyebode, R. Jamieson, J. Mullaney, K. Davison: Koro and schizophrenia in Singapore.
British Journal of Psychiatry, 1987, 150, 106–107.

It is a case report of Koro in a 75-year-old immigrant Chinese to Singapore who also had a concurrent schizophrenia diagnosis. Two points in the clinical note are essential: (1) precipitation of Koro after eating a banana—which the patient regarded as a "cold" food (traditional belief) and (2) presence of reducible inguinal hernia. The authors stress the importance of careful history taking in elderly Koro patients to exclude any local or systemic disease contribution. They provide a nosological scheme for the classification of Koro syndrome.

[34]. M. Scher: Koro in a native born citizen of the US.
International Journal of Social Psychiatry, 1987, 33, 42–45.

It is a Koro case report of an unmarried Caucasian man in his mid-twenties who came to the hospital for loss of erectile power and fear of abdominal disappearance of both testes and penis, at the background of depression with suicidal contemplation and long-standing learning disability. Masturbatory guilt (for religious grounds) was present, but there was no fear of death in this case. He drank an average of six bottles of beer per day. The patient recovered with benzodiazepines.

[35]. K. M. Mo, L. S. Li, L. W. Ou: Report of koro epidemic in Leizhou Peninsula, Hainan Islands.
Chinese Journal of Neuropsychiatry, 1987, 20, 232–234. [In Chinese]

This is a Koro epidemic report of May 1987 in the Leizhou Peninsula around the Haikang country area of Guangdong Province, involving 300 subjects.

[36]. T. J. Holden: Koro syndrome associated with alcohol-induced systemic disease in a Zulu.
British Journal of Psychiatry, 1987, 151(5), 695–697.

It is a case report of genital retraction syndrome or Koro in a 38-year-old married Zulu immigrant male, with a background of alcoholic hepatitis, avitaminosis, and urinary tract infection, from Kingston, Canada. The patient had the firm conviction that his penis had been shrinking into his abdomen for the past three days, and he is apprehensive that he would die when it disappears completely. A course of ampicillin, diazepam, and vitamin supplementation resulted in the penile symptom's complete remission. The author discussed the various diagnostic options for this non-culture bound secondary (to physical illness) Koro symptoms, like Atypical Psychosis—monosymptomatic delusion of bodily change (DSM-III: 298.90) or Psychogenic Paranoid Psychosis (ICD-9: 298.4) or Organic Delusional syndrome (DSM-III: 293.81). The author asserted that Koro might be a reaction to various psychological or physical stressors than solely a culture-bound manifestation.

[37]. T. Mukherjee: Koro-like states.
British Journal of Psychiatry, 1987, 150(6), 881. (L)

It is a case report of a Koro-like state in a 25-year-old white male from Kent, UK. There was a history of anxiety state and reactive depression at age 21. In 1983 after the breakdown of his relationship, he first showed this symptom of retracting penis and testicles into the abdomen. Three years later, he had hypomania, which eventually subsided, but he maintained his faith in retracting genitalia. He developed depression and was treated with amitryptiline and stelazine and recovered, but his belief regarding genitalia remains unaltered. No cultural factor is noted in this case.

[38]. H. V. Kumar: Koro in an Israeli man.
British Journal of Psychiatry, 1987, 150, 133. (L)

It is in response to Modai et al.'s Koro publication (BJP, 1986, 149: 503–506). The author corrected the number of reported Koro cases in Non-Chinese subjects: 22 as of 1987.

[39]. E. M. Kendell, P. L. Jenkins: Koro in an American man.
American Journal of Psychiatry, 1987, 144(12), 1621. (L)

This is a case report of "delusion of Koro"; in a 35-year old black American male from Columbia, USA. In his sixth hospital admission due to schizophrenia, he expressed his delusional belief concerning sex organs and sexuality like: "had the largest penis in the world"/ "being turned into a bitch" along with the fear and anxiety of penile retraction. He applied a cloth ligature around the base of the penis to prevent retraction. He responded to rapid treatment with neuroleptics. This case is an example of Secondary Koro.

[40]. J. Money, C. Annecillo: Body-image pathology: Koro, the shrinking-penis syndrome in transcultural sexology.
Sexual & Marital Therapy, 1987, 2(1), 91–99.

This is a significant first research paper on a Koro-like case report (from Baltimore, USA) with optical measurement and projective drawing of a shrinking penis. The case is the father of a boy treated by the authors for idiopathic panhypopituitarism. The father made a self-referral to an already known physician (authors) about his problem as follows: "shrinkage of my penis and genitals." He further clarified that: "shrinkage had begun about 3 months earlier, was visibly obvious, represented approximately a 75% decrease, and applied to the diameter as well as the length of the penis." He also complained of depression and guilt over this problem. Further history revealed that he was also suffering from erectile failure.

Shrinkage evaluation: All investigations, including urological, laboratory tests, diabetes tests, hormonal levels including testosterone, and physical examination of scrotum and testes—all were within a normal range. One important finding was: "The penis length was difficult to measure because of a localized suprapubic and lower abdominal fat pad that enveloped the root of the penile shaft, and held it retracted within." The maximum stretched-length measurement (corresponds to the erected length) was 5 inches (13 cm). The average standard for regular stretched penis length is 6.57 inches with an sd of 0.77 inches (authors' previous work). An interesting observation is made on the projective drawing of the penis by the patient. The patient did two pictures—before and after the shrinkage: one on the flaccid state and the other on the erect state. The authors very nicely described the patient's perceptual estimates through these drawings:

> At the outset he had difficulty and made two false starts, one on the reverse of the page, and one visible as an abandoned glans penis. He miscalculated the after-shrinkage size of the flaccid penis and had to do it again, smaller, and labeled 'actual length after shrinkage'. The dimensions of the erected penis before and after shrinkage do not differ appreciably from those of the flaccid penis. This discrepancy, together with

> the false starts and size miscalculation are consistent with the perceptual and ideational errors that typify a body-image syndrome. (p. 95)

The patient was treated successfully with medication and a joint discussion involving his wife. The authors discussed the different possibilities of penile shrinkage from the viewpoint of neurovascular control of penile erection and flaccidity, and in this case, the role of suprapubic fat. The authors also highlighted the immense importance of active listening to the patient's complaints and empathic intervention, both of which prevent the expansion of conviction of penis shrinkage to complete penis-disappearance delusion.

1988

[41]. S. T. C. Ilechukwu: Koro-like syndromes in Nigeria.
Transcultural Psychiatric Research Review, 1988, 25, 310–314.

This is a report of a few fascinating epidemics of 1975–1977 and 1978 in Nigeria where the main complaint was the sudden vanishing of the penis.

The author describes two cases from Kaduna, an urban area in northern Nigeria in 1975, relating to penis vanishing cum theft. In 1975–1977 there was an epidemic of penis disappearing among the newer migrants into Lagos. In 1977, the author examined Lagos's case, a 20-year boy who tied a string to his penis shaft to prevent further shrinkage. There were reports of epidemics of vanishing breasts and pregnancies also. The author mentioned a criminal syndicate behind this "fake" penis vanishing drama and rob the victim, and eventually, Police were involved in smashing these syndicates. The author discusses the traditional beliefs and phallic values of the various ethnic groups of Nigeria and the social cognition in the interpretation of retraction of tongue or penis as equivalent to imminent death.

> In Nigeria, it seems that one must look to popular myths for possible explanations. Various ethnic groups in Nigeria ascribe high potency to the external genitalia as ritual and magical objects to promote fecundity or material prosperity to the unscrupulous. Ritually murdered persons are

often said to have these parts missing. These speculations may be fertile ground for unconscious cultural symptom construction. (p. 313)

The author tried to find the reason for this public display of personal distress in the prevalent Nigerian psyche of "shame culture": "This construct would allow the projection of perceived individual sexual inadequacy into alien aspects of the environment." This is a valuable short paper to understand the socio-cultural background of African penis-vanishing episodes.

[42]. R. Durst, P. Rosca-Rebaudengo: Koro secondary to a tumor of the Corpus Callosum.
British Journal of Psychiatry, 1988, 153, 251–254.

This is a case report from Jerusalem, Israel; the authors presented a case with a diagnosed tumor in the genu of the corpus callosum, displaying typical Koro symptoms. The patient had a history of acute anxiety attacks for which he was hospitalized two years ago. He complained of impotence, vague physical symptoms, and frontal headache with dizziness and depression in the current situation. His principal reason for fearful concern was the shrinkage of the penis into the abdomen and fear of death. The tumor was inoperable, and electroconvulsive therapy offered adequate relief.

The presence of premorbid fear of sexual inadequacy, intense guilt, and shame of "excessive masturbation," marital conflicts, attacks of acute anxiety and complaints of impotence, and depressed mood with suicidal intentions and the tumor "which had probably been present for an extended period of time" are the important issues here. The authors believe that all these provide sufficient ground for the psychosexual pathology, leading to the perception of penile shrinkage rather than the tumor's contributions. The tumor is probably a coincidental finding. In this event, the heading of the paper may be misleading.

[43]. H. V. Kumar, E. Moloney: Koro secondary to a tumor of the corpus callosum.
British Journal of Psychiatry, 1988, 153, 711–712.

This is a short letter objecting to Durst and Rosca-Rebaudengo's (1988) report, who associated tumor of the corpus callosum with Koro. The authors showed with clinical scrutiny that the Koro was not associated with tumor in the case at all. On the other hand, they claimed from the patient's clinical detail that the Koro was a manifestation of depressive illness.

[44]. W. S. Tseng, K. M. Mo, J. Hsu, L. L. Shuen, O. L. Wah, C. G. Qian, D. W. Jiang: A socio-cultural study of Koro epidemics in Guangdong China.
American Journal of Psychiatry, 1988, 145, 1538–1543.

It is a comprehensive account of the Koro epidemics of Guangdong, China, in 1984–1985 and 1987. It reports an affectivity figure of 2000 in Guangdong's Hainan Island and Leizhou Peninsula between November 1984 and May 1985. In May 1987, several hundred subjects were affected by Koro in the Leizhou Peninsula around the Haikang country area.

They provided an excellent and brief account of the area's socio-cultural background. It reveals that people are poorly educated, lack modern city life, and have deep faith in magico-religious worldviews about health and disease because of the site's geographical isolation and remoteness. The traditional Chinese theory of yin-yang imbalance causing disease is a well-rooted belief in the population. There is a robust popular myth that ghosts of the dead (who have no penis) hunt for penises to become alive again. This myth is extended to the cult of a disguised spirit in the form of a female ghost fox (Hu-li-jing) or a fair lady who would come to collect penises for this purpose. The authors believe that it was probably the most influential social cognition operating at the root of Koro's mass outbreak in this region.

The detailed report of the epidemic is a valuable addition to the Koro literature. Sporadic Koro cases occurred in August 1984, culminating in a massive outbreak in November 1984, and a second wave started in May 1985. The prediction of a fortune teller that the year 1985 would be a bad year and people would suffer from many diseases was a key triggering factor (social cognition and supernatural beliefs) in the epidemic's background. The news of "disaster" brought by a beggar from Hainan Island to the Leizhou Peninsula was the cause of the second epidemic wave there. In May 1987, another epidemic broke out in Haikang town.

A report from Haikang County showed 232 cases (males 195, females 37). The males were mostly between 10 and 25 years of age, single, student or farmer, and had only elementary school education. Most of the females were single and between 15 and 20 years of age.

All the patients had the folk belief that the female fox spirit caused Suo-yang. Above 76% had their attack at night, and 69% of men had a prodromal phase of chills. The clinical features include acute anxiety (100%); palpitation (65%); tremor (69%); fear (68%); and feeling of impending death (62%) with disturbance of consciousness (9%); paleness (51%); and heavy perspiration (34%). The social treatment offered by local people included manual penile traction, and in females—the subject's head is covered with a fishing net. She is then severely beaten with tree branches, and her fingers are painfully cramped with a chopstick to exorcise the ghost. The Chinese traditional healing was applied by offering specific yang foods to the sufferer like red pepper jam or black pepper powder, ginger juice, or liquor for combating the yang (male) deficiency. Several casualties are identified due to maltreatment from over-zealous social rituals. There was a death of a one-year child from asphyxia during forced-feeding of pepper juice, several cases of penile injuries, nipple injuries (due to insertion of a pin), and several girls being beaten as they are targeted as fox-maidens in disguise.

There are two case reports: one a 28-year-old single male and the other a 20-year-old female for whom there were no genuine Koro complaints from her side, yet the villagers attributed her depressive and fainting spells to Koro. The girl's story is quite interesting, especially her regular ritual crying before the marriage. The coincidental Koro epidemic triggered a mass response to identifying it like a ghost possession and Koro. Many local elderly believe in ghosts' role (stealing penises) as ghosts have no penises and need human penises for returning to human form.

The authors think that Koro can be designated as "genital retraction panic disorder in sporadic cases." However, individual psychosexual issues (e.g., lack of masculine identification, lack of confidence and experience in heterosexual relations, misconceptions about sexual practice, or presence of castration anxiety) also play an essential role. The Koro contagion model in epidemics depends on some socio-cultural and community factors like socio-cultural stress and socially shared beliefs and a conducive social atmosphere that accepts and maintains the morbid cognition, thus helping the spread. The map relating to the tracing of Koro spread in the Islands is valuable for the paper. Some important historical information about the past Koro epidemic was also provided: epidemic 120 years ago (probably 1865), in 1948, 1955, 1966, and 1974.

[**Note**: This paper was presented at the Conference of the Society for the Study of Psychiatry and Culture, Quebec City, on September 16–19, 1987.

This paper was abstracted and discussed by R. H. Prince in the Asia section, *Transcultural Psychiatric Research Review*, 1988, 25, 74–77. He concluded by mentioning two crucial issues of this research as: the absence of any significant socio-political stress like fear of genocide (as was in the Singapore or Thailand epidemic) in this epidemic and secondly, the role of fox-spirit imagery as a vital folk belief in the Koro symptomatology.]

[45]. C. S. Mellor: Depersonalization and self-perception.
British Journal of Psychiatry, 1988, 153(Suppl. 2), 15–19.

This paper describes depersonalization's phenomenology and focuses on the relationships between depersonalization, self-perception, and body image. Different concepts of depersonalization are discussed. Koro is cited as an example of depersonalization, which leads to body image disturbances. The depersonalization in Koro is said to be somatic and localized to the genital area. The author states that Koro's condition "differs from more usual manifestation of depersonalization by the presence of apparent delusions and the absence of the experience of having no emotions."

[46]. R. M. Hawley, J. H. Owens: Koro: Its presentation in an elderly male.
International Journal of Geriatric Psychiatry, 1988, 3, 69–72.

It is a case report of Koro in an 81-year-old British male, may be termed as chronic Koro, from Bristol, England. The predominant presentation was the symptom of a firm conviction that his penis is steadily retracting into his abdomen, and eventually, he will die. This belief was maintained for three months and was associated with clinical depression. He had a diagnosis of recurrent depression from the age of 51 and had ten hospital admissions. The authors described a detailed history of multiple hypochondriacal complaints and somatic symptoms. He responded well with a combination of tricyclic antidepressants and antipsychotic major tranquilizers. The patient had no link to Asian culture. The author made an excellent review of the 22 published Koro cases in non-Asian subjects.

[47]. H. R. Kranzler, P. Shah: Atypical Koro.
British Journal of Psychiatry, 1988, 152, 579–580. (L)

It is a case report of "Atypical Koro" in a 36-year-old Jamaican male from Connecticut, USA. The patient was diagnosed with paranoid schizophrenia nine years earlier. His current presentation was "testicles are swollen and bothered me" for the last year. He was fearful if the testicles retract into the abdomen, then he will die. He responded well with oral fluphenazine treatment during his five-week hospital stay with a modest reduction of his testicle fear. From the short description, it seems that he was suffering from somatic delusion as a part of his schizophrenic process rather than a Koro-like (no concern with the penis) state.

[48]. N. Fernando: Monosymptomatic hypochondriasis treated with a tricyclic antidepressant.
British Journal of Psychiatry, 1988, 152, 851–852.

This is a significant case report of a 26-year-old male European from New Zealand. He was diagnosed with monosymptomatic hypochondriasis with Koro-like symptoms. This paper is notable for three definitive insights it offers to understand Koro's phenomenology. These are:

1. The relationship of Koro-like symptoms with hypochondriacal health concern of dysmorphophobic nature (asymmetrical body) is well illustrated. The patient has perceived "his penis and testicles were reducing in size and gradually disappearing into his abdomen." It was not an acute episode as it happens in Koro, but a chronic perception and this perception, coupled with other bodily abnormalities (asymmetrical body, excessive growth of hair in the pubic area, penis and both legs, which are "alive") persisted for over six months. Some researchers have seen genital concern (about shape, size, and shrinkage/retraction) in Koro as a hypochondriacal concern with hidden obsessive color. It also touches on the clinical criteria for body dysmorphic disorder.
2. The second important issue is the diagnosis of monosymptomatic hypochondriacal psychosis (because of the delusional conviction of genital deformity). So, the Koro perception here may be termed either "Secondary Koro" (related to other mental disorders) or "incomplete Koro", as it lacks the classical features. Another crucial issue to be noted is the severity of the dysmorphic distress—he attempted suicide by therapeutic drug overdose.
3. Third important issue is the treatment response with clomipramine—an antidepressant drug with known efficacy on OCD symptoms. The patient did not respond to pimozide, but improved with clomipramine and has remained symptom-free for 1.5 years. This response highlighted Koro's OCD flavor, keeping in mind that the DSM-5 (2013) placed Koro under "Other specified Obsessive–Compulsive and Related Disorders" (300.3).

[49]. J. Maslowski: Koro-like syndrome in Maltese subject on the basis of chronic schizophrenia.
Bulletin of Maritime & Tropical Medicine in Gdynia, 1988, 39(1–2), 108–110.

It is a case report from Mount Carmel Mental Hospital of Malta of a 26-year-old single Maltese male having a history of schizophrenia from the age of 19. The patient complained of continuous upsetting thoughts about his ill health and thought that his penis shrank in size. He was going to die, along with other features of schizophrenia and mixed mood of anxiety-depression. The author suggested that this may be defined as somatic hallucination and hypochondriacal delusions. Hence, it is a Koro-like symptom at the background of a psychotic process or maybe termed "Koro-delusion." It is an excellent report to understand how the penile delusion may mimic Koro symptoms.

1988–1989

[50]. H. V. Perera: Two cases of koro-like states occurring in Sri Lanka.
Journal of the Ceylon College of Physicians, 1988–1989, 21–22, 33–35.

It is a case report of Koro-like symptoms from Sri Lanka. Two cases are described. The first one is a 21-year Sinhalese male who developed a firm conviction that his penis was shrinking into the abdomen, and he would die. He has an acute excited schizophrenic episode (thought of interference and broadcasting and strong paranoid ideas-being spied and poisoned, ideas of control, and auditory hallucination). Large doses of chlorpromazine and 4 ECTs resulted in a very successful resolution of symptoms. After discharge, he was advised by a local healer that a demon possesses him, and he discontinued his neuroleptic medications. Two months later, he committed suicide by jumping from a high-rise building.

The second case was a 22-year Muslim male who showed a clinical pattern of chronic Koro-like symptoms. It has started after he contracted venereal disease from homosexual contact. He complained that during the last three weeks, his penis was slowly drawn up into his abdomen. Subsequently, he was preoccupied with the obsessional doubt that his penis would disappear inside the belly. He repeatedly checks, holds, and observed the organ almost on a half-hourly basis. He also had clinical depression. He responded well with clomipramine 50 mg twice daily.

Observation: The first case is an example of Koro in the background of acute psychotic episodes' delusional content. The second case exemplifies Koro-like symptoms at the background of psycho-sexual pathology and depression with obsessive rumination and compulsive behavior.

1989

[51]. E. Hollander, M. R. Liebowitz, R. Winchel, A. Klumker, D. F. Dlein: Treatment of body-dysmorphic disorder with serotonin reuptake blockers.
American Journal of Psychiatry, 1989, 146, 768–770.

The authors describe five patients with body dysmorphic disorder who responded preferentially to serotonin reuptake blockers. They review the literature and analyze how patients with excessive concern about body abnormalities lie along a spectrum of doubt and certainty and discuss the similarities and differences between this and obsessive–compulsive disorders.

They describe a case of body dysmorphic symptoms with obsessive rumination and cannabis smoking. A 24-year-old single male had a childhood diagnosis of minimal brain dysfunction. An adolescent, he had a history of two long-term hospitalizations diagnosed with a borderline personality disorder, Tourette's syndrome, obsessive–compulsive disorder, and marijuana abuse. He developed an obsessive rumination regarding a small and ugly penis at the age of 20. He showed marked improvement with clomipramine (60 mg/day) and was symptom-free for three years, but had a relapse/recurrence at the age of 24 when he discontinued the medicine and started to reabuse marijuana. He showed improvement by re-treatment with clomipramine (60 mg/day). His mother was also a patient of obsessive–compulsive disorder.

[52]. D. De Leo, P. Mauro, C. Pellegrini: An organic triggering factor in koro syndrome? A case report.
European Journal of Psychiatry, 1989, 3(2), 77–81.

This is a Koro-like case report in a 39-year-old separated male from Padua, Italy. After an attempted suicide (superficial cuts to left wrist), he was admitted to the hospital because of the fear of retracting his penis and testicles into his abdomen. There was an idea of reference for the last two years, and an examination showed traits of borderline personality disorder, hypochondriacal fears, and a moderate degree of phimosis. He responded well with perphenazine (24 mg daily) and clomipramine (100 mg daily) treatment for four weeks of his hospital stay. The authors suggested that an organic condition (phimosis) affecting genitals may precipitate Koro among Western Europeans.

[53]. J. Westermeyer: A case of koro in a refugee family: Association with depression and folie a deux.
Journal of Clinical Psychiatry, 1989, 50, 181–183.

It is a sporadic Koro case report in a 31-year-old married Homong refugee in the USA, in association with psychotic depression. The clinical description is fascinating: "…2 months before evaluation, a pronounced worsening in his condition was marked by the patient's perception that his penis and scrotum are now 'disappearing back inside my body.' He had the sensation that his testicles were migrating around inside his abdomen and thighs and causing pain. At times, he thought he saw his testicles moving under the skin of his legs and trunk." Also, there were all the physical and emotional symptoms of depression with paranoid delusional ideas and suicidal thoughts. There was also a marked symptom of anxiety.

The person had several investigations, and all were normal. He was diagnosed with major depression with mood-congruent psychotic features. The author described the different aspects of acculturative stress to adjustment of isolated Homong refugee families in the USA and thus stressed the importance of familial and socio-cultural factors in developing Koro symptoms. There was family stress related to the marriage negotiation of their daughter. His wife was also suffering from major depression and shared the belief that her husband was undergoing genital retraction with potentially fatal outcomes (folie a deux). At the end of the paper, the author described Koro's nosological relation with different psychiatric disorders. He stressed the differences between phobic fear and psychotic perception in a clinical context as follows:

> It is important to distinguish between a patient's fear that the genetalia might retract and possibly cause death (a phobia) and a patient's actual perception or belief that the genitalia are retracting and the death is imminent (a hallucination and/or delusion). The former is analogous to cardiophobia or cancerphobia in somatoform but nonpsychotic patients. The later is analagous to psychotic delusion and/or hallucination in severely disabled patients, such as those who are convinced that they suffer a fatal cancer or heart disease despite assurances to the contrary. In sum, koro may involve phobia with acute anxiety or panic or somatic hallucinations, delusions of a fatal illness—just as with nonsexual symptom foci, such as heart disease or cancer. (p. 183)

The last part of the paper draws some clinical and psycho-social differences between sporadic and epidemic Koro cases. He mentioned female Koro's lack as a sporadic case and noted that only 5–33% of the epidemic population sample was female. Different forms of folk therapy are used to treat epidemic cases, but psychotropic medications and ECTs are used to treat sporadic cases. Socio-political tension or conflict is operative behind epidemics, but individual psychopathology and familial factors are critical in sporadic cases. This paper provides a good insight into personal risk factors and cultural stress in Koro phenomena.

Observation: Two issues deserve mention here: firstly, the symptoms of disappearing penis and scrotum are not like that of acute penile retraction in Koro (more appropriately may be termed as Koro-like symptom), and secondly, the moving scrotum under the skin reminding a somewhat similar culture-bound syndrome in India—Gilhari (Lizard) syndrome—it is believed that a small swelling move under the skin from back to the neck and may cause airway obstruction and death.

1990

[54]. W. F. Sheeley: Koro or hysteria?
Journal of Clinical Psychiatry, 1990, 51, 39. (L)

It is a response to the case reported by J. Westermeyer (JCP, 1989, 50: 181–183) where the author suggested that the patient was suffering from hysteria and presented Koro symptoms ("theatrical malady") for some secondary gain and family (wife and daughter) was utilized as a supportive role.

Dr. Westermeyer's Reply: ***Journal of Clinical Psychiatry*****, 1990, 51, 39. (L)**

He disagreed with the suggestion of Dr. Sheeley that the patient was suffering from hysteria. He thinks that this supposition reflects the ethnocentric approach for discarding more comprehensive world views.

[55]. L. Turnier, G. Chouinard: Effect anti-Koro d'un anti-depresseur tricyclique.
Revue-Canadienne de Psychiatrie, 1990, 35, 331–333. [Article in French].

The authors here are reporting a case of Koro in association with major depression. The case was treated with trimipramine (150 mg/day), bromazepam. Besides, the patient received psychotherapy, which allowed him to deal with the situation and eliminate guilt feelings. It is hypothesized that the tricyclic antidepressant had a curative effect on Koro syndrome by simultaneously treating depression.

[56]. D. N. Anderson: Koro: The genital retraction symptom after stroke.
British Journal of Psychiatry, 1990, 157, 142–144.

This is a Koro's case report in a 73-year-old Briton who developed psychotic depression following a non-dominant temporoparietal stroke. The patient presented with acute urine retention after believing that penile shrinkage would obstruct urine outflow. The author suggests that the term "genital retraction syndrome" should be avoided as it may cause semantic confusion about Koro's etiology, which may be cultural, and also psychophysiological.

[57]. R. L. Bernstein and A. C. Gaw: Koro: Proposed classification for DSM-IV.
American Journal of Psychiatry, 1990, 147, 1670–1674.

This is an excellent paper devoted to the nosological analysis of the past research findings and a new diagnostic proposal for Koro for DSM-IV. This is a must-read paper for all Koro researchers.

It also contains a case report of Koro in a 25-year-old Cantonese of Boston. The patient complained of pain in the penis and insomnia following intercourse with a prostitute a month ago. After a 3-day intermittent burning pain in the penis, he had an acute anxiety attack with fear of shrinking the penis and consequent death. The patient migrated from China and knew about *suk-yang* illness. As compensatory proof, he tried masturbation to convince himself that his penis was not shrinking. He also avoided sleep for fear of death.

The authors provided a short historical review with different diagnostic terms used for Koro by various researchers systematically. They also specify the role of cultural beliefs in Koro symptom development. They strongly argued in favor of the category "culture-specific disorder" for Koro in DSM-IV. Their argument is:

> … one must differentiate culture-specific cases of koro from koro-like states. Furthermore, a person influenced by a folk belief in koro should not be considered psychotic or delusional, unless the person's ego functions are severely impaired. The presence of a folk belief in koro or other culturally shared beliefs is a key factor in understanding the koro phenomenon as well as in elucidating the genesis and perpetuation of koro epidemics. It is in this relation to the cultural set which makes koro distinctive and its presentation dramatic. To allow clear and adequate consideration of this cultural factor, the concept of a culture-specific disorder would have to be added in DSM-IV, since this category is clearly missing. (p. 1672)

Then they provided prevalence and cultural considerations. They also raised the question:

> It appears obvious that the cultural belief in the concept of koro is an important factor in the genesis of the syndrome, yet the question of whether koro is a unique cultural syndrome or merely the cultural expression of a universal phenomenon has been raised. (p. 1671)

They try to delineate the difference between Koro and Koro-like syndromes and assert that Koro can occur in the right setting and stimulus even in non-Chinese cultures. Ample examples of Koro-like symptoms associated with drug withdrawal, brain tumor, epilepsy, and syphilis provide a firm ground for a primary physiological substratum in Koro.

Following the philosophy of DSM-IIIR, under the "Proposal for DSM-IV," they formulated a clinically useful flow chart for a diagnostic decision tree with four diagnostic options: (1) Physical condition; (2) A specific Axis I disorder (other than somatoform disorder); (3) Genital Retraction disorder, culture-specific (either single or epidemic); and (4) Genital Retraction disorder, not culture-specific. Then they discussed the definition of Koro and Koro-like symptoms. They also discussed the different steps and clinical situations in the proposed classification and suggested the following diagnostic criteria for genital retraction disorder for inclusion in DSM-IV classification:

* * *

A. A feeling of overwhelming panic associated with the sensation of or the belief in genital retraction.
B. A fear of impending death, should the genitals be allowed to fully retract.
C. A tendency to prevent retraction by holding onto the penis, enlisting help in doing so from friends or relatives, or using devices attached to the penis.
D. Aside from the belief and its ramifications, behaviour is not obviously is odd or bizarre.
E. Has never met criteria for any axis I disorder other than somatoform disorder, and it cannot be established that an organic factor initiated and maintained the disturbance.

Specify Type:

Whether in a cultural context or not in a cultural context. Whether a single case or an epidemic.

* * *

They also provide a beneficial summary description of Koro for DSM-IV in the appendix: definition, associated features; age at onset; course; complications; prevalence; predisposing factors and sex ratio; family pattern; cultural background and differential diagnosis.

In Appendix 1, they define Koro as follows:

> The essential feature of this disorder is a complaint of genital retraction with a fear of impending death, occurring where culturally sanctioned beliefs of folk disease or pathology are present. Among males, the most common complaint is that of the penis shrinking into the abdomen and resultant death; among females, the shrinking of the labia or breasts and resultant death. The person may appear to be in a state of acute distress and attempt to pull his penis, have family members or friends hold onto the penis, or use clamps or string tried to the penis to prevent retraction. (p. 1673)

The differential diagnosis includes Delusional disorder—somatic subtype, body dysmorphic disorder, panic disorder, schizophrenia, organic delusional disorder, and sexual disorder not otherwise specified.

[58]. A. M. Cortell: Apropos the first case of koro syndrome in Spain.
Medicina Clinica (Barcilona), 1990, 95(9), 358–359. [Article in Spanish]

Comments on that article: **L. Caballero, L. Iruela, P. E. Munoz, E. Baca: Koro syndrome: 1st case in Spain.**
Medicina Clinica (Barcilona), 1990, 95(13), 519. [Article in Spanish]

[59]. M. Amering, H. Katschnig: Panic attacks and panic disorder in cross-cultural perspective.
Psychiatric Annals, 1990, 20(9), 511–516.

It is a fascinating clinical paper based on epidemiological surveys, clinical data on the panic disorder (PD), and literature survey on culture-bound syndromes to examine whether panic attack exists in other cultures (English, Spanish, and German). They referred to the clinical data from a study of 1168 PD patients in 14 European and North and South American countries, which showed that PD occurred in all the nations. Still, there were differences among cultures concerning its symptomatologic expression. Interestingly they observed similarities between Western PD and panic attacks and the "culture-bound" syndromes of Kayak-Angst (in Greenland and Polar Eskimos) and Koro (in Southeast Asia).

Kayak-Angst is a clinical condition known in East and West Greenland and Polar Eskimos (Gussow, 1963). An acute anxiety state affects hunters when they are out in the sea in their one-person boat hunting for seals, especially on a sunny day with a calm sea. Suddenly the person experiences a violent vegetative reaction, characterized by helplessness, a loss of orientation, and a fear of drowning. The situation subsides if they reach near the shore or when fellow hunters offer help. The authors commented that panic attacks' expression depends on specific cultural patterns of norms and values, culture-specific concepts of time, and emotional labeling states' semantic issues. Disentangling many of these components is the task of future cross-cultural research on panic anxiety.

KORO LITERATURE: From 1991 to 2000

Preamble: A total of 68 Koro and related publications are discussed in this time frame, thus indicating the increasing medical and academic psychiatric concern regarding Koro. Among these, the significant issues are:

1. Koro is reported from new geographical regions like the Middle East (Amman, Riyadh, Jeddah, Qatar); Nepal, New Zealand, Ireland, Russia, Sri Lanka, and South Korea.
2. Contribution from Urology—there are few Koro case reports from urogenital clinical facilities that strengthen our insight about the diverse presentation of Koro in association with organic pathology.
3. There are eight letters in response to the article by Bernstein and Gaw (1990). These letters unfold many exciting facts regarding Koro viz. body dimorphic disorder, secondary psychiatric morbidities, and

Koro's nosological status, including one proposition of Koro being a "cultural variant of hysteria."

4. Relation of Koro with forensic presentation—two case reports reviewed—one from the USA and the other from New Zealand. After Palth's similar Koro report in 1937, these two repotting focused on the forensic significance of Koro.
5. The report of an epidemic of "penis-loss" in Nigeria by Dr. S. T. C. Illechukwu is a finding with a far-reaching transcultural significance in this field. It may be regarded as a Koro-variant presentation of a Mass Psychogenic Illness.
6. The discussion paper by Dr. Raymond Prince on the cultural cognition of fox-spirit and Koro in Hainan Island (China) gives a new impetus in favor of the culture-boundness of Koro and provides a unique conceptual bridge between psychiatric morbidity and traditional beliefs of anthropological interest.
7. The paper by Dr. Laurence J. Kirmayer on the castration theme and Koro sheds light on this universal phenomenon's transcultural aspect.
8. Koro presentation involving tongue (Malaysia) is a very valuable reporting in this decade.

1991

[1]. A. A. M. Zain, M. Subramanian: Sporadic Koro and material disharmony.
Psychopathology, 1991, 24, 49–52.

It is a case report of Koro in a 36-year-old Malaysian Chinese man in the setting of marital disharmony and sexual rejection. The most unusual feature of the case was the episodic "feeling that his penis was being sucked into his body," occurring once or twice in a week for a year. Each episode, accompanied by the fear of impending death, lasted for about 30 minutes. The authors tried to offer a psychoanalytical explanation for this penile symptom choice from the psychological reaction of disturbed marital relations, namely the defense mechanism of repression and dissociation. Two clinical observations are important here: the continued maladjustment with heightened anxiety that triggered the Koro perception, and the fear of "insanity" as an ideational component in addition to death. They suggest a scheme of classification of genital retraction symptoms to distinguish between epidemic and sporadic forms of Koro and Koro as a symptom (of mental illness) and Koro syndrome (with underlying psychiatric illness). The authors assert that the present case is a unique example of how marital disharmony and associated conflicts like the perception of adultery (of wife) could precipitate the Koro syndrome in a person with a preexisting anxiety state in a conducive culture that endorses Koro as severe sexual morbidity.

[2]. E. Chen: Drug-induced Koro in a non-Chinese man.
British Journal of Psychiatry, 1991, 158, 721. (L)

It is a Koro case report of a 69-year-old married Englishman referred from a surgical ward with urethral trauma. "He had inserted a knitting needle into his urethra in the belief that his penis was shrinking into his abdomen, thus obstructing urine flow." The patient was on L-dopa therapy for his idiopathic Parkinsonism. The author presented this case as a Koro symptom complex in the context of an organic psychosis (depression with auditory and visual hallucination) caused by L-dopa therapy. The delusion of genital shrinkage was present for about two months. Koro's ideational component was the blockage of urinary flow from the shrinking penis, not the usual "fear of death." The author suggested that the belief that the penile shrinkage would lead to obstruction of urine outflow may reflect a pathoplastic effect on the aged Koro patient (also referred to as the same concept reported by Anderson (BJP, 1990, 157: 142–144).

[3]. R. Durst, P. Rosca-Rebaudengo: The disorder named koro.
Behavioural Neurology, 1991, 4(1), 1–13.

It is a well-written, good descriptive paper on Koro from Israel. The authors discussed Koro's culture-boundness in South-East Asian countries and compared them to the sporadic cases in the Western hemisphere concerning psychiatric, systemic, and neurological disorders. The account is very informative to all Koro researchers. The authors discussed the topic with essential sub-headings: Definition and symptomatology, Etymological and geographical background, Historical root, Cultural pathogenesis, Personality predisposition, Epidemics, Sporadic cases, and Therapeutic modalities. It also contains an exhaustive reference list. It is a valuable review of Koro and would be helpful to all Koro researchers.

[4]. R. C. Simons: Mechanism and classification of Koro.
American Journal of Psychiatry, 1991, 148, 959. (L)

In response to the article of Bernstein and Gaw (1990), in this letter, the author corrected the quotes of the citation: "a self-incrementing causal loop" in place of "a self-incriminating causal loop," erroneously referred to by Bernstein and Gaw (AJP, 1990).

[5]. A. Lipschitz: Mechanism and classification of Koro.
American Journal of Psychiatry, 1991, 148, 959. (L)

It is a letter in response to the paper of Bernstein and Gaw (AJP, 1990). As Bernstein and Gaw proposed, the author opposes Koro's distinct categorization as a "genital retraction disorder, culture-specific" for DSM-IV. He feels that Koro's categorization would not be within scope when it occurs with other disorders, such as body dysmorphic disorders or dysmorphophobia, or obsessive–compulsive disorders. In support of the placement of Koro under obsessive–compulsive disorder, he said:

> … Koro may well be a form of obsessive-compulsive disorder; segregating it into a unique class would obscure its unity with other somatoform disorders that also occur in sporadic, epidemic, and endemic fashion and would inhibit its response to the serotonergic drugs that are effective in treating other diseases of the obsessive-compulsive disorder spectrum. (p. 959)

[6]. W. F. Sheeley: Mechanism and Classification of Koro.
American Journal of Psychiatry, 1991, 148, 959. (L)

It is a letter in response to the article by Bernstein and Gaw (AJP, 1990). The author is against a new culture-specific category for Koro in DSM-IV and believes that: "Hippocrates would presumably have called Koro a cultural variant of hysteria," and that can nicely be fitted into the present DSM classification.

[7]. R. L. Bernstein, A. C. Gaw: Mechanism and Classification of Koro.
American Journal of Psychiatry, 1991, 148, 959–960. (L)

It is a letter in response to the criticisms and suggestions of Simons (AJP, 1991), Lipschitz (AJP, 1991), and Sheeley (AJP, 1991) on the authors' article. The authors had earlier discarded Koro's proposal as an example of body dysmorphic disorder because they asserted that in body dysmorphic condition, the primary preoccupation is "with some imagined defect in appearance." In contrast, in Koro, the central concern is the fear of genital retraction/dissolution and eventual death, not with the genital appearance. Despite the presence of a hysterical component in Koro, they rejected the view to label Koro as hysteria because this term has been deleted from the current classification system.

[8]. B. Kennedy, G. R. Flick: Classification of Koro.
American Journal of Psychiatry, 1991, 148, 1278–1279. (L)

It is a letter in response to the article by Bernstein and Gaw (1990). The authors point out the association between panic disorder and Koro. They illustrated the case of a 21-year-old Caucasian male who had Koro symptoms at the background of a history of six-month-long episodic anxiety attacks (both somatic and psychological components with fear of death). He also had a one-month history of severe depressive symptoms, a mitral valve prolapse diagnosis, and "lazy-eye" syndrome. The patient was put on imipramine for depression when he developed hesitancy and strain on urination and pain (on day 12), along with fear of penile retraction. He had also had similar genital retraction fears six years earlier when he used a vibrator two to three times for masturbation. He had intense masturbatory guilt and a history of panic-like symptoms while masturbating 3 to 4 years earlier.

The authors argue that the fear of genital retraction, in this case, was not culture-bound. They think, "The symptom was related to conditions that increase sympathetic tone, i.e., guilt and anxiety about sexual practices, penile manipulation, anticholinergic medication, and a predisposition to high-anxiety states." So, the proposed classification by Bernstein and Gaw (1990) may be overly restrictive because the "genital retraction might be a multifactorial symptom rather than a specific disorder."

[9]. S. H. A. Sajjad: Classification of Koro.
American Journal of Psychiatry, 1991, 148, 1279. (L)

This is a letter in response to Koro's classification for DSM-IV proposed by Bernstein and Gaw (1990). Given Koro's occurrence in different parts of the world, the author rejects the plea of treating Koro as a culture-bound illness. In support of this, the author analyzes the Koro orthography and cultural belief differences between China's social systems and the Malay Archipelago and between the East and West. The author prefers the term "genital retraction syndrome" in place of Koro. He also argues against Bernstein and Gaw's (1990) comments that "fear of impending death" should not be the only inclusion criterion for Koro diagnosis since other fears are relatively common, like fear of sex change or severe illness. Finally, he differs from the proposition of Bernstein and Gaw (1990) that fear of genital retraction or death is primary and anxiety is secondary in Koro since he asserts that:

> In most of the cases described in the Western literature, the patients have been under considerable stress and anxiety before developing the syndrome. The focus of anxiety is directed onto the genital area for various psychological or organic reasons, and this then predominates the clinical presentation. (p. 1279)

So he proposes that the Axis I diagnosis should be that of primary disorder, and the genital retraction syndrome should be a secondary diagnosis if the criteria are met.

[10]. D. J. Stein, M. Frenkel, E. Hollander: Classification of Koro. *American Journal of Psychiatry, 1991, 148, 1280.* (L)

This is a letter in response to the article by Bernstein and Gaw (1990). The authors think that there already exists a proper category in DSM-IIIR for the inclusion of Koro., viz. body dysmorphic disorder or delusional disorder-somatic type, depending on whether it is of delusional intensity or not.

The authors favor dual diagnosis if so warranted, e.g., if fear of genital retraction fits into body dysmorphic disorder or somatic type delusional disorder and is independent of another axis I disorder, then both the diagnosis should be recorded. For example, if a case of obsessive–compulsive disorder develops viral encephalitis, then both the diagnosis is recorded. They criticized the possible diagnostic options for Koro by Bernstain and Gaw (1990) as (1) A physical condition; (2) A special Axis I disorder, (3) Genital retraction disorder, culture-specific, and (4) Genital retraction disorder, not culture-specific. They doubted that whether there is any need for a separate berth for "genital retraction syndrome, not culture-specific" at all, because in their opinion:

> It appears that further research is required to establish the validity of this entity as distinct from body dysmorphic disorder, delusional disorder, somatic type and obsessive-compulsive disorder. (p. 1280)

They also raised a question with the label "culture specific" as Bernstein and Gaw (1990) suggested. They think that the symptoms may have different implications and meanings in a different culture and other disorders not with a tag of cultural specificity, for example, anorexia nervosa, then escapes its culture-dependent body image perception. They support neither the validity of the entity "genital retraction syndrome, cultural-specific" as a distinct diagnosis nor the implicit meaning of "culture-specific" as advocated by Bernstein and Gaw (1990). The critical suggestion they provided for Koro is noteworthy:

> the authors work on koro makes an important contribution to the evolving conceptualization of the spectrum of body dysmorphic disorder.... Conversely, the literature on body dysmorphic disorder and delusional disorder, somatic type, may be helpful to those interested in koro. The response of body dysmorphic disorder to serotonergic medications (Hollander et al., 1989), for example, suggests that such medication may be useful in treatment of koro. (p. 1280)

[11]. R. L. Bernstein, A. C. Gaw: Classification of Koro.
American Journal of Psychiatry, 1991, 148, 1280. (L)

This is a letter of clarification by the authors about the points raised by Kennedy and Flick (AJP, 1991), Sajjad (AJP, 1991), and Stein et al. (AJP, 1991).

The authors support Kennedy and Flick's (1991) contention that a concurrent diagnosis of panic disorder is justified in genital retraction syndrome associated with panic disorder. Notwithstanding the universality of genital retraction complaints suggested by Sajjad (1991), the authors highlight the unique cultural situation where Koro occurs in endemic or epidemic proportions by the descriptive term "culture-specific." They also believe that although anxiety is an essential component in Koro, the form and content of the disorder's dramatic presentation appropriately justifies the nomenclature "genital retraction disorders."

The authors are against the proposition of placing Koro under body dysmorphic disorder (BDD). In BDD the primary psychopathological concern is with a "static appearance" (imagined defect in physical appearance in a normal-appearing person), while in Koro, the central preoccupation is with an "active transformation" (active sag or dissolution of the genitals) of a body part. Moreover, they believe a marked disruption of social and occupational functioning in genital retraction disorder but it is not so markedly common in body dysmorphic disorder. They object to the inclusion of Koro under delusional disorder, somatic type, as the perception of penile shrinkage in Koro is not delusional. Still, it occurs in persons having clear insight and with intact ego functions.

[12]. Koro classification and case reports.
American Journal of Psychiatry, December 1991, 148(12), 1765–1767. (L)

Three letters were published in response to Bernstein & Gaw's (AJP, 1990, 147: 1670–1674) proposal on Koro classification for DSM-IV.

The first letter was by D. A. Fishbain from the USA (pp. 1765–1766) and offered valuable insight into Koro's classification. The author argued with the reference of 26 Koro cases reported from non-Chinese/non-Indonesian patients about the significance of the clinical difference between culture-bound Koro in Chinese/Indonesian culture and Koro in Western culture. He pointed out at least two criteria: attempt of mechanical restraining of retracting penis and fear of death, are cardinal signs for culture-boundness. In Western culture—the feeling of penile retraction offers several clinical options. It may be a delusion or an overvalued idea or symptom of other psychiatric disorders like depression, anxiety, and any of these could be a monosymptomatic hypochondriacal psychosis. He believes that placing Koro under somatoform disorder offers more flexibility to explore these dimensional symptom differences.

The second letter was by J. L. Fabian from Canada (p. 1766): He reported a Koro case from a non-Asian culture (though the exact ethnicity of the case was not mentioned) and argued against the culture-boundness of Koro. The case was a 38-year married man referred for evaluation of sexual dysfunction. He previously consulted a sexologist and a urologist for his premature ejaculation complaints, from which he was suffering for many years. In the last two years, he developed erectile difficulties that heavily impacted his marital relation. He also recently noticed (no timeline was given) that his penis was shrinking and penetrating his abdomen. This caused him highly anxious with the fear of "serious physical damage." A diagnosis of delusional disorder, the somatic type was made. He did not continue his psychiatric follow-up. After two years, he developed a major depressive episode without any complaints of Koro symptoms' and responded well with desipramine (300 mg/day).

In this case, the author stressed the importance of non-culture boundness (of Asian culture) and raised the doubt that the diagnosis of affective disorder was probably missed in the first consultation.

The third letter was by R. K. Chadda and S. Shome from India (pp. 1766–1767). They reported a 20-year older adult with episodic and situational penile shrinkage at the background of depressive disorder NOS. Penile shrinkage occurred only during exercise and during the act of micturition and returns to normal after 10–15 minutes. He was also having guilt over masturbation and was very fearfully preoccupied with the thoughts of losing his masculinity. The authors pointed out the role of physiological factors in penile morphology and consequent psychosexual anxiety reaction in sporadic Koro-like cases, which very definitely differs from the classical presentation of Koro.

1992

[13]. I. Heyman, T. A. Fahy: Koro-like symptoms in a man infected with human Immunodeficiency virus.
British Journal of Psychiatry, 1992, 160, 119–121.

It is a Koro case report in a 32-year older adult with a depressive illness (suicidal ideas, BDI score at admission was 34) and infection with human immunodeficiency virus. The history of depression was of a recurrent nature of five years duration. The relationship within the family was strained because the patient had disclosed his teenage homosexual habit. Since the age of 16, he has had multiple male sexual partners. Premorbidly, he showed an extreme concern with his physical appearance and health. During the first week in the hospital, he developed dysmorphic concern about an imaginary skin eruption, which a dermatologist could not substantiate. He also had a transient belief that his brain was dehydrating. He had a firm conviction that his penis had gradually been shrinking over the previous three months. He felt that it might disappear altogether, for which he made several visual scrutinies of the penis daily. He responded reasonably well with dothiepin (150 mg/day) and cognitive psychotherapy. On discharge, his BDI score was 14, and follow-up for eight months showed no recurrence of penile shrinkage belief.

The authors state that the patient's hypochondrial belief's prominence had a pathoplastic influence on the Koro-like symptom manifestation. They propose that somatic awareness and health consciousness may be the common clinical feature in patients who suffer from Koro or Koro-like symptoms. In classical Koro, these concerns are exaggerated and molded by culture-specific ideas, whereas in Koro-like syndromes, the final presentation is generated by psychotic or anxiety-related beliefs.

[14]. W. S. Tseng, K. M. Mo, L. S. Li, G. Q. Chen, L. W. Qu, H. B. Zheng: Koro epidemics in Guangdong, China, A questionnaire survey.
Journal of Nervous & Mental Disease, 1992, 180, 117–123.

It is a very valuable survey of Koro patients of the Guangdong epidemic about symptom manifestation, personality profile, life problems, and folk beliefs of the cases. The authors compare the findings of 214 Koro cases (173 men and 41 women) with a clinic group ($n = 56$) of neurosis cases (neurasthenia and anxiety disorder) and 153 normal subjects. They use the following tools: symptom checklist for minor psychiatric disorders of Derogatis et al. (1971), Cattell's 16 personality factor test, and life problem questionnaire. The last one contains three sections with 14 questions, viz. sex-related beliefs, Koro-related beliefs, and supernatural beliefs. The study results revealed that the anxiety and phobic subscale values in Koro patients were considerably elevated than those of the control group.

Regarding personality traits, Koro patients showed less intelligence and no significant life problems in males. There were higher scores on economic issues and disease and death in female cases than in the other two groups. Sex-related beliefs showed no significant difference among the groups. Still, in Koro-related thoughts, the Koro patients showed substantial positive endorsement on ideas of penile shrinkage and death and also in the existence of supernatural beliefs.

The authors believe that Koro's primary clinical feature is anxiety, which expresses a panic reaction because of their folk beliefs. They note some risk factors, e.g., young age, unmarried men, and low education.

The authors try to postulate a theory of social stress as the root cause of Koro's mass expression in the Guangdong area. In support of this contention, they identified some concomitant social disturbances with each Koro outbreak. For example, the 1952 epidemic was related to land reform after Communist liberation. The 1962 epidemic was concurrent with the economic changes associated with the "Great Leap Forward" movement. The 1966 epidemic occurred during the high point of the Cultural Revolution, and the 1974 epidemic was related to an outbreak of encephalitis. The authors suggest that community mental health education focusing on high-risk groups may minimize Koro's epidemic occurrence.

[15]. M. G. Smyth, C. Dean: Capgras and Koro.
British Journal of Psychiatry, 1992, 161, 121–123.

It is an unusual case report of Koro with Capgras syndrome with an underlying affective disorder in a 23-year-old West Indian. He was diagnosed as a case of an acute psychotic state with features of paranoia, Capgras misidentification, and Koro. The patient identified his father as an "imposter" and clutched his penis to fear its disappearance into the abdomen. Besides the delusional misidentification, he also had a depressed mood and threatening second-person auditory hallucination and hypomania history three years earlier. He responded favorably to thioridazine.

The authors attempt to explain the commonality between Capgras and Koro in respect of depersonalization and body image disturbances. They state that depersonalization is partial in Koro while it is projected in Capgras. From the broader perspectives of body image disorder, they postulated that in Koro, the disturbance is in the localized body part, while in the misidentification syndrome, it involves the "internal and external change in physical or psychological identity" of a person. They also point out that the non-culture bound Koro cases to lack the classical presentation, viz. penile retraction, and concurrent disappearance of it into the abdomen and fear of death. They also stress the importance of mood disorder in the background of both Koro and Capgras syndrome.

[16]. M. Hotopf, R. Mullen: Koro and Capgras syndrome in a non-Chinese subject.

British Journal of Psychiatry, 1992, 161, 577. (L)

It is a short letter in response to Smyth & Dean's report (BJP, 1992) on "Capgras and koro." The authors argued the difference between the Koro as a culture-bound illness in South-East Asia and China (with its solid cultural predilection) and Western societies. They cautioned that it would be "misguided to use a sporadic case-report from the Western literature to challenge the basis for Koro as a distinct nosological entity in the Far East."

[17]. S. T. C. Ilechukwu: Magical penis loss in Nigeria: Report of a recent epidemic of a Koro-like syndrome.

Transcultural Psychiatric Research Review, 1992, 29, 91–108.

This is an excellent report of an epidemic of "magical penis loss" from Nigeria in the last part of 1990. The affected subjects complained that their external genitalia had simply vanished, and the author described this entity as a "Koro-like syndrome." This epidemic case's spectacular clinical expression was the sudden perception of the sufferer that the penis (sometimes breast in females) had vanished because they were "taken" by magically influential persons or their agents. A four-stage sequence of this genital loss phenomenon has been identified: cue, flash, cheek, and alarm. They provided the most spectacular description of this African penis vanishing saga. In the author's colorful description, the sequences are as follows:

The "cue" (usually a stranger asking for time or seeking a conversation) followed by "flash" (sudden feeling like an electric shock affecting the genitals) and "check" (personal checking to discover the loss of genitalia). The last one is the calling alarm for help, where others jumped him to recover his genitals. In Lagos, the typical alarm was "*ole! Oko mi ti too!*" (*"Thief! My genitals are gone!"*). This sequence of events is very nicely drafted by the author as follows:

1. Cue represents the cortical limbic phase and is influenced by cultural beliefs, social class, and personal pathology.
2. Flash represents the vegetative phase and is characterized by the fear response and vegetative signs like cardiovascular, visceral, cremasteric, and dartos muscle reflexes.
3. Check which represents the focusing phase and is characterized by heightened arousal and elaboration of genital sensations.
4. Alarm which represents the final manifest phase, is characterized by stereotypical reporting and behavior.

Others also mishandled this issue. The syndrome was believed to be a supernatural event where the affected were robbed of their genitalia to benefit interested people. People, usually a "lynch minded mob," identified the genital thief, who were commonly "prosperous looking strangers" or women, and they were maltreated (beating, clubbing, or even burning), which caused even bodily severe injuries. "It was held that the rougher the treatment, the more likely it was that the 'thief' would relent and return the seized genital." The crowd response helped the spread of the message of penis loss from Lagos to other urban centers like lbadan, but skipping the rural areas, and people in the streets were so afraid of genital theft that:

> Man could be seen in the streets of Lagos holding on to their genitalia either openly or discretely with their hands in their pockets. Women were also seen holding on to their breasts directly or discretely by crossing the hands across the chest. It was thought that inattention and a weak will facilitated the 'taking' of the penis or breasts. Vigilance and anticipatory aggression were thought to be good prophylaxis. This led to further breakdown of law and order. (p. 96)

This epidemic took place in the background of severe economic depression amidst speculation about currency change and the election of a non-military government. The author hypothesizes that this epidemic was the mass expression of male resentment over women's success during a period of social turmoil and strain and "the symbolic equation of masculine sexuality with economic-social and creative prowess in many cultural myths."

The author also provides four typical case histories, of which two had preexisting psychopathologies. The first one is a police constable; the alleged thief was a butcher. The second one was a 17-year-old Igbo trader's apprentice, and the alleged thief was an unknown person. The third one was a 23-year single Igbo businessman with preexisting sexual anxiety. The fourth one was a 24-year-old engineering student (had preexisting depression). The alleged thief was an older woman. The analysis of the epidemic reveals that there were both genuine and fictitious cases. The latter was part of a deliberate plan of well-organized gangs to rob affluent persons. The actual cases had the subjective feeling of the disappearance of the penis with a mark of the influence of magico-supernatural faith in mysterious touch or of accumulation of personal power by taking others' sex organs or sorcery. There is a short discussion on the psycho-anthropological and mythological significance of male dominance and phallic symbolism in the Nigerian psycho-social belief system. Lastly, the author attempts a phenomenological correlation between Koro and the magical penis-loss event. He believes that both express a common denominator, viz., the genitally focused primordial anxieties.

[18]. R. H. Prince: A symposium on the Vulnerable Male: Cultural Variations on the Castration theme, Introduction.
Transcultural Psychiatric Research Review, 1992a, 29, 87–90.

It is an introductory paper on the objectives of a symposium devoted to the discussion on the castration theme and the male vulnerability, held by the McGill Division on Social and Transcultural Psychiatry, Montreal, June 20, 1991.

The author provides a brief transcultural account of male sexual anxiety syndromes like Koro or suk-young in China and Dhat or Jiryan in India. He asserts that the male fears of penis loss or loss of potency are prevalent. It usually takes the clinical expression at par with the cultural meaning of any given society. He stresses that despite an age-old emphasis on the male castrator's construct, the female castrator is much more common in different socio-cultural themes. He cites examples in this favor, viz., the implications of females in witchcraft of fifteenth-century Germany, the attribution of fox spirit in the disguise of a woman in Koro in Hainan Island, China, the mythological construct of Adam in the middle-east and the fantasy of a "poisoned maiden" of Indian and Persian cultures. He cites an extraordinary example of a female castrator in the form of "vagina dentate" (the vagina with teeth) fantasy of the Amerindian culture. Many authors discussed Koro as a castration fear, so these introductory comments help all Koro researchers.

[19]. R. H. Prince: Koro and the Fox Spirit on Hainan Island (China).

Transcultural Psychiatric Research Review, 1992b, 29, 119–132.

It is an outstanding discussion paper with a wealth of information on Koro's cultural dynamics, especially in the context of the Chinese Yin-Yang philosophy. The first part gives a brief overview of Koro symptomatology that ranges from Dr. Slot's previous report on the Celebes to the recent one of Hainan Island, China. He also analyzes the Indonesian and Chinese Koro expressions' phenomenological differences and their ritualistic healing methods. The second part summarizes the recent Koro epidemics of Singapore, Thailand, India, and China, emphasizing the concurrent geopolitical stresses in each country.

The first part is devoted to the detailed analysis of the Hainan Island Koro epidemic, emphasizing the cultural construct of fox spirit in causing Koro. The author provides an excellent anthropological account of the fox-spirit theme in Sino-Japanese folklores and attempts to corroborate its significance with Hainan's cases' Koro cognition. With citations from van Gulik (1961), he analyzes the traditional folk beliefs that animals like foxes, badgers, and tortoises are endowed with long lives and supernatural abilities because of their contact with the "cosmic vital essence" of earth. A detailed description of the magical and mystic powers of the fox has enumerated in one of the Tang dynasty (618–906 AD) records as follows (Gulik, 1961):

> When a fox is fifty years old, it assumes the ability to change itself into a woman. At a hundred it can assume the shape of a beautiful girl, or that of a sorcerer, or also that of an adult man who has sexual intercourse with women. All that age a fox knows what is happening at a distance of one thousand miles, it can derange the human mind and reduce a person to an imbecile. When the fox is one thousand years old, it is in communication with Heaven, and is when called Heavenly Fox *(t'ien-hu)*. (p. 210)

The folk belief regards that the fox is a yin creature who wants to transform into a celestial fox (*tengu*) for entry into heaven. The most crucial thing for this is collecting a male or yang principle, the penis being one such suitable object. Hence, the fox spirit desperately searches the penis for its necessity.

The Japanese fox lore also endorses the belief that at the age of 500, the fox will change its colour from red to white, and at 1000 years, it will disappear from the earth, although it may return to cause natural havoc in the form of thunder and lightning. The author traces a symbolic similarity between this Sino-Japanese folklore and the name of the "Leizhour" peninsula of Guangdong province. Leizhou means "thunder region."

The author analyzed the Chinese Yin-Yang humoral theory and folk beliefs of fox spirit and the Indonesian and Malaysian cultural beliefs in vengeful female ghosts. He concludes that there is "a pan-human male dread of castration and sexual importance" where the female figure represents the threat as castrator rather than the male figure depicted in the oedipal myth. This unconscious fear has a crucial psychodynamic significance in the symptom choice of genital retraction and its accompanying fear of death.

This discussion is an elegant masterpiece that provides a conceptual bridge between psychiatric morbidity and traditional anthropological beliefs. This is more so because, for the first time, Koro—an illness very often cited as a culture-bound syndrome—is analyzed in the background of specific cultural content in the real sense, viz., belief in the evil fox spirit. This discussion on the fox spirit's cultural beliefs highlights and readdresses the Koro phenomenon as really a culture-bound illness. This is a unique theoretical reinforcement to the weaning cultural significance attached to Koro.

[20]. L. J. Kirmayer: From the Witches' Hammer to the Oedipus Complex: Castration Anxiety in Western Society.
Transcultural Psychiatric Research Review, 1992, 29, 133–158.

This is an elegant and comprehensive analysis of the theme of castration anxiety, including its universality, variability, and meaning across the cultures. In his attempt to explore the dynamics of castration anxiety and sexual identity in culture-related illnesses of oriental societies like Koro, Dhat syndrome, or magical penis loss, the author also cites an equivalent clinical entity in Western culture. In the elucidation of these similarities, he mentions four critical dimensions of socio-cultural cognitive constructs as follows:

1. Cultural differences in modes of thought;
2. Different ethno-physiological theories regarding specific bodies vulnerabilities and the meaning of distress;
3. Universal psychodynamic principles at the background of unconscious fantasies and fears of castration, and
4. The contribution of socio-cultural male role in creating gender-related anxiety in vulnerable individuals.

The author stresses the role of conversion and its changing symptom profile about the perception of penis loss and Koro. He argues that with the advent of bio-medical care, the classical hysterical symptom manifestations only changed in presentation but not in prevalence. The dynamics of dissociative psychological mechanisms of conversion disorder is changing or replaced by "physiological dysregulation due to emotional conflict or social stress." "This process," he further adds, "would tend to affect both men and women equally." The author mentioned various forms of somatization or hysterical equivalents, irrespective of "medical legitimation and delegitimation," reflecting sexual anxiety. He cites the example of the North American epidemic of chronic fatigue syndrome in this context, which is a reflection of fear or loss of potency by the individual in the broadest sense. Thus, sexual-distress perception and its clinical presentation depending on the cultural reference of beliefs and practices in a society.

The author provides a rich discussion on various ethno-physiological influences on castration anxiety expression in different cultures. He cites examples of semen-conservation doctrine, sexual restraining, masturbatory guilt, and psychosexual anxieties in support of the cultural specificity. The "mythic wound" section contains a thoughtful discussion on phallic symbolism in mythology and iconography. The author forwards the most exciting and academic argument is the mother's primal fear or the theme of "castrating female" unlike the commonly accepted theory of male (father) castrator in the genesis of male sexual anxiety. This valuable insight of "fear of the feminine" is a research endeavor necessary for a meaningful understanding of sexual tension in vulnerable males and the varied forms of a male predicament in the present-day world. Like the psychoanalytical theme, Kirmayer also attaches equal importance to social roles in male sexual anxiety genesis. He asserts a dual influence, i.e., the castration anxiety and male social role in the genesis of male sexual anxiety. He maintains the masculine existential concern as follows:

> What polarizes the sexes may be partly biology but it is also surely the asymmetry in social roles. Both sexes have similar existential concerns: the struggle to bind a balance between active and passive, aggressive and receptive, containing and being contained. But social roles privilege one side for each sex and force the individual to hide his or her conflicts with role-appropriate behaviour. Thus, the man who feels his own passivity too clearly is ashamed and struggles to regain his own phallic power. The bedrock of castration anxiety then is not only a psychodynamic problem but a social problem – his disqualification or disavowal of the feminine. (p. 146)

The author explains the theme of castration anxiety in its broader perspective ("power, potency, and physical endowment") in North American society. He critically analyzes the male gender anxiety from the developmental and upbringing perspectives of Western societies. A father's absence is becoming a harsh reality in the typical family unit of technologically advanced societies. That prompts the author to say,

"The American male then is doubly bereft: he lacks his father to initiate him into the male role and lacks male mentors to nurture and validate his manhood." A stepwise analysis shows how the psychodynamic relevance of Oedipal anxiety has changed with the changing socioeconomic pattern of society. The expanding orbit of Oedipal anxiety, in this process, eventually equates sexual fear with death.

In conclusion, the author discusses the role of ethno-physiological ideas in culture-specific syndromes. He stresses the dual influence of psychodynamics and the social-interactional dispositions on the cultural cognition of culture-bound syndromes. He interprets the male vulnerability toward sexual anxiety in the post-traditional society as the "anxiety of influence," a desperate attempt of the male to free from his father image for easing the expression of his individual spectrum in its totality.

[21]. S. B. Menezes: A case of Koro and folie a deux in a Shona family.
South African Medical Journal, 1992, 82(6), 483.

It is a Koro case report of a 31-year-old black man from a Shona family, a Zambian immigrant in London. Six years earlier, he made pregnant a teenage girl and fled from Zambia to Zimbabwe to avoid civil marriage. Subsequently, he married another woman. For a considerable period (the time not mentioned), he consulted various traditional healers (*nyangas*), general practitioners, and churches because he felt that his penis was being pulled into his abdomen. On the advice of a traditional healer, he returned to Zambia, where he had a mental breakdown, and then returned to the UK and was hospitalized. On examination, he was found with depression, paranoid features with depersonalization, and auditory hallucination. He was very anxious and holding his penis to prevent shrinking into the abdomen. His wife was also very worried and shared the same belief. He was diagnosed with psychotic depression and was treated successfully with thioridazine and amitriptyline. At three months, he was symptom-free, and his wife was happy to have normal sexual relations.

Analysis of the psychodynamics of this case unfolds a rich cultural element. In Shona culture, there is a strong belief that extramarital sexual activity may lead to the disappearance of the male sex organ. To prevent that, one has to compensate the wronged woman with some traditional rituals. The patient believed that his former traditional wife cast a *kusunga* (a protective lock from infidelity), and his penis was shrinking now as a consequence of his second marriage. It is a belief in Shona culture that *kusunga* might be reactivated after crossing a river. The patient had a mental breakdown soon after crossing the Livingstone Bridge to enter Zambia. This case may alternatively be labeled as Secondary Koro, but the cultural ideational element is quite exciting and offered a rich explanatory framework for "Shona Koro" perception.

[22]. H. Montaser: Koro-like symptoms in Saudi patient.
Arab Journal of Psychiatry, 1992, 3(1): 56–60.

It is a case report of Koro-like symptoms in a 20-year, single Saudi national from Riyadh. He has a very complex psychosexual history. At age 16, he developed the belief that his penis is smaller than average. This conviction compelled him to visit many clinical facilities without any benefit. After reading an article on hermaphrodism, he felt that his penis is shrinking into the abdomen (but with no fear of death). This idea leads to a "delusional" belief that his gender is changing: developing a womb and a "vaginal entrance at the site of his shrinking penis." A psychometric test showed a high psychotic score, average IQ, and schizoid type premorbid personality. Initial treatment with trifluoperazine 5 mg yields no result. He was admitted, and the dose of trifluoperazine was increased to 30 mg, and after four days of treatment, all symptoms disappeared. He was diagnosed as a case of atypical psychosis as per DSM-IIIR. He had no previous knowledge of Koro nor had any contact with people of Chinese culture. The author pointed out the prevailing Saudi cultural stress on fertility and masculinity and commented that small sexual organ complaints are common among Saudi males.

1993

[23]. R. Durst, A. Teitelbaum, S. Cohen, P. Rosca-Rebaudengo: Koro syndrome-clinical and cultural aspects.
Harefuah, 1993, 124(11), 673–676, 740. [Article in Hebrew]

It is a general descriptive account of Koro similar to their previous publication in 1991. They discussed the epidemic form seen in South East Asian countries and sporadic cases observed in Western societies. They informed that 6 cases of Koro is reported from Israel.

[24]. W. Zeng, G. Mo, G. Chen, L. Li, R, Wen, T. Liu: Social psychiatry and epidemic koro. Comparison of folk belief among young men in Taiwan, Jilin, and Guandong Provinces.
Chinese Mental Health Journal, 1993, 7(1), 38–40. [Article in Chinese]

It is a comparative study about Koro's folk beliefs in three regions of China and Taiwan, at the background of the Koro epidemic in Guangdong Province during 1985 and 1988. The China Koro Research Cooperative Group carried out the investigation by using a "Folk Belief Questionnaire." It was a 14 item questionnaire with multiple-choice items addressed: attitude toward Koro, Koro epidemic, sexual issues, and folk beliefs. The test subjects were as follows: 326 normal male Chinese adolescents (aged 17–20 years) in Taiwan; 128 in Guangdong city; 100 in Jilin province and 98 in Gaoxiong city. Regions and social and cultural factors made comparisons. They noted that both the groups in China (Jilin and Guandong) held the traditional belief in sexual activity related to masturbation and semen conservation. Still, the Taiwan subjects have less faith in these conventional concepts. Regarding Suo-yang, Guangdong subjects, compared to Jilin and Taiwan sample, tended to believe more in the idea of the illness.

[25]. J. K. Zhang, M. X. Zhu: Three case reports of children Koro.
Chinese Journal of Mental Health, 1993, 7, 40–41. [Article in Chinese]

1994

[26]. K. L. Goetz, T. R. Price: A case of koro: treatment response and implications for diagnostic classification.
Journal of Nervous & Mental Disease, 1994, 182 (10), 590–591.

It is a report from Pennsylvania, USA. It is an interesting case of a sporadic Koro at the background of several psychiatric diagnoses and repeated hospital admissions. The patient was a 29 year single white male. He was admitted at the age of 13 after a hit on the abdomen in a fight. Then he developed a conviction that he had developed a hernia, contrary to clinical evidence. Then he developed an extreme preoccupation with the belief that his penis would disappear into his body and that will kill him. He then experimented with different substances like hallucinogens, amphetamine, and heroin. At age 19, he was admitted with a diagnosis of schizophrenia, still with the same complaint. After two years, he was admitted for detoxification with a diagnosis of drug dependency and latent schizophrenia. He continued to have his penile conviction. Then he was treated with several medications, including neuroleptics, benzodiazepines, and tricyclic antidepressants, but without any benefit. Then again admitted for his continuous ruminations regarding his genitals. There was no evidence of psychosis at this admission, and he responded significantly with clomipramine (100 mg p.o. qHS), including resolution of anxiety and significant "decline in his genital preoccupation." The authors suggested that this case is an example of non-culture bound Koro and may be regarded as a body dysmorphic disorder variant. However, the question remains why it is not an example of a solitary obsessive–compulsive disorder that responded well with clomipramine.

[27]. R. A. Adeniran, J. R. Jones: Koro: culture-bound disorder or universal symptom?
British Journal of Psychiatry, 1994, 164(4), 559–561.

It is a case report of Koro from Britain, associated with a depressive illness in a 31-year-old male Briton. It is an exciting account to show how sex guilt culminated in a belief of delusional proportions. The events' sequences were as follows: 18 months history of clinical depression, stopped medications for six weeks and deteriorated and admitted. At the workplace, he was teased by some workmates about being feminine. He discovered that he has homosexual feelings. He started to masturbate and felt depressed. He also believed that a curse is placed on him for his "evil" masturbatory acts. He was agitated, depressed with a delusion of guilt, persecution, and ideas of reference on admission. He was convinced that his penis was retracting and would ultimately disappear, and in that case, he would lose his gender. His penile delusion was further elaborated as his penis had irretrievably retracted, which made him "no longer a real person" and impotent with dead testes. He responded favorably after a course of ECT, in addition to antidepressant and neuroleptic medications.

Observation: The authors very elegantly analyze this Koro-like symptom with the psychodynamic formulation: here, the operating force behind the symptom choice is the masculine power and potency at the background of depressive, negative self-image. Interesting to note the symptoms of "no gender," "no sperm," or "dead testes" are like nihilistic delusion. This case is an excellent example of sporadic Koro-secondary in nature from Western culture.

[28]. G. Wolff, K. McKenzie: Capgras, Fregoli and Cotard's syndromes and Koro in folie à deux.
British Journal of Psychiatry, 1994, 165(6), 842. (L)

This is a fascinating and rare report where all five clinical syndromes (Capgras; Koro-like symptoms, Fregoli's syndrome; folie a deux, and Cotard's syndrome) were present in a 58-year-old man with evidence of cognitive impairment, including impairment of facial recognition. He had a conviction that the penis is shrinking and would disappear inside the abdomen, and he would die with a feeling that his head was also shrinking. Initially, he responded with antipsychotic medications (misidentification syndrome) but developed depression with prominent nihilistic delusion—believing his body parts are not working (Cotard's syndrome). He has improved with ECTs and antidepressants.

[29]. G. S. Ungvari, R. S. Mullen: Koro: The delusion of penile retraction.
Urology, 1994, 43(6), 883–885.

It is a sporadic Koro-like chronic case report from Dunedin, New Zealand, at the background of delusional disorder, somatic type. A 66-year-old man presented with a variety of hypochondriacal symptoms with "vague persecutory delusions." He has a firm conviction that his penis had been gradually shrinking into the abdomen for the last six months, and that indicates a "fatal somatic illness." There was no acute presentation of classical Koro. He was treated with low-dose haloperidol (1.5 mg/day) and showed good improvement by two months. One year follow-up showed no recurrence of symptoms. The authors stressed the importance of clinical evaluation of Koro-like symptoms in diverse clinical associations like psychiatric disorders or urological illness.

[30]. R. E. Bartholomew: The social psychology of "epidemic koro."
International Journal of Social Psychiatry, 1994, 40(1), 46–60.

This is a paper elaborating on the sociological approach toward the Koro epidemic. The author argued that the Koro epidemic is the collective manifestation of the social, cultural, cognitive, and physiological context of Koro-related beliefs. In that sense, it is the expression of mass psychopathology or irrationality. He also questioned the contextual term culture-bound and stressed the non-psychopathological explanation as an attempt to reclassify the Koro epidemic. He postulated that "koro is a rational attempt at problem-solving which involves conformity dynamics, perceptual fallibility and the local acceptance of Koro-associated folk realities, which are capable of explaining such episodes as normal within any given population."

1995

[31]. C. N. Chin, K. H. S'ng: "Koro"—Like syndrome affecting the tongue—A case report.
Medical Journal of Malaysia, 1995, 50(2), 175–177.

It is a fascinating case report of Koro-like symptoms affecting the tongue from Kuala Lumpur, Malaysia. A 52-year married Malay man reported sudden, episodic retraction of his tongue before he is about to fall asleep.

Given two years' duration, it can be termed as a "chronic Koro-like" symptom. This retracting feeling evoked a startle reaction, with intense anxiety and fear. Fear is about potential death; in the event of falling back of the tongue, he would choke and die from suffocation. He prevents this by grasping the tongue with his fingers and often bites the tongue with his teeth. After 10–20 minutes, things become normal, and the retraction stops. The first episode was after work-related stress, and subsequently, it occurs when he has a very talkative day. His wife also believes that this tongue retraction may lead to death, and there is a similar incident in one of his relatives. He had no prior knowledge of Koro. The author adds a new item to the proposed classification by seven "taxon" by Simons (1985) as "tongue retraction taxon."

[32]. A. Puranik, J. Dunn: Koro presenting after prostatectomy in an elderly man.
British Journal of Urology, 1995, 75(1), 108–109.

It is a case report from Kent, UK. A 76-year-old Caucasian man presented with recurrent depressive disorder, who developed Koro symptoms after transurethral resection for prostatic hypertrophy. He had difficulties passing water and believed that his penis would shrink inside the abdomen and die. He was treated with ECTs and fluoxetine. The authors discussed the penile symptoms concerning other urological complaints and mentioned the other three cases of Koro in older men, reported in the English literature: Hawley and Owens in 1988; Anderson in 1990 and Chen in 1991.

[33]. A. Gerlach: Castration anxiety and oral envy in sexual relations. Analytic studies with ethnological observations.
Psyche (Stuttg), 1995, 49(9–10), 965–988. [Article in German]

It is a psychoanalytical paper that tried to explore the psychodynamics of Koro (in an epidemic setting), by using Ethno-psychoanalysis (the study of the unconscious in a foreign culture). According to the author, the repeated Koro epidemic among young unmarried men in Hainan Island, China, is the collective manifestation of overcoming castration anxiety resulted from covert gender envy. He stated: "… the epidemic is in effect a species of rite of passage in which a group of young males makes the communal attempt to overcome castration anxieties which are themselves the product of covert gender envy." He also reported a case from Germany that displayed Koro symptoms.

[34]. S. Cohen, S. Y. Tennenbaum, A. Teitelbaum, and R. Durst: The koro (genital retraction) syndrome and its association with infertility: A case report.
Journal of Urology, 1995, 153(2), 427–428.

It is an interesting case report of Koro associated with infertility at the background of organic pathology and cultural-religious-immigration stress. A 44-year-old man of Jewish Ashkenazi descent presented with an acute psychotic state with heightened anxiety because of his firm conviction that his penis gradually shrinks and disappears inside the abdomen, and eventually, he will die. He also tried to prevent the retraction by pulling the organ repeatedly. He immigrated to the USA. There he had problems of sexual potency and performances with a frequent habit of masturbation. He had bilateral varicoceles and oligoteratoasthenospermia syndrome, and infertility. During the development of his fear of penile retraction, he became paranoid about his family and wife and believed that he was poisoned and robed out of his sexual vitality. He returned to Israel and was hospitalized. His psychiatric diagnosis was acute paranoid psychosis with depressive features associated with Koro syndrome. He is treated with a combination of antipsychotic and tricyclic antidepressant medications, and his Koro symptom is resolved after three weeks and psychotic symptoms after six weeks of treatment. No remission is reported at a 1 year to follow up.

The authors discussed the role of organic pathology, especially urogenital pathology in the development of sporadic Koro cases. They provided a helpful summary table of 6 such reported cases (including this one) as follows: 56 years (Great Britain) with micropenis; 75 years (Singapore) with Inguinal hernia; 38 years (Zululand) with urinary tract infection; 36 years (Jamaican) with swollen testicles; 39 years (Italy) with phimosis and 44 years (Israel) with oligoteratoasthenospermia and varicocele.

[35]. W. M. Schleidt, R. Hamerlinggasse
Journal of Urology, 1995, 154(4), 1484. (L)

In response to: The koro (genital retraction) syndrome and its association with infertility: a case report. By S. Cohen, S. Y. Tennenbaum, A. Teitelbaum, R. Durst. Published in: *Journal of Urology*, 1995, 153(2), 427–428.

It is a short letter citing the case report of the penis' retraction published in Lancet in 1886. The authors discussed the role of temperature and adaptation of the penis from pre-historic ages. The authors also described the evolutionary development of penile signaling in male–male communication as preverbal and nonverbal signaling in pre-historic periods. They shed light on the relationship between stress and infertility, facilitating the link between urology and psychiatry.

[36]. G. M. Mo, G. Q. Chen, L. X. Li, W. S. Tseng: Koro epidemic in Southern China.
In, Chinese societies and mental health (Eds. T. Y. Lin; W. S. Tseng; E. K. Yeh), 1995, pp. 231–243, Oxford University Press, Hong Kong.

This is a chapter (No. 17) in the above book. It is very informative, with a wealth of new information on Koro or *Suo-yang* in China, especially in the Hainan and Leizhou islands. There are many subheadings in the article packed up with lots of information.

They described a detailed history of Suo-yang in China. They cited that the earliest description of *Suo-yang* is in the ancient Chinese medical text *Huangdi Nei Jing* (Yellow Emperor's Classic on Internal Medicine). That described *Suo-yang* as a fatal disease caused by retraction of the *body's yang parts* (protruding organs like penis, breast, nose, tongue, or ears). In another reference from *Yanfang Xinbin* (New Collection of Remedies) written by Pao Siann-Ow in 1834, they mentioned the conceptual component of death fear in *Suo-yang* as: "During intercourse, the man may be seized suddenly with acute abdominal pain. The limbs become cold and the complexion dusky, the penis retreats into the abdomen. If effective treatment is not instituted at once, the man will die."

Subsequently, many Chinese medical texts stressed the dangers of *Suo-yang* and described many associated symptoms very much, similar to panic attacks. They also highlighted different sexual activities (too much intercourse or masturbation) as triggering factors for the development of *Suo-yang*. This construct is closely related to the yin-yang dichotomy—shrinkage of the penis represents an excessive loss of the *yang* element or vital force, causing a severe *yin-yang* imbalance.

In the next chapter, the authors provided a beneficial chronological and historical description of past Koro or Suo-yang epidemics in Hainan Island. These can be summarized as follows:

1. 1862: In *Yazbou Zhi* (local chronicle of Ya state, Hainan) recorded that: "In the eleventh year of the *Xinyou* regime in the Qing dynasty (1862) suo illness had spread; men's genitalia shrank, female's breast, ears, tongues, or other parts shrank. To rub with ginger or set firecrackers off will stop it. Some died from the shrinkage."
2. 1864: In *Dan Xian Zhi* (local chronicle of Dan county, Hainan) recorded that:

> In the second year of the *Tongzhi* reign in the Qing dynasty (1864), a *suo* illness was prevalent in this region. Such patients complained of retraction of ears, noses, hands, feet, male genitalia, and female breasts, with loss of consciousness. It helped if many people beat gongs and drums, pulled the retracted part, fed the patient with ginger soup, then the patient would be cured immediately. This is a strange illness. (p. 232)

3. 1920: French physician L. Legendre, described an "epidemie mentale" from Sichuan, in which many schoolboys had genital retraction. He called it collectively or individually as "Asiatic psychosis" and thought that impotence or inability to reproduce might be an aftermath of this disorder.

After World War II, at least five epidemics took place in this region, and each was associated with some type of socio-economic tension.

4. 1952: *Suo-yang* epidemic took place during the period of land reform.
5. 1962: *Suo-yang* epidemic took place after the Great Leap Forward movement.*
6. 1966: *Suo-yang* epidemic took place during the Cultural Revolution.**
7. 1974: *Suo-yang* epidemic took place along with an outbreak of encephalitis.
8. 1984–1985: *Suo-yang* epidemic took place in an atmosphere of fear when a fortune-teller predicted a bad year. It involved eight counties in Hainan and seven counties in Leizhou—at least 3000 people were affected.
9. 1987: small epidemic involving a few hundred victims
10. 1988: epidemic in Warring county, Hainan involving about 100 patients. A case of tongue retraction was also reported.

Next, they described the physical and population demography of the region. Population-wise it is inhabited by Han nationals and two minority groups—Li and Miao. Most of the population is peasants and fishermen. People are very religious and believe in yin-yang's Traditional Chinese medical concept with sex-related codes and behaviors. They also believe in ghosts searching for the penis, and as fox spirits, ghosts may steal the *yang* force (penis) of men. There are many folklore and community legends regarding mysterious penis stealing stories.

They provided every detail of the epidemiological data of the 1984–1985 epidemics. One interesting fact from Haikang County was the male (84%) and female (16%) distribution among the 195 Suo-yang victims.

Mode of attack: The authors provided a detailed nature of the clinical presentation. 73% *Suo-yang* attacks occurred at night coincided with the prevalent community belief that ghosts often hunted at night. 69% of attacks were preceded by a sensation of chills over the body. Nipple retraction was the sole presentation among the females. No vaginal symptoms were reported. All cases manifested various anxiety symptoms like palpitations (65%), tremors (69%), pallor (51%), and excessive sweating (34%). 62% had a fear of impending death, of which 68% shouted out in fear. 9% of cases had brief disturbances of consciousness. In 60% of cases, the episode lasted about 20–60 minutes. 22% had two attacks; few had more than three attacks. No death was reported.

Community Reaction: A very lively description was given about the different fascinating ways people reacted in the community. Some important details are:

1. At the onset, all people around tried to resuscitate the patient—attempted to pull the penis, suck the nipple or tie the penis with string or the stem of a green yam (full of *yang* force).
2. The female victims were suspected of being possessed by a female ghost or fox spirit (*huli jing*). The victim was covered by a fishing net and severely beaten by a peach tree branch. As a last resort, she might be dipped in the sea for an exorcism.
3. Fatality from folk intervention: Nine fatalities were reported. A child died of asphyxia, a young woman was beaten to death, another woman was drowned at sea, and numerous men suffered penile injuries due to mechanical handling to pull the penis. Some women sustained injury and infection after an iron pin was inserted through their nipples.
4. The whole community became "hysterical" in behavior. Some large groups strike drums, gongs, and made large noises with firecrackers or shoot guns to scare the evil ghosts. Many with swords, knives, or other weapons patrolling the streets, block the village entry point so that no outsider can enter (ghosts might enter the village in the disguise of a human being).

The authors very nicely described the atmosphere of a tense social environment that helped spread the epidemic. The belief in supernatural evil forces among the rural communities helped the epidemic set in, compared to no incidence in urban settlements. They provided a fascinating account of public reaction when ten persons were attacked simultaneously with *Suo-yang*, and miraculous intervention is done by a wise medical man in a Wangwu commune of Dan County in the 1974 epidemic.

The authors then described three research work sets—personality, life problems, and folk beliefs of the victims with control groups. These studies are published elsewhere. They concluded from these researches that:

> … the victims of *koro* are not potentially psychiatric patients. They are ordinary people who, may have slightly less intellectual endowments than average. They are more familiar with and tend to believe in the *suoyang* folk belief and are more susceptible to *suoyang* than their counterparts living in the same community. (p. 240)

They provided pieces of very important research study by comparing folk beliefs (by using 14 items Folk Belief Questionnaire) among three groups of people—one in Jilin in the north-eastern part of China, Guangdong, and Taiwan. They noted both the groups in China held the traditional belief in sexual activity (sexual activity should be carefully protected for health, excessive masturbation harms the body, semen needs careful conservation). Still, Taiwan subjects have less belief in these traditional concepts. Regarding Suo-yang, Guangdong subjects tended to believe more in the illness compared to Jilin and Taiwan sample.

The last part addressed "culture, belief, and epidemic" and compared Singapore, Thailand, and India's epidemic backgrounds. They opined that though some inter-ethnic conflict issues or racial tension were present in those countries, no such factor was observed in the Guangdong outbreak. They also stressed that the age-old social and cultural folk belief concerning sex and death probably provided the basis of the epidemic. They concluded the presentation by emphasizing the role of social intervention to prevent or mitigate such outbreaks.

[*The Great Leap Forward was an economic and social campaign by the Communist Party of China, PRC, from 1958 to 1962. That aimed to transform the country from an agrarian economy into a socialist society by industrialization and collectivization.

**The Cultural Revolution was a sociopolitical movement by the Chinese Communist Party, PRC, from 1966 to 1976, intending to preserve Chinese communism by removing capitalist and traditional elements from the Chinese society.]

[37]. M. Kesomaa, M. Lappi, P. Lehtonen, J. Sairanen, J. Anttila, T, Joutsi, J. J. Klockars: Koro: Cultural heritage from Southeast Asia.
Duodecim, 1995, 111(12), 1093–1095. [Article in Finnish]

This is a review paper on Koro, highlighting the differences in Koro presentation between Southeast Asian and Western countries. The authors discussed the epidemic form in Southeast Asian countries and the sporadic cases of Koro-like symptoms (*korotyyppisena*) in Western societies. They cited three case notes in this regard from the published literature. They stressed the importance of research of Chowdhury from India on dismorphophobic penile perception (*peniksenpiirtamistesti*a) of Koro patients. The authors expressed no Koro reported from Finland until now but given recent immigration, they wonder the situation may change.

1996

[38]. B. Y. Ng, E. E. H. Kua: Koro in ancient Chinese history.
History of Psychiatry, 1996, 7, 563–570.

It is a valuable research paper so far as Koro's cultural evolution in ancient Chinese medical classics. The authors trace Koro's historical evidence or Suo-yang (based on Yin-Yang's traditional concepts in Chinese medicine) from the Chinese texts. They stated that the earliest record of Suo-yang was from northern China, written more than 2000 years ago. They discussed in detail the different philosophical constructs of Yin and Yang polarities in health and disease. The penis is a protruding part of the body, is rich in yang elements, and thus the disorder is named Suo-yang. Some prefer Suo-yin for the female Koro name.

The earliest records of Koro or Suo-yang are found in the Yellow Emperor's Classic of Internal Medicine, written by a court physician Ch'I Po during 476–221 BC. In the first part of the paper, they outlined a short description of some related medical concepts according to Chinese Medicine: the philosophical construct of Yin-Yang duality; *Qi*- the life energy; *Zang-fu* organs where the vital substances are stored—kidney being one crucial for its role in reproduction and production of spermatic fluid; *Fing-luo* or meridians—invisible networks inside the body through which *Qi* and blood circulate. Three meridians—Kidney, liver, and "chong" meridians are implicated in Suo-yang and pathogenic environmental conditions like heat, cold, wind, dryness, fire, and other extreme climatic conditions that may have an aetiological role in a disease condition.

In the second part, the authors traced precious chronological time-line records with references of Suo-yang by the eminent medical personalities in each classical Chinese medical text in each dynasty as follows:

- *Han dynasty (206 BC–AD 200):* Suo-yang was described as a febrile disease caused by cold.
- *Fin dynasty (AD 265–420):* Suo-yang was described as "the penis ascending and entering the abdomen," and acupuncture was advised for treatment.
- *Sui dynasty (AD 589–618):* Intercourse in the post-febrile state is identified as a triggering factor for Suo-yang.
- *Tang dynasty (AD 618–907):* Elaborated on the causes of Suo-yang, like excessive sexual intercourse or intercourse during the recovery phase of an illness.
- *Sung dynasty (AD 960–1280):* First printed book described Suo-yang in a question–answer manner—101 questions regarding Suo-yang—designated as a cold-induced disorder.
- *Ming dynasty (AD 1368–1644):* Several physicians explain the illness in different ways.
- *Qing dynasty (AD 1644–1911):* Many eminent physicians explained Suo-yang. In his New Compilation of Tested Prescriptions (1846), Bao Xiang-ao collected 6000 prescriptions in 18 volumes and described Suo-yang as: "During intercourse, the man may be seized suddenly with acute abdominal pain. The limbs become cold, and the complexion dusky, the penis retracts into the abdomen. The disease is due to the invasion of cold vapours" (p. 567).

It is fascinating to note that Suo-yang descriptions were persistently the same throughout these long dynastic periods. More interesting is that the description of the symptomatology in these classical texts corresponds with the present-day construct of panic disorder. This paper sheds critical light on Koro or Suo-yang's medico-cultural background over the centuries in Chinese society. This paper has a high historical value to all Koro researchers to understand Koro's cultural legacy from a Traditional Chinese Medical perspective. One very important contribution of the article is the list of Chinese references in relation to Suo-yang, including a book chapter on Suo-yang by SY Gao [Suo-yang. *Clinical Therapeutics in Andrology* (Ed. F Lee) Beijing People's Health Press, 1991, pp. 366–372].

[39]. P. Rosca-Rebaudengo, R. Durst, Minuchin-Itzigsohn: Transculturation, psychosis and koro symptoms.
Israel Journal of Psychiatry & Related Science, 1996, 33(1), 54–62.

It is a general descriptive paper discussing the different associations of sporadic Koro cases with various psychiatric, neurological, and systemic disorders. They also reported a sporadic Koro case associated with paranoid psychosis or schizophrenia and discussed immigration's role in the pathogenesis. They also discussed the interrelation between psychosis, transculturation, and cultural influence in developing Koro symptoms.

[40]. D. Phelan, R. J. Daly: Koro-like syndrome associated with brief reactive psychosis in an Irish male.
Irish Medical Journal, 1996, 89(2), 75–76.

This is a case report of a Koro-like symptom in a 32-year-old single Irish male from Cork, Ireland. One week before his psychiatric hospitalization, on awakening, he felt mild discomforts in his genitals. He noticed that his penis and scrotum had contracted to a petite size and caused urination blocking. Over the next 24 hours, he was convinced that his genitals has contracted and lead to erection failure and felt that he became impotent. He further believed that some conspirators broke into his house and caused this sickness while he was asleep. After 48 hours, he identified IRA or *Gardai* as the conspirator who monitored him. Three days after, his genitals returned to average size. He was diagnosed with paranoid psychosis with a range of persecutory beliefs. The authors suggested that initial genital pain and difficulties in urination may aggravate the anxiety, and subsequently, symptoms were incorporated into the delusional system.

[41]. K. Dantendofer, M. Amering, D. Prayer, D. Maierhofer, P. Schinder, H. Katschnig: Treatment of Koro and panic attacks after stroke.
Anxiety, 1996, 2(1), 53–55.

It is a case report of a Koro-like state in a 43-year-old Caucasian male from Vienna, Austria. At age 41, he was diagnosed with a case of cerebral insult from idiopathic hypertonia. At age 43, he developed recurrent attacks of anxiety (typical panic attacks) with somatic sensations. After a month of panic attacks, he developed the associated feeling that his penis and scrotum are contracting and shrinking and retracting into the body. He estimated a visible reduction of penile size by 50% during panic attacks. Subsequently, he had multiple panic attacks with or without genital symptoms. The condition was further complicated by agoraphobic avoidance and erectile dysfunction. An MRI showed subcortical and cortical lesions in both temporal and frontal lobes and the right parietal lobe's postcentral region. Treatment was instituted with carbamazepine 600 mg daily and clonazepam 6 mg daily for two weeks, and he was symptom-free at two years follow up. The authors proposed that Koro and panic attacks are related to distinct brain structures' dysfunctions and may provide an organic explanation for the Koro perception, as parietal lobes play an essential role in body image disturbances.

[42]. M. Chiniwala, C. A. Alfonso, J. R. Torres, J. Lefer: Koro in an immigrant from Guinea with brief psychotic disorder.
American Journal of Psychiatry, 1996, 153(5), 736. (L)

It is a case report of a Koro-like symptom in a 41-year-old single West-African Muslim man (an immigrant from Guinea) at the background of paranoid schizophrenia, from New York, USA. He was admitted in a very agitated state after an attempt to kidnap a nursing home inmate, who he thought was his father. The psychiatric evaluation showed ideas of reference, thought broadcasting, and intense anxiety relating to his perception of the retracting penis. Two important clinical issues to note are: his obsessive preoccupation with a televised celebrity trial and racial conspiracy; and guilt relating to the cultural-familial sexual transgression of being "not-pure" as he had sex with a prostitute. Separation from the family of origin (Guinea) for three years was also a stress factor.

He responded favorably with rapid neuroleptization with 35 mg parenteral haloperidol over 7 hours. History showed that he had guilt over having sex with a prostitute, thoughts of racial conspiracy, and his breakdown coincided with Ramadan's holy month. He was treated with haloperidol 5 mg BD for ten days and was symptom-free. The authors pointed out that the cumulative stress generated from guilt over sexual relations, separation from family, immigration stress probably precipitated psychotic breakdown (with the delusion of genital retraction) in the holy month of prayer and fasting.

[43]. S. T. Cheng: A critical review of Chinese koro.
Culture, Medicine & Psychiatry, 1996, 20(1), 67–82.

An in-depth analytical paper focuses on the Koro (primary Koro) more as a social disorder than individual psychopathology. It is a precious analysis of Koro in Chinese society regarding the Koro epidemic in Southern China (Hainan Island) precisely and in the Chinese socio-cultural milieu in general. The article contains extensive references and is subdivided into a few essential headings like:

The Koro epidemics: General review of Koro illness, course and male–female distribution and differences between Asian and Western presentation.
Symptom manifestation: Discussed in detail the demography and ethnicity of the 233 koro victims of Haikang county. 85% were male.
Characteristics of Koro victims: Mostly, the victims were Han single, poorly educated with firm beliefs, and fear of supernatural force.
Cultural beliefs and indigenous treatment: Belief in fox folklore (possession by fox spirit), general Chinese world view about semen, sexual

restrain, and yang accumulation leads to a combination of treatment with exorcism and Chinese herbal traditional medicine.

Lastly, the author tried to answer the vital question: Why Koro epidemic occurred in Southern China. He analyzes the role of superstition (fortune teller's prediction/fox ghost). The hyper-vigilant community enhanced the chance of Koro victimization and facilitated the transmission of the epidemic from one area to the other. Deficient sex education, particularly among young unmarried adolescents in the Han community (in comparison to Li and Miao community), was more vulnerable to this socio-cultural collective anxiety.

This is a precious analytical paper on the Koro epidemic and addressed a few future research angles that would benefit the Koro researchers.

[44]. J. Tobin: A case of Koro in a 20-year-old Irish male.
Irish Journal of Psychological Medicine, 1996, 13(2), 72–73.

It is a very interesting case report of a Koro-like symptom of a 20-year-old Irish married male from England. He presented with agitation, psychomotor restlessness, recent onset impotence, and a belief that "his penis had been shrinking over the previous two months, up to his brain, and that this was going to kill him." As a preventive measure, he tied a fishing weight to his genitals. The author described this penile belief as of "delusional intensity." He has a strong family history of mental illnesses: father had schizoaffective disorder, mother had reactive depression, oldest brother has a manic depressive disorder with a learning disability, one twin brother had schizophrenia, and the other had sexual identity disorder with endogenous depression, and another brother had a severe psychotic episode. He was admitted to the hospital and responded favorably with depot flupenthixol. The author explained this presentation in light of substantial family psychopathology and familial stress.

1997

[45]. S. Wilson, C. Agin: Genital pain associated with genital retraction: A case of Koro syndrome.
Journal of Pain & Symptom Management, 1997, 13(3), 176–178.

It is an exciting Koro-like case report from New York, USA. A 29-year-old single white male complained of pain at the penis and scrotum root for 5-month. The pain was of mild variety and non-radiating. He also had the sensation that his penis and testicles are retracting into his belly. From time to time, he has to reaffirm manually or visually the presence of his genitals. These symptoms intensify upon prolonged walking, driving or sitting, hiking, fishing, and micturition. He had a history of episodic hyperventilation. Once, while traveling on a train he developed an acute exacerbation of the symptoms: severe pain and the feeling of full retraction of genitals inside the abdomen. He visited a hospital emergency where inguinal hernia, urinary tract infection, proctitis, prostatitis, and testicular disorders were ruled out by examination. Reassurance and bed rest was advised, with which his pain symptoms reduced significantly. Investigations like an ultrasound of prostate, testicle, pelvis, X-ray lumbosacral spine, sigmoidoscopy, CT, and MRI scan showed no abnormality. He was prescribed antibiotics, ibuprofen, and codeine.

Psychosocial evaluation at the pain management clinic reveals hypochondriacal traits as evinced by repeated "doctor shopping and frequent requests for laboratory investigations even after negative results. He also had compulsive traits in keeping a detailed daily record of fluctuations in his symptoms. He was diagnosed with anxiety disorder with Koro syndrome. He responded favorably with desipramine, and by two weeks, the genital perception disappeared, and the pain subsided significantly by two months.

Observation: This case is an excellent example of how genital shrinking or retraction perception mixed with hypochondriacal preoccupation or expressed as a part of obsessive doubts and compulsive checking–rechecking behavior.

[46]. C. F. Lewis, K. Ednie: Koro and homicidal behavior.
American Journal of Psychiatry, 1997, 154(8), 1169.

This is a case report of Koro-like delusion from Michigan, USA. A 25-year-old black American man was admitted to a forensic hospital after murdering a stranger, with a 6-year diagnosis of chronic Paranoid schizophrenia. He had the belief that his penis sometimes retracted into his abdomen, often wholly leaving behind the skin only. He was instructed in command hallucination to kill himself or others; otherwise, he will be punished by complete and permanent retraction of the penis and thereby death. He said, in self-defense, he murdered the stranger. He responded well with the fluphenazine decanoate regimen.

This is a critical case to show how sexual delusion mimics a Koro-like symptom. In a psychotic breakdown, sexual deception may lead to destructive, risky behavior like genital self-mutilation, suicide, or homicide. This is the second case report of Koro with forensic significance in the literature.

[47]. A. N. Chowdhury, R. Chaplow: Koro and offending behavior: A report from New Zealand.
Transcultural Psychiatry, 1997, 34(4), 528–529. (L)

This is a Koro-like case report from Auckland, New Zealand. A 25-year-old Pacific islander was arrested for "wilful damage" and "threaten to injure." He was present to the Court Liaison Psychiatric service as highly agitated, with incoherent speech, self-harming risk, and threatening "to string his penis up." On inquiry, it was revealed that he had a firm conviction that his penis has shrunk into his abdomen for the last couple of weeks, and his repeated attempts to "pull it out" failed. He felt helpless as his family could not understand his sickness, and his wife, family, friends, and police are ridiculing and laughing about his penile complaint. This caused him great anguish, frustration, and led to the alleged offense. He also accused his wife of infidelity. His sexual performances deteriorated because of impotence. Acute stress of delusion of penile retraction, in this case, leads to paranoid ideas and offending behavior. This is the third case report of Koro with forensic significance in the literature.

[48]. B. Y. Ng: History of Koro in Singapore.
Singapore Medical Journal, 1997, 38(8), 356–357.

This is a discussion paper focusing on the 1967 Koro epidemic in Singapore. The author described the general socio-political atmosphere about infected pork rumor as the triggering factor for the epidemic. The author very logically analyzed why death fear imagery is so crucial in the clinical presentation of Koro symptoms. He mentioned the historical importance of the "castration" theme in Chinese culture and suggested the Koro illness as a "form of 'psychological castration,' a symbolic loss of potency and power." This fear of penis-loss is culturally so ingrained that Koro or Suo-yang sometimes occurs during or after intercourse may be because the patient views the "vagina as a castrating device." He also very categorically pointed out the risk factors for the epidemic and sporadic occurrences of Koro. He suggested the nosological label of Koro as a form of panic disorder. As a preventive approach, he advocated health and sex education to the general public to clarify the myths and misconceptions about human sexuality.

[49]. S. T. Cheng: Epidemic genital retraction syndrome: Environmental and personal risk factors in Southern China.
Journal of Psychology & Human Sexuality, 1979, 9(1), 57–70.

This is a valuable research paper from Hong Kong. The author meticulously delineated the different environmental and personal risk factors for the Koro vulnerability in the Guangdong Koro epidemic. He very nicely showed how the socio-cultural environment promoted Koro behavior in Hainan Island and the Leizhou Peninsula and how individuals in those communities responded to this psycho-social demand of the environment. Among the environmental risk factors, he identified: (1) Positive cultural attitudes and beliefs regarding Koro phenomena, especially among the Han community (who were primarily affected), but not among Li and Miao communities. The crucial ingredients acted here were belief in fox spirit possession (of the victims), collective rescue operation (pulling out the penis) by the community, movement of the fox spirit from area to area to cause epidemic spread, and a high level of superstitious belief. (2) Role of rumors to increase social vulnerability to Koro and thus helping the spread of the epidemic. (3) The role of the anxious neighborhood to perpetuate and potentiate Koro attacks. Among the individual risk factors, he stressed: (1) low level of education and low intelligence level; (2) Younger age—(adolescents and young adults, mostly 10–29 years); and (3) Unmarried status (deprived of correct sexual information). The author concluded in the discussion that "Koro in China is best conceived as a social malady supported by cultural myths which tend to affect young people who are deprived of proper sex information to explain their physical development."

[50]. J. Sandford: Koro in a Caucasian male with panic disorder.
International Journal of Psychiatry in Clinical Practice, 1997, 1(4), 295.

It is a report of a Koro in a white 25-year-old English male from Bristol, UK. He has a 7-year history of panic disorder and agoraphobia. He also had a hypochondriacal concern that excessive masturbation had damaged his penis. He discovered that he has a complete penile retraction during the panic attack and had an acute fear of imminent death. Though his panic symptoms subsided, his fear of "penile loss" remained for further two weeks. After reviewing similar cases, the author proposed a psychophysiological mechanism (vasoconstrictive penile changes and consequent cognitive misinterpretation) for Koro pathology.

[51]. B. M. Sackey: The vanishing organ phenomenon in the context of Ghanaian religious beliefs.
African Anthropology, 1997, 4(2), 110–125.

This is a very valuable cultural anthropological research paper on "Vanishing Sexual/genital Organ Syndrome (VSOS)" from Ghana. It very elegantly analyzed how cultural myth and belief in supernatural power enacted to cause vanishing or disappearing of genital organs in culturally vulnerable individuals.

> In January 1997, there were widespread reports in Ghana about people possessing spiritual powers that could cause the sexual organs of other persons, namely, penises, breast and vaginas to vanish, shrink or to be sealed respectively either by a handshake or a touch on any part of the body. This phenomenon, ... resulted in a 'ritual' of instant mob lynching and burning of the alleged culprits. In Accra, seven suspects were reported to have been publicly lynched in the first two days of the genital vanishing scare and an undisclosed number of people in different parts of the country were executed this way. (p. 110)

This VSOS became a focal epidemic and spread through other African countries like Cameroon, Ivory Coast, and Senegal. The author described five case reports from local newspapers and analyzed these in terms of Ghanaians religious, cultural beliefs, a high premium on male sexuality and sexual organ, and provided the serious forensic consequences of mob violence in each incident. He also compares VSOS and Koro, where the former is spiritually (or magically) induced and the latter by cultural beliefs. The author also listed many risk factors as precipitators like political and economic stressors, religious stressors, ethnicity, and lawlessness.

1998

[52]. E. Witztum, Y. Bersudsky, H. Mayodovnik, M. Kotler: Koro-like syndrome in a Bedouin man.
Psychopathology, 1998, 31(4), 174–177.

This is a case report of Koro-like symptoms in a single 34-year-old Bedouin (Arab nomadic tribe) man from Negev desert, Israel. The patient was admitted in an agitated state and was diagnosed with psychosis NOS with voyeurism and mixed personality disorder with paranoid and antisocial traits. History reveals that 5 or 6 years ago, he visited a prostitute, and after that, he developed impotence and felt that his penis was shrinking and receding into his abdomen. The patient has also had hypochondriacal health concerns (contracting AIDS or syphilis) and social stress and hostility related to his Bedouin community culture. It is not clear from the report how long he had this Koro-like perception.

But the moral transgression of visiting a prostitute may have some role in developing impotence and Koro-like penile perception. He had no fear of death.

[53]. A. Kovács, P. Osváth: Genital retraction syndrome in a Korean woman: A case of koro in Hungary.
Psychopathology, 1998, 31, 220–224.

This is a very interesting case report from Hungary. It highlighted a unique culture-bound sexual ideational component with a transient acute psychotic episode with depersonalization. Though the authors labeled it as Koro, many questions remained open to designate this presentation as real Koro. The case was a 29-year-old married South Korean lady who was an immigrant in Hungary for two years and showed acculturative stress during this period. The index episode was as follows: police brought her because she was running naked along the highway at night. She said that she had a love affair with one of her music teachers, which recently split up. She came to this town previously with her lover, and this time she came alone, "hoping that she might meet her lover spiritually" The description follows as:

> Walking on the street she became tense, she stopped feelings her leg, and experienced itching and tingling in her thighs. The numbness spread upwards in her body, she felt that she was becoming less and less a woman: her breast were shrinking and she was gradually transforming into a man. This imagined sexual metamorphosis became increasingly threatening to her, because she believed that by becoming a man she would lose all her energy and finally die. She thought she heard her lover's voice trying to tell her what to do. She took off all her clothes, because it eased her mind and made her 'feel something' in her legs. She was convinced that she would be able to remain a woman only if she had sexual intercourse with someone, and by doing so she would receive 'penis and energy'. Her fear of physical transformation and her sexual impulses gradually took possession of her. She was begging the male members of staff to have sexual intercourse with her to save her life. (p. 221)

Afterward, her husband gave a history of her recent social isolation and paranoid ides—"being watched by police," and police may assault her children. Later she had two other psychiatric admissions in Hungary.

Observation: There are some anomalies in this case report's heading as there was no complaint of genital retraction in the description. The whole episode, bodily feelings and running behavior on the motorway at night, in an unknown town for "spiritual union" with alleged lover—all indicate loss of reality testing and psychotic episode. In fact, the authors diagnosed her with Acute polymorphic psychotic disorder (ICD 10 code—F23.00). Three issues are important here:

1. It is not a Koro symptom. Koro's sign in a female constitutes three cardinal features—(a) perception of inward retraction/shrinkage of vagina/vulva toward the abdomen and/or retraction/shrinkage of nipple/breast into the chest fear that and all these will lead to death. The vaginal symptom here is absent, and the breast symptom mentioned is very well the part of the delusion of sex change. The feeling around the thigh probably indicated transposing of a male sexual organ rather than a retraction of the vagina or vulva into the abdomen.
2. The ideational component of death expressed here was because of sex change-into male and cure she believed would be by intercourse. This has some cultural relevance to the Yin-Yang dimension of sexual exchange in Chinese culture (maybe the same Taoist concept is also prevalent in Korean culture).

   Gulik (1951) described the importance of intercourse for a woman in traditional Chinese teaching. The semen contains the Chi—"the universal spirit of life," which has Ching—the sexual energy, the Yang essence of man. In sexual intercourse, the woman draws the precious Yang essence of man, strengthening the woman's Yin or tiger quality (Evola, 1991).
3. The ideational component of Koro anxiety instead of death has been reported in the literature as the fear of sex change or turning into a eunuch is by male Koro patients. In female cases, the perception of loss of or devalued the concept of womanhood or fear of sterility (Chowdhury, 1994) plays a similarly important role. Perception of

loss of sexual identity, potency, and attractiveness is the potential contributory factor for Koro expression in males and females (Srivastava & Pandit, 2013). But demand for intercourse by a male to cure the disorder is not a part of Koro illness.

[54]. A. Kovács, P. Osváth: Koro (genital retraction syndrome): A symptom or a disease?
Psychiatria Danubina, 1998, 10(1), 45–51.

It is a discussion paper on Koro's nosological complexity. Koro may have various associations with other medical and psychiatric disorders and express in incomplete or complete presentation. The authors supported the terminology in favor of "genital retraction syndrome." They also presented two cases—one is already reported previously (*Psychopathology*, 1998, 31, 220–224), and the other is a 35-year-old male with a history of paranoid schizophrenia.

[55]. A. N. Chowdhury: Hundred years of koro: The history of a culture-bound syndrome.
International Journal of Social Psychiatry, 1998, 44 (3), 181–188.

This paper describes the last 100 years' history of Koro's publication in the Western medical press. Koro was first reported in 1895, and during a century, Koro's culture-bound specificity lost its ground and is renamed as "genital retraction syndrome." The world literature review showed that Koro is reported from various geographical locations and diverse ethnic populations. The author tried to trace the historical track of the Koro illness as a distinct entity associated with other psychiatric morbidities. Gradually it earned a new nosological dimension like monosymptomatic hypochondriacal psychosis or body-dysmorphic disorder, or penile dysmorphophobia besides its culture-bound definition. It also highlighted Koro's cultural tag regarding fox spirit in the Guangdong Koro epidemic in China. This is a brief and concise review of the then global status of Koro.

[56]. S. P. Chand: Koro associated with phobia for AIDS.
International Journal of Psychiatry in Medicine, 1998, 28(3), 353–356.

This is a case report from Oman. A 30-year-old single Muslim Jordanian male had a Koro-like perception in the background of phobia for AIDS. The author designated the case as an incomplete form of Koro as the patient had a perception of a shrinking penis and reduced penis size over a long period. The symptoms of anxiety and fear of contracting AIDS started after a sexual experience with an American girl. Subsequently, he developed typical doubts, checking and rechecking a blood test for AIDS and fearing losing his sexual potency. He responded well with cognitive-behavioral therapy. The clinical description shows that the patient has a high degree of hypochondriacal health concern with obsessive traits. He has specific obsessive characteristics of being a perfectionist. The genital symptoms may be more suitably designated as close to the Chronic Koro presentation.

[57]. R. H. Ramos, C. L. Budman: Emergence of koro after abrupt cessation of olanzapine.
Journal of Clinical Psychiatry, 1998, 59(2), 86–87.

It is a very interesting Koro-like case report from New York, USA. A 19-year-old white man was admitted to the hospital after a suicide attempt. He had a history of recurrent depression with persecutory and auditory hallucinations. At admission, his olanzapine treatment was stopped for the preparation for ECTs. His depression has improved after 4 ECT treatments, but he started overwhelming fear and anxiety that his penis and left testicles shrank and receded into his abdomen. Repeated reassurances, physical and urological examination fail to diminish his anxiety and penile symptoms. Olanzapine 5 mg q,d started after five days, and his Koro symptoms were subsided without further recurrence. This finding focuses on the role of olanzapine that whether it has a curative effect on Koro perception or has a placebo effect or antipsychotic (anti-delusional) effect.

[58]. V. V. Marilov: Koro syndrome.
Zhurnal Nervologi Psikhiathrii Im SS Korsakova, 1998, 98(1), 52–53.
[Article in Russian]

It is a Koro case report from Russia.

[59]. R. E. Bartholomew: The medicalization of exotic deviance: A sociological perspective on epidemic koro.
Transcultural Psychiatry, 1998, 35(1), 5–38.

This is a long paper where the author argued against labeling the Koro epidemic as a medical phenomenon. The author believes that the Koro epidemics "should be reclassified as a sociological phenomenon involving mass social delusions." The author argues that in epidemic Koro, the victims are not "psychologically disturbed or exhibiting somatoform reactions, but are experiencing the physiological consequences of anxiety generated by a false belief, and the cognitive consequences of altered perceptual sets." In his opinion, the present medical model represents detachment from the local socio-cultural context and meaning. This proposition is inviting more debate regarding the medical categorization and conceptual framework of Koro.

[60]. C. S. Estcourt, B. T. Goh: Koro presenting to genitourinary medicine services.
International Journal of STD & AIDS, 1998, 9(3), 175–176.

This is a case report of a recurrent Koro-like symptom in an 18-year-old single male, born in the UK from Greek parents. He developed the acute feeling that his penis was disappearing in different situations and contexts on three occasions. No acute anxiety or fear of death was reported. No details of the Koro presentation are described, but because of the nonpsychotic background, it seems like a hypochondriacal response to some underlying stress relating to sexuality.

1999

[61]. N. Al-Hmoud: Koro-like syndrome in a Jordanian male.
Eastern Mediterranean Health Journal, 1999, 5, 611–613.

It is a case report of a Koro-like symptom of a 24 year single Jordanian male from Amman. He had a two weeks history of sleep disturbances, social isolation, apprehension, and fearfulness. During this episode, he developed acute fear that his penis was shrinking and asked for help to check the organ, and he was pulling his penis to prevent it from being sucked into his pelvis. He was very anxious and awake the whole night with this condition. He had no fear of death from this organ shrinking but preferred death if he loses his masculinity. At age 19, he had an orchidopexy operation for torsion of the left testicle, after which he developed the idea that he would be infertile and would lose his manhood. He had a heterosexual experience with a prostitute one month before this event, for which he developed guilt and embarrassment. He was diagnosed with anxiety disorder and panic and responded well with imipramine and alprazolam. He was asymptomatic in 3 months, and ten months follow-up showed no recurrence of symptoms. Psychopathosexuality, operation on the testis, and a strong emphasis on masculinity in Jordanian culture are underlying psychodynamic forces in this symptom formation.

[62]. Flores Post, Indonesia, October 1999.

A Koro epidemic involving hundreds of cases (school children) occurred in Ende, the southern coast of Flores, Indonesia, as reported in a local newspaper Flores Post, from 5 to 7 October 1999 (Mitchell, 2018).

2000

[63]. J. E. Hallak, J. A. Crippa, A. W. Zuardi: Treatment of koro with citalopram.
Journal of Clinical Psychiatry, 2000, 61(12), 951.

This is a Koro case report from Sao Paulo, Brazil, and probably the first Koro report from a South American man. A 56-year-old single white male presented with a firm belief that his penis shrank inside the abdomen and caused great anxiety. He pulled his penis to prevent retraction. He also holds his penis through the trouser pockets while he is in social situations like visiting a church. He had a similar episode when he was 19, and after pulling the penis, retraction stopped. Currently, he had no other psychiatric diagnosis. He responded favorably with citalopram 10 mg/day and showed remission of penile symptoms after a month. The authors discussed the Koro symptom presentation in non-Asian culture and the different diagnostic options as per DSM-IV criteria.

[64]. J. M. Caballero, A. Avila, X. Cardona, F. Sastre, P. Maho, J. Bello: Genital pain without urogenital pathology: The koro-like syndrome.
Journal of Urology, 2000, 163(1), 243.

It is a Koro-like case report from Barcelona, Spain. A 78-year-old man presented with left scrotal pain, which started 18 months earlier. He had feelings of penile retraction into the abdomen with intense anxiety. Later he developed burning scrotal pain and believed that it was due to the left testicle drawing up the penis into the stomach. He had Parkinsonism and was on antiparkinsonian medications—750 mg levodopa and 3 mg pergolide. Left epididymectomy was done, followed by anesthesia infiltration of the left testicle but without any relief of pain. The urological examination was normal. Psychiatric assessment put a diagnosis of psychotic depression with Koro-like symptoms. The dosage of levodopa was reduced, and pergolide was stopped, but there was no result. He responded favorably with ECTs, which resolved his scrotal pain as well as fears of penile retraction. The authors stressed the importance of Koro-related knowledge of the Urologists as Koro-like symptoms are reported more and more with urogenital pathologies.

[65]. K. A. Kuruppuarachchi, J. A. Ratnayake, N. A. Dasanayake, R. R. Rajakuruna: The Koro syndrome.
Ceylon Medical Journal, 2000, 45(4), 182–183. (L)

These are two case reports from Sri Lanka. The first case was a 19-year-old man with symptoms of primary Koro attack: high anxiety, intense fear of death due to retraction of the penis, which started after a penile injury during masturbation. He had mild depressive symptoms as well. He responded well with anxiety management and thioridazine treatment. The second case was a 42-year-old man who presented with a depressive episode and delusional conviction that his penis was retracting into the abdomen. He responded well with treatment with imipramine and a small dose of trifluoperazine.

[66]. R. E. Bartholomew: Exotic Deviance: Medicalizing cultural idioms from strangeness to illness.
Boulder, University Press of Colorado, 2000.

This is a book with extensive sociological explanation (opposed to medical reason) of three distinct mass psychogenic illnesses, viz: Latah, Koro, and dancing episodes of medieval Europe. The author suggested that culturally specific idioms should be understood in the context of society's local cultural meaning. He explained that the three different grades of Latah—mild, moderate, and severe in other age groups-are seen differently in society. He believes that Latah's medicalization was a colonial expression or even a racist way of medicalization that undermined Malay people. For Koro in the epidemic form, he postulates a theory of collective delusion (social) where a shared misperception of penile size spreads through the vulnerable community. He also offered a sociological explanation of Europe's dancing episodes and discussed the mass conversion reactions in school settings. It is a valuable contribution to understand mental epidemics from a sociological lens and enables medical experts to examine human behavior by an alternative approach.

[**Note**: This book is reviewed by R. J. Barrett—Ocenia (2002), 72(4), 299–300.]

[67]. J. Kim, M. Kim, N. Lee, Y. Park: A case of urethrocutaneous fistula with koro syndrome.
Journal of Urology, 2000, 164(1), 123.

This is an interesting case report from South Korea. Practically it shows the genito-urinary complication of folk treatment (a mechanical procedure to prevent penile retraction). The Koro attack or illness details are not described, neither was it acute or chronic told. It appears from the description that he probably has recurrent Koro attacks. He was a 65-year-old Korean man who presented with penile pain of three months duration. He had the feeling or believed that his penis would shrink and retract into the abdomen (Koro-like symptoms). He put an "anti-retraction device" around the glans penis seven months ago to prevent this disorder. This was a steel bottle cap with a hole in the center. The steel cap had penetrated to penile tissue and caused severe infection with inflammatory granulation tissue on the penile shaft's ventral side. Strangely he was diagnosed with delusional disorder, not with Koro. The title of the paper should be reversed—Koro syndrome with urethrocutaneous fistula.

[68]. R. S. Bayer: Koro-like symptoms and transient post-ictal psychosis.
Qatar Medical Journal, 2000, 9(2), 68–69.

It is a case report of a Koro-like symptom in a 32-year married Jordanian male from Jordan. Complex functional factors were present: acute schizophrenia-like features including persecutory delusion, ideas of reference, second and third-person auditory hallucination, somatic hallucination, and thought broadcasting at the background of temporal lobe epilepsy for ten years. He was on anti-epileptic medication (Tegretol 400 mg/day), which he stopped recently, and had two epileptic fits three days preceding the psychotic episode. During this acute episode, he felt that his penis was retracted inside the abdomen, which prompted him to search whether the organ was in place repeatedly. There was no fear of death present. He was treated with haloperidol 15 mg/day with the commencement of Tegretol 400 mg/day. After seven days, he showed complete recovery. He was diagnosed with transient post-ictal psychosis and follow-up for one year showed no recurrence of symptoms. This case is a valuable addition of sporadic Koro-like cases with organic and functional backgrounds, not culture-bound.

References

Anderson, D. N. (1990). Koro: The genital retraction syndrome after stroke. *British Journal of Psychiatry, 157*, 142–144.

Chen, E. (1991). Drug induced Koro in a non-Chinese man. *British Journal of Psychiatry, 158*, 721.

Chowdhury, A. N. (1994). Koro in females: An analysis of 48 cases. *Transcultural Psychiatric Research Review, 31*, 369–380.

Derogatis, L. R., Lipman, R. S., Covi, L., & Rickels, K. (1971). Neurotic symptom dimensions as perceived by psychiatrists and patients of various social classes. *Arch General Psychiatry, 24*(5), 454–464.

Diagnostic and statistical manual of mental disorders (3rd Rev. ed.). (1987). American Psychiatric Association. American Psychiatric Press Inc.

Diagnostic criteria from DSM-IV. (1994). American Psychiatric Association. American Psychiatric Press Inc.

Diagnostic and statistical manual of mental disorder (5th ed.). (2013). American Psychiatric Association.

Edwards, J. G. (1970). The Koro pattern of depersonalization in an American schizophrenic patient. *American Journal of Psychiatry, 126*, 1171–1173.

Edwards, J. W. (1984). Indigenous Koro: A genital retraction syndrome of insular South East Asia: A critical review. *Culture, Medicine & Psychiatry, 8*, 1–24.

Evola, J. (1991). *Eros and the mysteries of love: The metaphysics of sex*. Inner Traditions International.

Gulik van, R. H. (1951). *Erotic colour prints of the Ming period*. Tokyo.

Gulik, van R. H. (1961). *Sexual life in ancient China*. E. J. Brill.

Gussow, Z. (1963). A preliminary report of kayakangst among the Eskimo of West Greenland: A study in sensory deprivation. *International Journal of Social Psychiatry, 9*, 18–26.

Gwee, A. L. (1963). Koro—A cultural disease. *Singapore Medical Journal, 4*, 119–122.

Gwee, A. L. (1968). Koro—Its origin and nature as a disease entity. *Singapore Medical Journal, 9*, 3–6.

Hawley, R. M., & Owens, J. H. (1988). Koro: Its presentation in an elderly male. *International Journal of Geriatric Psychiatry, 3*, 69–72.

ICD-9. (1978). *Mental disorders: Glossary and guide to their classification in accordance with the ninth revision of the international classification of diseases*. World Health Organization.

ICD-10. (1992). *Classification of mental and behavioural disorders. Clinical description and diagnostic guidelines.* World Health Organization and Oxford University Press.

Ifabumuyi, O. I., & Rwegellera, G. G. C. (1979). Koro in a Nigerian male patient: A case report. *African Journal of Psychiatry, 5*, 103–105.

Legendre, J. (1908). Une curieuse epidemic. *Annales De Medicine Coloniale, 11*(2), 280–281.

Mitchell, D. (2018, June 27–30). *Is shrinking penis syndrome a delusion or real thing?* Paper presented at the 'History of Medicine in Southeast Asia Symposium' at the Indonesian Academy of Sciences. https://theconversation.com/is-shrinking-penis-syndrome-a-delusion-or-a-real-thing-99631

Murphy, H. B. M. (1982). *Comparative psychiatry: The international and intercultural distribution of mental illness* (pp. 269–277). Springer-Verlag.

Ngui, P. W. (1969). The Koro epidemic in Singapore. *Australian & New Zealand Journal of Psychiatry, 3*, 263–266.

Raven, T. (1886). Retraction of the penis. *Lancet, 2*, 205.

Read, B. E. (1926). Gleanings from old Chinese medicine. *Annals of Medical History, 8*, 16–19.

Rin, H. (1966). Two forms of vital deficiency syndrome among Chinese male mental patients. *Transcultural Psychiatric Research Review, 3*, 19–21.

Simons, R. C. (1985). Introduction: The genital retraction taxon. In R. C. Simons & C. C. Hughes (Eds.), *The culture-bound syndromes: Folk illnesses of psychiatric and anthropological interests* (pp. 151–153). D. Reidel.

Srivastava, M., & Pandit, B. (2013). Koro—A case report and review. *International Journal of Physiology, 1*(1), 37–40.

Wong, K. C. (1918). An inquiry into some Chinese sexual diseases. *National Medical Journal of China, 4*, 26–31.

8

Western Publications: Part Three—From 2001 to 2020

KORO LITERATURE: From 2001 to 2010

Preamble: A total of 52 publications are reviewed in this section. The "penis theft" epidemic from Nigeria and Congo, Africa, is also included. Association of drug abuse (cannabis, amphetamine, and steroid) with Koro are reported. Japan, Pakistan, Oman, Spain, Greece, Turkey, Check Republic, and Poland are the new geographical territory, reported Koro. Two unusual but related topics are included: vanishing testis syndrome and one on sudden death during sexual activity.

2001

[1]. M. Earleywine: Cannabis induced Koro in Americans. *Addiction, 2001, 96 (11), 1663–1666.*

This is an interesting case report from Los Angeles, California. The paper has a transcultural flavor as similar findings are also noted from India. It was a telephonic survey among 70+ men who reported adverse reactions after smoking cannabis. 3 (4.29%) of them (Caucasians, aged

A. N. Chowdhury, *Koro*,
https://doi.org/10.1007/978-3-030-87962-4_8

22–26) reported Koro symptoms after cannabis intake. All of them had had prior knowledge of cannabis-induced Koro. Two of them had body dysmorphia. The author implicated three factors for this Koro presentation among men from non-Eastern cultures: prior knowledge, cannabis-induced heightened panic reaction, and poor body image.

[2]. G. O. Krizek, R. Honzak: Psychiatric syndromes observed after damage of the right hemisphere.
Prakticky Lekar, 2001, 81(9), 507–510. [Article in Czech]

The authors discussed the psychiatric manifestation of right cerebral hemisphere damage. They may manifest as delusions of place and persons or somatic and sexual delusions. They also mentioned two culture-bound syndromes—Koro and Dhat syndrome.

[3]. C. D. Carmaciu, C. Sanderson, H. R. Markar: Secondary koro with unusual features in a Briton.
Transcultural Psychiatry, 2001, 38(4), 528–533.

This is an exciting Koro case report from the UK, with sound academic logic and explanation. The authors provided a short overview of Koro's earlier history and geographical distribution. They then drew attention to its two clinical types: "complete" or classical cultural form and "incomplete" or non-cultural form, along with a short discussion of its psychopathological interpretations.

The case report is really unusual in its presentation. The subject was a 53-year-old single Briton, laboratory technician by profession, having a long history of "concern that his penis was shrinking." He believes he had a long period of sexual arousal with six months of feeling depressed with hearing derogatory voices (probably pseudohallucination) with a very negative self-image. He has a symptom-free period of 20 years, and when he has lost his job, that triggered the re-emergence of penile symptoms. The authors described his behavior and ideational component behind the Koro perception very nicely:

> When going to the toilet he would sometimes find it difficult to get his penis out of his pants leading to thoughts of his penis shrinking, disappearing into the abdomen and causing death through compression of the urethra, i.e. through not being able to pass any more urine. (p. 529)

He was diagnosed with psychotic depression, and sertraline was prescribed. Despite poor compliance, his depression, anxiety, and genital preoccupation symptoms gradually disappeared over six months.

Another two very unusual features present were his last contact with psychiatric service 25 years ago with the complaints of "blood was draining away from his penis, which was getting smaller from muscle wasting." As a consequence, he developed paraphimosis with excessive scaling around the penile region. He also developed a fear that water may enhance the blood draining from his penis, for which he avoided bath and washing the pubic area for two months. He was admitted, and phenelzine and trifluoperazine were prescribed, and he responded well and was symptom-free for a further two years.

Family and personal history showed some critical issues: Father had a paranoid schizophrenia diagnosis and possibly a pedophile. At age 16, he had orchitis, had a history of migraine, irritable bowel syndrome, hypertension (on metoprolol), and non-insulin-dependent diabetes mellitus (on gliclazide).

Observation: It is a matter of further research whether any of his medical conditions (or treatment thereof) may contribute to his penile perception. The behavior of avoiding bath for months may be an example of phobic avoidance or extreme hypochondriacal behavior (which in some cases may reach a psychotic proportion).

In the strictest sense, this case may be called Koro-like as there was no perception of penile pull from inside the abdomen; instead, he complained of a shortening of the penis. Given his schizoid personality traits, the firm conviction of "blood draining from the penis to abdomen" amounts to delusional perception.

2002

[4]. M. Nakaya: Fluvoxamine treatment of a Japanese patient with koro.
Journal of Clinical Psychiatry, 2002, 63(12), 1182–1183.

This is a Koro-like case report from Mibu, Japan. A 36-year-old Japanese man had hypochondriacal cardiac complaints and was treated with benzodiazepine (12 mg/day), and treatment was continued for two years. His symptoms remitted after five months. At age 40, he developed a sudden experience that his penis was shrinking, and it would recede into his abdomen. That perception leads to "continual compulsion to manually pull his penis" to prevent the disappearance of the penis into the abdomen during wakening hours. At night, a cloth was tied around the base of the penis. After treatment failure with bromazepam and risperidone, he was put on fluvoxamine. Initially, 100 mg/day and then 150 mg/day for one year, and the symptoms remitted. When the dose was reduced to 50 mg/day, there was a recurrence of penile symptoms, and with an increment of an amount to 150 mg/day, the symptoms remitted. This was continued for one and half years without any relapse. The author discussed the different nosological options to classify Koro and indicate the efficacy of SSRI medication in Koro's treatment.

[5]. A. Gobel: Men these days, They are a problem: Husband-taming herbs and gender wars in rural Zimbabwe.
Canadian Journal of African Studies, 2002, 36(3), 460–489.

This is not a Koro paper. This intensive ethnographic research is based on rural Zimbabwe's socio-anthropological and cultural perspective (among Shona women in Sengezi Resettlement in Wedza district). The author focused on using husband-taming herbs (*mupfuhwira*) dispensed by traditional healers *(n'angas*). The author did a detailed analysis of women's role in a male-dominated society, their economic and relational crisis, the fear of HIV/AIDS infection, the threat of divorce and husbands' infidelity, and domestic violence. A new social change due to an economic reason was observed. This is the changing local community population with more migrant females, which increases the scope of gendered exploitation and facilitates the use of husband-taming herbs by many married women. This is the only acceptable (but confidential) way to deal with this rapidly spreading gender exploitation. For Koro researchers, these incidents help develop insight regarding the broader socio-cultural atmosphere where suspicion of being herbed (also by witchcraft and sorcery) may be operative at the background belief of fear of penis loss or vanishing penis in vulnerable males in African society. There are "magical penis loss" epidemics that hit at least ten countries in Africa.

[6]. N. Kennedy, M. McDonough: Koro: A case in an Eastern European asylum seeker in Ireland.
Irish Journal of Psychological Medicine, December 2002, 19(4), 130–131.

It is a Koro-like case report from a 30- year- old Eastern European asylum seeker in the background of depression for four months. "He felt that his penis had shrunk over the last month and believed it would eventually retract into the abdomen." This perception triggered a lot of anxiety and compelled him to regularly check his penis to ensure that it had not disappeared inside the abdomen. The ideational component was not fear of death but sexual dysfunction. He responded well with fluoxetine 20 mg daily, and Koro-like symptoms resolved after four weeks of treatment and depression after ten weeks. The authors discussed the symptom pattern in the non-culture bound variant of Koro illness.

[7]. M. Wang, F. Wang: Conceptualisation and treatment of Koro in traditional Chinese medicine.
The Chinese Journal of Human Sexuality, 2002, 11(1), 559–561. [In Chinese]

2003

[8]. P. Garlipp, W. Machleidt: Koro–discussing a transcultural psychopathological phenomenon.
Fortschritte der Neurologie-Psychiatrie, 2003, 71(2), 103–107. [Article in German]

It is a discussion paper highlighting the transcultural aspect of Koro from the global reporting perspective. The authors also discussed a case of paranoid hallucinatory psychosis that developed Koro-like symptomatology.

[9]. D. Laguna, D. Napiorkowska-Laguna: Koro—Culture-bound or universal syndrome? Review of the literature and case report.
Advances in Psychiatry & Neurology 2003, 12 (4), 457–468. [Article in Polish]

It is a general discussion paper on Koro with a helpful review of the literature. The authors presented a Koro case- probably first from Poland: a 45-year-old Polish married farmer who had feelings of genital retraction in the background of an anxiety attack and depressive episode. It seems that he had his first attack at age 18 when he abused a lot of alcohol as self-medication, and then 15 years ago, he had another episode and seeks medical treatment. Last three years, he was in psychiatric treatment and responded well with fluvoxamine 100 mg daily for five months.

[10]. D. Mitchell: Shrinking penis disease.
Inside Indonesia, July–September, 2003 [http://insideindonesia.org/edit7513mitch2.html]

This is a very informative short report on Koro from Indonesia. Some new information available is: the Indonesian name of Koro is *kerut*. People in Indonesia only recognize Koro when it is said as *koro laso* (shrunken penis). In South Sulawesi and Flores, Koro is known in the Ende language as *mbaze*. On the island of Sumba, it is called *hidu tama (*going inside disease*) or hei lulu* (everything pulled up). The author also provided a very firsthand report of the traditional healing method for Koro in rural Indonesia.

The author described his recent visit to a traditional healer or *dukun* Hina Panjara (in East Sumba), who has an impressive track record of successful treatment of many Koro cases. *Dukun* has special massage oil prepared from roots and barks from the forest trees, a recipe handed down from his ancestors. He gave a vibrant account of his treatment procedures as follows:

> He vigorously rubs the oil into the legs and the abdomen of his patient, ...treatment is always effective and the penis returns to its normal state within 15 minutes to half an hour. If the condition occurs again the patient may apply the oil themselves directly to the affected part. The dukun himself avoids massaging the penis but the patient is encouraged to do so.

Hina described the tonic as a *kebal* (immunity) medicine, taken orally in small amounts. It also contains a clove of garlic and other kitchen herbs to make it more palatable. He believes that the potency of his oil rests with the goodwill of God.

2004

[11]. D. Mitchell: Curing Koro, the shrinking penis disease. Proceedings of the 1st Annual Conference of the Monash Asia Institute, Mumbai, India, February 9–13, 2004.

It is an extended version of the author's previous paper of 2003. The article covers a brief review of Koro's history, including some specific cultural names used in Indonesia's Flores and Sumba region. Indian scenario of Koro epidemic and his field experience in Flores with a local healer- who treats Koro patients, was discussed. This paper's most valuable contribution is Koro's cultural concept and traditional novel healing methods (herbal oil massage of the penis) in cases of penile retraction by a local healer. The particular technique of rapport with the patient also has a therapeutic effect. This research unfolds the Indonesian cultural context of Koro illness.

[12]. R. N. Bloor: Whizz-dick: Side effect, urban myth or amphetamine-related koro-like syndrome?
International Journal of Clinical Practice, 2004, 58(7), 717–719.

It is a fascinating paper from Staffordshire, UK, highlighting a new direction in Koro research. The author reported a case of a 17-year-old male patient referred to urology services. His main complaint was "uncomfortable sensation in his groin and a feeling that his penis was being sucked into his abdomen." He has had a history of regular use of amphetamines and cannabis for the past two years. He reported that penis shrinkage is a widespread phenomenon in amphetamine use and is known as Whizz-Dick. He responded well with reassurance and supportive counseling.

It is suggested that Whizz-Dick is an acute and temporary penile shrinkage secondary to amphetamine use. The author also cited another name, "Speed Willy" in the North of England, to describe the shrinking-penis effect of amphetamines. Unfortunately, there is no detailed description of this penis shrinkage episode except the victim's observation and perception. The author labeled it as a "koro-like syndrome" and suggested that in drug-induced Koro, the drug might heighten a panic reaction and induce an abnormal body image that facilitates Koro-like perception and, as a consequence, may generate secondary neurotic symptoms and psychosexual dysfunction. The author suggested further research to examine the effects of amphetamine on penile morphology.

[13]. C. R. Altable, A. R. Urrutia: Koro-misidentification syndrome in schizophrenia? A plea for clinical psychopathology.
Psychopathology, 2004, 37(5), 249–252.

It is a very interesting clinical paper with a Koro case report from Spain. The authors very logically discussed the pitfalls of diagnostic procedures in psychiatry by referring to the concept of "surface grammar" (similarity in symptom) and "deep grammar" (different psychopathology). For example, they cited a case of acute psychosis with Koro perception and questioned the diagnostic confusion as per the usual rules of descriptive psychopathology.

They presented a case of a 23-year-old Caucasian male who suffered from:

> ... coenesthetic, gustatory, and olfactory hallucinations as well as from nonhallucinatory distortions in the perception of colours and a persecutory delusion, in which delusional perceptions and delusional interpretations were prominent. Depersonalization and derealization were also intense and severely affected body experience. Nevertheless, they seemed somewhat less prominent since the beginning of the persecutory-misidentification delusion. He suffered from thought withdrawal and passivity phenomena and experienced time as fragmented and devoid of direction. (p. 250)

Two days before admission, he complained of a sudden shrinkage of his penis and testicles that seemed to be pushed into his abdomen at this symptomatic clinical background. There was no fear of death. He also perceived that his neighbors and the medical staff who attended him were the same people in disguise. The authors discussed the controversy in diagnostic precision- whether the Koro perception is a part of abnormal body experiences of a schizophrenic perceptual abnormality or coexistence of Koro and misidentification syndrome (Fregoli subtype).

[14]. S. Sarró, V. Sarró: Koro syndrome: A case report.
Transcultural Psychiatry, 2004, 41(4), 558–560.

It is a Koro-like case report from Spain. The patient is a 49-year-old Moroccan married male who complained of pain in his penis and "spontaneous shrinking toward the abdomen with a persistent sensation of strain, forcing him to adopt certain postures to alleviate the discomfort." He has a long history of several medically unexplained somatic complaints that compelled several hospital visits. He has a history of hospitalization at age 43 for a paranoid disorder (against wife and daughter). All laboratory investigations were negative, except persistently positive urine tests for cannabis. He responded favorably with depot injection (zuclopenthixol decanoate, 200 mg, IM) and after that with added citalopram 30–60 mg daily.

[15]. M. MacLachlan (Ed.): Mass Hysteria.
In, Embodiment: Clinical, critical and cultural perspectives on health and illness. Open University Press, McGraw-Hill Education, 2004, England.

This book has a new approach to psychiatric phenomenology incorporating neuroscience, psychology, sociology, and anthropology. In a sub-chapter on Mass Hysteria (pp. 62–65), a brief discussion on Koro symptom formation (mainly epidemic form) and the role of fox spirit in the context of Chinese folk belief is described. It is suggested that "Koro cannot be adequately understood from the perspective of individual's (psycho) pathology, but should be approached from the perspective of expression of a community anxiety" (p. 64). Kirmayer and Santhanm (2001) suggest that in Koro "as with other epidemics of hysteria, social stresses create widespread feelings of vulnerability in a population or in group, and combine with individual vulnerabilities to anxiety to give rise to symptoms that follow culturally available symptom schemas."

2005

[16]. C. Mather: Accusations of genital theft: A case from northern Ghana.
Culture Medicine & Psychiatry, 2005, 29(1), 33–52.

It is a valuable research paper with high ethnographic quality. The author, a Canadian anthropologist, described his firsthand experience of genital theft and mob lynching phenomena ("instant justice") during his fieldwork at a village Zorse, in Northern Ghana. He also attempted to compare the genital theft of West Africa and genital involution and disappearance in South Asian Koro. After a descriptive and historical account of these two disorders, he stressed the two disorders' local meaning and cultural context. Citing the example of his observation of one such penis snatching episode at Zorse, he linked the etiological explanation of genital theft with the local cultural construct of "strangers and external threats." This mass psychology produces strong beliefs in witchcraft, diviners, magic and supernatural power, and misfortune causes. Magical power and knowledge influence personal and collective identity. The local power structure and social-political organization of communities demarcate *insider* and *outsider*. The latter is a threat to individual and collective identities and independence in many different ways. Also, the broader national climate of social transformation, the impact of rapid socio-political and economic changes, and its resultant threats of losing personal and collective identity are evident and impact local communities. In terms of psycho-social dynamics of genital theft and accusation, the author concluded that:

> Genitals are the means of procreation. Loss of genitals amounts to loss of the capacity to self- perpetuate. The victim of the crime experiences at the personal level what the Kusasi are experiencing at the level of the community and the region. Resolution of a case of genital theft, whether in the courts or by mob justice, reasserts the community's self-autonomy and ability to self-identity. (p. 49)

The concept of outsider-insider and external threat (with associated magical beliefs) explained the mass psychogenic response and behavior in "penis vanishing" epidemics in Africa.

[17]. V. A. Dzokoto, G. Adams: Understanding genital-shrinking epidemics in West Africa: koro, juju, or mass psychogenic illness? *Culture Medicine & Psychiatry, 2005, 29(1), 53–78.*

This is an extensively researched article on the penis-snatching episodes of six Western African nations. The authors analyzed 56 media reports of penis snatching/theft incidences between January 1997 and October 2003. They attempted to explain cultural psychology and compared these with Koro of South Asian settings. They believed that these episodes might represent culturally grounded idioms of distress or somatic response to panic. They also discussed other possible reasons for this epidemic behavior, like the folk construct of penis napping and money juju, deliberate acts of intentional deception, and social tension.

The common complaints in males were shrinking penis (20 cases) and vanishing or disappearing the penis (15 cases). It is interesting to note female victims' complaints, which ranged from shrinking breasts, changes to their genitalia, or both. One complained of "private parts sealed." And another complained that her genital organ vanished. One very serious and issue of forensic interest is "instant justice"—a social term for immediate beating and lynching of the alleged suspect. The authors documented at least 36 deaths from different African countries. The authors pointed out how the official and police system identified the complaints (and the victim) as a criminal offense instead of providing psychological assistance.

They discussed at length the cultural and local social context as a cause of these genital stealing phenomena. The authors pointed out the concept of "Money Juju"—a syndicate earning money through ransom and folk beliefs in witchcraft, sorcery, or juju and the role of local and regional social-political tension. They identified these episodes as "a culturally grounded idiom of distress or somatic response to panic." There is a good deal of discussion on Koro, and they compared this "genital shrinking disease" across four geographical areas: West Africa, South East Asia, Europe, and North America. This is a beneficial cross-cultural comparison. Lastly, they discussed Mass Psychogenic Illness (MPI) model and analytically discussed culture-bound syndromes and genital theft epidemics.

Observation: It seems confusing as the authors used the term genital shrinkage throughout the paper for genital theft. Ilechkwu (1992) described this as "magical penis loss." Still, in reality, the African incidences were related to the sudden vanishing of genitals (rather than shrink), allegedly by theft by a malevolent snatcher. In that sense, it is not Koro (or at best a variant of Koro), relatively a different African phenomenon altogether.

[18]. R. W. Freudenmann, C. Schönfeldt-Lecuona: The syndrome of genital retraction from a transcultural psychiatric point of view. Chinese Suo-yang, Indonesian koro and non-Asian forms (koro-like symptoms).

Nervenazrt, 2005, 76(5), 569–580. [Article in German]

This is a case report of Koro-like symptoms (KLS) in a 47-year-old German man associated with a major depressive episode. He had a terrifying perception of a shrinking penis. In his previous depressive episode, he had a similar penile perception as well. He responded favorably with lithium and venlafaxine treatment. The general discussion reviews the syndrome of genital retraction (SGR) from the transcultural perspective. The authors described the Koro expression in Chinese culture, which is mainly in epidemic form. But in the Western world, SGR is an isolated phenomenon usually associated with other neuropsychiatric illnesses and without any underlying cultural construct. This is called, Koro-like symptoms (KLS). They compare both forms of presentation, i.e., Asian Koro and Western KLS, and provided an account of their specific symptoms, cultural aspects, and therapeutic strategies. The authors provided the clinical distinction between the classical form of a syndrome of genital retraction (SGR) and the koro-like symptoms (KLS), which are less dramatic and without any cultural context. They commented that KLS is not a distinct entity in Western countries but represents an unspecified clinical entity related to other neuropsychiatric illnesses. The paper has a helpful review of the literature with 91 references.

[19]. R. W. Freudenmann, C. Schonfeldt-Lecuona: Koro-like symptoms in a recurrent depressive disorder.
Nervenarzt, 2005, 76(7), 883, 885–887. [Article in German]

It is a case report of a Koro-like symptom (KLS) in a German male with a recurrent major depressive disorder background. He had a terrifying perception that his penis was shrinking. He had a similar penile perception in his previous depression episode and then had a symptom-free interval. He responded favorably with treatment with venlafaxine and lithium. The authors concluded that "KLS is not a distinct clinical entity in Western countries but represents a concomitant syndrome that requires treatment of the underlying illness."

[20]. H. H. Deng, H. B. Zhen, J. Li, X. Huang, W. J. Xu, X. X. Peng: Report of Koro endemic in primary school students of Yangxi county, Fuhu school in Guandong.
Chinese Journal of Behaviour Medicine Science, 2005, 5, 451–452.
[Article in Chinese]

2006

[21]. C. K. Kalaitzi, A. Kalantzis: Cannabis-induced koro-like syndrome. A case report and mini review.
Urologia Internationalis, 2006, 76(3), 278–280.

This is a Koro case report in association with cannabis use, the first report from Greece. The case was a 32-year-old Caucasian male who presented to the Urology clinic because his penis had shrank for 2–3 days. There is a history of high work stress and smoking cannabis every weekend for the previous five years. Still, recently the frequency of cannabis smoking had increased to 3–4 joints daily. Toxicological urine screening showed a high cannabis level. His symptoms gradually reduced, and subsequently, he was diagnosed with a generalized anxiety disorder and treated with sertraline 100 mg/day and cognitive psychotherapy.

The discussion is an excellent global literature survey on Koro, secondary to neurological and urological pathology, and illicit drug use. The author suggested that: "serotoninergic effect of cannabis could underlie the emergence of cannabis-induced Koro-like syndrome, but only in individuals predisposed to dysmorphophobic apprehension by means of personality traits, cultural beliefs or psychopathology" and thus classify this "as a distinct form of substance-induced depersonalization disorder."

[22]. W.-.S Tseng: From peculiar psychiatric disorders through culture-bound syndromes to culture-related specific syndromes.
Transcultural Psychiatry, 2006, 43(4), 554–576.

This is a scholarly paper with heavy academic value. This article reviews the historical evolution of "exotic disorders" nosological concept and culture-bound Syndromes' (CBS) journey to Culture-related syndromes. He provides a short historical account of atypical or exotic psychiatric disorders during the 1890–1970 period. It contains many historical references and incidents of naming and identifying mental disorders from non-European societies and cultures. Though Yap (1951) referred to these folk mental illnesses as "peculiar to certain cultures," they were termed mainly as "exotic, rare, uncommon, extraordinary" or unclassifiable by the Western psychiatrists.

He then analyzed the trend to identify CBS in different rubrics during the period from 1970 to 1980. He devoted a lengthy discussion regarding the need for categorical grouping and place in the current classificatory system. A good conversation is dedicated to "Culture bound to Culture related" disorders with extensive referencing. Then he discussed the changing clinical pattern of many of the CBSs over time. He also touched on the culture-related syndromes in Western societies. The discussion section opened with a few important academic questions in Cultural Psychiatry in general and CBS in particular. These are: Symptom or Syndrome? Folk label or discrete disorder? Need for clinical observation and psychiatric examination; Clinical understanding versus social interpretation. In conclusion, he stressed the need for scientific research on culture-related syndromes and reminded the health professionals of the essential role of cultural psychiatry:

> It is time to move from merely studying the cultural aspects of psychopathology (fascinated by peculiar or exotic syndromes) to the provision of culturally competent care for all people of diverse cultures, in order to fulfill the contemporary mission of cultural psychiatry. (p. 571)

It is a quite extensively researched article of historical and practical value with a long list of valuable references.

[23]. M. Parzeller, R. Bux, C. Raschka, H. Bratzke: Sudden cardiovascular death associated with sexual activity. A forensic autopsy study (1972–2004).

Forensic Science, Medicine & Pathology, 2006, 2:2, 109–110.

This is not a Koro report. As coital death and Koro are mentioned in Traditional Chinese medical texts (Gwee, 1963), all Koro researchers should understand the real epidemiology. Gwee (1963) inquired about this association and found only 4 sudden deaths in Singapore. Three were due to coronary thrombosis. One was due to cerebral hemorrhage, and none were associated with Koro.

This is a 33 years forensic autopsy report (1972–2004) from the Frankfurt University Hospital, Germany. The findings among 32,000 autopsies were: 0.22% (68) of natural death occurred during sexual intercourse. 92.6% were men (average age 59.1 years), and 7.4% were women (average age 39.8 years). The most frequent cause was myocardial infarction- MI (41.2%), followed by coronary artery disease (29.4%). In 19 cases, there was a history of previous MI. 10.3% had cerebral hemorrhages. The authors calculated the annual incidence of sudden cardiovascular death during sexual activity to be 1.9 per 1000 autopsies for men and 0.16 per 1000 autopsies for women.

[24]. J. L. Powell: Culture-Bound Syndromes: Koro.
In, Encyclopedia of Multicultural Psychiatry. Y. K. Jackson (Editor), Sage publication, Thousand Oaks, California. 2006.

It contains a discussion on Koro (pp. 138–139) under the heading Culture-bound Syndromes in the chapter (pp. 130–147), which is a quite rich entry of the most prevalent culture-bound syndromes. On Koro's culture-boundness, the author commented: "Because koro (or at least its symptoms) is a universal disorder, it has been termed genital retraction syndrome, indicating that it may not be culture-bound but rather a culture-related psychiatric disorder" (p. 139).

[25]. J. Porta-Etessam, D. A. Pérez-Martínez. A. Martínez-Salio, A. Berbel-García: Syndrome Koro.
Revista de Neurologia, 2006, 43(10), 639–640. [L] [Article in Spanish]

It is a short discussion paper with a Koro case report of a 57-year single Spanish man. The authors also provided a summary table on 16 culture-bound syndromes.

2007

[26]. C. Buckle, Y. M. Chuah, C. S. Fones, A. H. Wong: A conceptual history of Koro.

Transcultural Psychiatry, 2007, 44(1), 27–43.

This well-researched article systematically described Koro's conceptual history development by citing examples from global reporting. They started with a broad triad of Koro's clinical components, viz., perceptual, cognitive, and emotional features of Koro's presentation. They missed to include the fourth dimension, i.e., behavioral. The paper is divided according to four major perspectives: Traditional Chinese Medicine (TCM), Psychoanalytical propositions, Psychiatric or biomedical observations, and Sociological construct. Each section has tried to highlight how Koro illness' construct develops over time and helps create more confusion than consensus. They asked a serious ontological question that whether Koro is objectively or subjectively real (*emic* perspective of TCM) or an *etic* (outsider) perspective (Western). They also discussed the different schools' different propositions regarding the definition and classification of Koro and the difference between sporadic and epidemic Koro. They discussed the inherent conflict between etiological and phenomenological classification, as is surfaced by recent sporadic Koro reporting with varied pathology and epidemic Koro in different cultural settings other than Chinese. They concluded:

> …it is clear that no single existing classification system can adequately integrate the various conceptualization of Koro….. The focus on phenomenological criteria, with limited consideration of etiology, can obscure important aspects of behavioral disorders, as exemplified by the difference between epidemic and isolated types of Koro. … one of the main purposes of consistent, rational disease classification system is to facilitate the grouping of disorders that may share a common etiology, with one potential benefit being the identification of homogenous diagnostic groups for research into the etiology of these disorders. (p. 39)

This paper helps Koro researchers develop an insight into Koro's phenomenological approach over time and the inherent contradiction and controversies in each nosological category.

[27]. I. Saman, N. Siddiqui, W. Yosafzai: Koro in a 13 years old boy of interior Sindh- a mistreated cultural syndrome.
Journal of College of Physicians & Surgeons of Pakistan, 2007, 17(1), 60. (L)

Probably it is the first report of Koro from Pakistan. The authors presented a 13-year-old boy from interior Sindh province, having a two-month history of absence from school, restlessness, clinging behavior, crying spells, and fear that his penis is retracting into the abdomen and he would die. He was diagnosed with a moderate depressive episode with Koro syndrome. He had several investigations and consulted many specialists, including spiritual treatment, without any benefit at all. He responded well with dothiepin 25 mg at night and education about the illness to the father. The authors discussed the Asian tendency to express mental health issues in terms of somatic problems. In that sense, Koro may be considered a form of somatization of the castration fear.

Observation: Given the two months' duration, the case may be labeled as chronic Koro, and constant preoccupation with anxious thoughts of penile shrinkage points toward the thought content's obsessive quality.

[28]. H. Atalay: İki koro sendromu olgusu veya genital organlarin geri çekilmesi korkusu ile birlikte olan anksiyete bozukluğu (Two cases of koro syndrome or anxiety disorder associated with genital retraction fear).
Türk Psikiyatri Dergisi, 2007, 18(3), 282–285. [Article in Turkish]

This is an excellent short paper where the author supported the contention that Koro is a form of anxiety disorder. First, he showed how the Koro nosology changed from a regional construct to a universal formulation, with the Koro reporting from different parts of the globe. From the standpoint of the anxiety spectrum, he postulated that it involves an anxiety reaction with the ideational component of fear of death from genital retraction at an individual or sporadic level. At the collective or epidemic level, it is expressed as mass-panic. Moreover, it is mainly with another comorbid neuropsychiatric condition in the former, but it has a specific cultural undercurrent in the latter. Analyzing the global data and his two cases, he questioned that: "… whether the genital retraction is one of many symptoms of anxiety rather than a specific symptom of the culture-bound Koro syndrome." He presented two Koro cases from Turkey and suggested that the anxiety spectrum was the primary presentation rather than any cultural predisposition.

Case 1: A 20-year-old Turkish male, while he was in an African country, one night had an experience of genital shrinking associated with fear of death. After his anxious return to Turkey, he was assessed and diagnosed with anxiety disorder NOS and responded well with antidepressants. He has only this solitary attack.

Case 2: A 36-year-old single Turkish male presented himself anxiously to a hospital emergency. His complaint was: "… not being able to feel his penis at night. He masturbated to be sure that his penis was intact, but he did not feel it again in the morning and thought it was retracting into his abdomen." There is a history of a feeling of numbness in his arms, and he thought he had a heart attack. Subsequently, a psychiatrist was consulted when he was worried about the recurrence of the penile experience. He was diagnosed with anxiety disorder NOS and responded well with antidepressant treatment for a month.

Observation: It appears from the case description that the first case may have some study stress in a foreign culture and country, and the second case, a possible diagnosis of hypochondriasis. In both situations, anxiety has a definite role to play. A longitudinal follow-up would be interesting to see whether there were any further similar attacks.

[29]. J. J. Mattelaer, W. Jilek: Koro- The psychological disappearance of the penis.
Journal of Sexual Medicine, 2007, 4, 1509–1515.

This is a scholarly written historical review of Koro phenomena with an ethnomedical focus on different world cultures. In the first part, the authors traced the early history of Koro reporting from Indonesia and then predominantly from the Chinese in Singapore. They maintained two clinical types- Primary Koro, where shared cultural beliefs play an essential role. The Secondary Koro, mainly from Western countries where Koro symptoms are secondary to mental or somatic disorder or drug-induced condition.

In the second part, they briefly described the Koro epidemics in Singapore (1967), Thailand (1976), Southern China (1984–1985), and India (1985). They tried to provide some local socio-economic and political tensions that impose a survival threat to the local population in each instance.

Then they described genital disappearance episodes in Africa. They noted few small-scale epidemics of "magical robbing of genitals" in some West African nations like Ivory Coast, Ghana, Senegal, and Nigeria. Several persons were lynched and killed by violent crowds for allegedly making male genitals shrink or disappear. Referring to the report by Prinz (1998) they cited a fascinating culture-bound syndrome as:

> ....*kaza basolo* syndrome among the Azande in the northeastern Congo, which is assumed to lead to a painful death after magical theft of the clitoris or penis by members of a secret society who rob these parts through handshake, then burn them and apply the ashes to their hunting gear for success in the hunt. (p. 1512)

They also described the loss of membrum virile by the magical attacks of witches in Europe in the middle ages. From this historical analysis, they concluded that the psychological disappearance of the penis is a universal syndrome. The extra credit for this paper is the presentation of five photos. Two of Koro patients of South China epidemic, one of a drawing showing the Zande sorcerer of DRC Congo who removed the penis of a boy; one of a phallus tree and one medieval woodcut showing a witch is taking the phallus of a man.

Note. In their similar publication, the authors provided a fascinating photograph relating to "Exorcism treatment" of Koro from the 1985-South China epidemic, which shows a traditional healer is extracting the possession of a female fox spirit from the middle finger of a koro patient:

Jilek W. G., Mattelaer J. J. Koro: The psychological disappearance of the penis. *De Historia Urologiae Europaeae,* 2006; 13, 57–73.

[30]. E. Stip, T. Bergeron, C. Lavigueur, J. L. Fabian, A. Bentaleb: Koro syndrome.
Medico Psychological Annals, 2007, 165(3), 147–153.

It is a handy clinical paper on Koro with a general discussion and exciting six cases from Quebec, who presents Koro-like symptom at the background of psychotic illness.

Case 1: A 31 year, Quebec man having difficulties with premature ejaculation and hypo-erection with "growing anxiety relating to the loss of physical integrity, namely penis shrinks and trying to enter his stomach." He was diagnosed with major depression and responded well with desipramine 300 mg daily.

Case 2: A 32-year-old Native American (Algonquin), having a history of alcoholism and solvents inhalation, with a delusion of persecution and self-talking. A very interesting symptom was the shouts of animal call (wolf).# He had a homosexual relationship with his brother. He tied his penis with laces or strings to prevent the shortening and disappearance of his penis into his belly. CT scan showed frontotemporal atrophy. He was diagnosed with cerebral organic syndrome and partially responded with a low dose of antipsychotics.

Case 3: An 18-year-old Quebecer had a history of repeated hospitalization for his paranoid schizophrenia. There are histories of aggressive behaviors, persistent discord with alcoholic father, broken love affairs that lead to repeated masturbation, and prostitute visits with resultant guilt. During his last hospitalization, after threatening behavior toward his mother, he expressed his extreme anxiety "to see his penis diminish and curl up and said the penis is like a piece of ice that is melting in the heat and would disappear." He expressed his conviction that masturbation and prostitute visits may prevent this penile condition.

Case 4: A 25-year-old man diagnosed with paranoid schizophrenia since age 16 presented at emergency with extreme anxiety and olfactory hallucination of genital origin (odors) and stated: "rape of his brain" and sex is about to disappear inside the abdomen, and he will die.

Case 5: A 25-year man with paranoid schizophrenia presented with an auditory hallucination of death threats and fear that his penis would be removed by magic (of satanic origin). His anguish took an obsessive form during his hospital stay to check and recheck his genitals frequently in the bathroom. He poorly responded with risperidone and venlafaxine for a two weeks trial.

Case 6: A 31-year-old man, diagnosed with paranoid schizophrenia since the age of 19, had several admissions (20 times), presented with command hallucination that orders him to kill him and predict the disappearance of his penis and testicles. So he always felt that his penis narrowed in and invaginated in his lower abdomen. He was obsessed with this eventuality; he repeatedly stood near the toilet to check his penis dimensions. He responded well with quetiapine 800 mg daily dose.

The authors discussed the delusion of genital disappearance in terms of psychoanalytic constructs. They also drew attention to the difference in these clinical presentations from Asian variants. This paper is full of clinically rich histories of the patients. It helps us understand the nature and degree of genital loss/disappearance delusion in the psychotic process.

This reminds me of a hysterical epidemic in a tribal village in Tripura, India. The victims there were mimicking different animal calls (Chowdhury, 1992a).

[31]. G. Adams, V. A. Dzokoto: Genital-shrinking in Ghana: A cultural-psychological analysis.
Culture & Psychology, 2007, 13, 83–104.

This unique psycho-social research on "Genital Shrinking Panic" (GSP) was conducted in Ghana, Africa. The authors tried to examine this epidemic in terms of a psycho-social framework of "mutual constitution" (MC)—a dialectical process by which cultural realities and psychological experience reciprocally orient themselves. They analyzed 52 incidents reported in 13 different news media articles (in two prominent Ghanain daily newspapers) in January 1997. It was observed that most of the alleged perpetrators were men, including one woman who caused genital shrinking. Most of the alleged victims were men, but a news report of women complained of genital organs or breasts shrinkage was also there. In addition to that, they interviewed 22 people in the community in local vernacular (Dagomba) following a pre-designed interview format.

The authors analyzed GSP's media interpretations as either "criminal tampering" or "false accusation." Then they, based on their findings, proposed the conceptual framework of 'mutual constitution. They summarize their theoretical framework as follows:

> To summarize, occurrences of GSP draw attention to an important process: the role of psychological activity in the reproduction of cultural reality. Beyond the classic ethnographic perspective that seeks to explain how episodes of genital-shrinking panic make sense given local beliefs, a cultural psychological analysis explores how beliefs in genital shrinking might be or become true. The focus of the analysis is not the invention of culture at the level of macrolevel structures, but instead the microlevel reproduction of cultural worlds through ordinary psychological activity. (p. 96)

Observation: The only concern in this research was the case definition—whether the victims had the genital organ in situ, be it shrunk or retracted, or their complete disappearance of the genital organ due to theft. Psychologically the presence or absence of organs makes a significant phenomenological difference in the construction of psychopathology. I think this area should clearly delineate the exact nature of the perceptual genital abnormality.

[32]. W. G. Jilek: Koro—el sindrome multicultural.
In, Villaseáor-Bayardo, Sergio J.; Fernández, Francisco A.; Garrabé de Lara, Jean (eds.) La psiquiatría en el siglo XXI: realidad y compromiso. Universidad de Guadalajara, Centro Universitario de Ciencias de la Salud: Guadalajara, Mexico 2007; pp. 189–197.

It is a scholarly written extensive overview of Koro illness from a transcultural perspective. From the very root of the first publication by Blonk in 1895, the author discussed the various epidemics covering different geographical regions to the examples of "loss of membrane virile" of medieval Europe. The author stressed the geopolitical and psychosocial stress in the background of the epidemics. The author also discussed the African phenomena of "penis-loss" epidemics from a transcultural perspective. The extra credit of this highly informative paper is its 61 references.

2008

[33]. H. Al-Sinawi, S. Al-Adawi, A. Al-Guendi: Ramadan fasting triggering Koro-like symptoms during acute alcohol withdrawal: A case report from Oman.
Transcultural Psychiatry, 2008, 45(4), 695–704.

This is a clinically interesting paper where the authors reported a case of 48-year-old Omani married man from Muscat. The patient has a long history of alcohol abuse. The case showed the impact of Ramadan fasting (which included abstention from alcohol) and complained of erectile dysfunction, which he believed to be related to the vicious act of his past lover who drugged him and amputated his penis in a private clinic as an act of revenge. The delusion of genital amputation is the predominant psychotic feature in his alcohol withdrawal delirium tremens. Family members believed that he was possessed by a *Jinni* of a "non-Muslim origin." His psychotic excitement was resolved successfully with diazepam, olanzapine, and other medications. The authors suggested that the chronic abuse of alcohol and resulting depressive disorder, erectile dysfunction, and withdrawal probably triggered his psychotic episode. They also discussed alcohol use in Omani culture.

Observation: One crucial question remains why the authors addressed this issue as "Koro-like symptom" when there is no penile shrinkage or retraction complaint or any fear of death. The delusion of penile amputation is in no way resembles Koro's symptom. There is ample description of his elaborate paranoid delusion and psychotic features of delirium tremens that best described his alleged genital amputation as a psychotic symptom. This delusional anxiety and other withdrawal symptoms are definitely not "conceptually and phenomenologically, similar to koro."

[34]. P. Garlipp: Koro–A culture-bound phenomenon: Intercultural psychiatric implications.
German Journal of Psychiatry, 2008, 11(1), 21–28.

It is a very extensively researched discussion paper on Koro, where the author surveyed 131 Koro publications between 1954 and 2006. He very elegantly discusses Koro's different clinical aspects, including aetiological or predisposing factors, various associated mental or physical disorders, and the psychodynamic construct (psychological castration) and psychophysiological changes. Finally, the types of treatment. He provided a useful long table depicting authors (year), patient's origin, diagnosis, age, duration, and treatment in each report. He discusses at length the different diagnostic provisions. From the 84 case reports analysis, he found two common features: the diversity of the cases and fear as a leading symptom. He mentioned the different types of medications used to treat Koro symptoms. He questioned that: "...whether the disappearance of the Koro-like symptoms reported can always be explained by the drug treatment or instead may be a natural course of the illness remains unanswered."

The author recommends using the term Koro with some restrictions to those who display socio-culturally rooted phenomena, as seen in epidemics. All cases with secondary pathology should be referred to as genital retraction syndrome. He also stressed the importance of knowledge of different medical faculty members about Koro, as many cases may present in clinics other than psychiatry. The article has a long reference list that is useful to any Koro researchers.

[35]. A. N. Chowdhury: Cultural Koro and Koro-like symptom (KLS).
German Journal of Psychiatry, 2008, 11, 81–82. (L)

The author wrote this letter to add a few essential missing issues in Garlipp's Koro paper (GJP, 2008). The first issue was the Koro in females, which has a passing mention in his writing. The author cited here the 146 female Koro cases from 1969 to 1988—all are epidemic cases. This paper also reports the interfamilial occurrence of Koro—21 patients from 9 families. It also added some research data on Koro with another psychiatric diagnosis: Schizophrenia (4 male cases); Paranoid schizophrenia (7 male patients), Affective disorder–(1 male first episode depression, two male bipolar depression, one female neurotic depression; 2 female psychotic depression and one female bipolar depression) and nine female conversion hysteria cases. This article also described the criteria for the clinical use of the term Koro and Koro-like symptom (KLS). He also pointed out the phenomenological difference between Koro and penis snatching/theft epidemics of Africa. He supports the contention that for proper clinical management, other faculty members should be adequately aware of this psycho-physical penis pathology of Koro or KLS.

[36]. V. R. J. Kondan: A case of koro in a Caucasian man.
Progress in Neurology & Psychiatry, 2008, 12(4), 25–27.

Koro's case report is a 43-year-old Caucasian man of Italian origin with a longstanding complaint of generalized and persistent anxiety and panic attacks from the UK. During his typical autonomic arousal episodes, he developed the feeling that his genitals were retracting into the abdomen. He then rushed to the toilet to check whether the retraction is occurring. It seems that these episodes were frequent for the last ten years, which means he had multiple Koro perceptions. The attacks occurred only for a few minutes every two to three weeks. He believed that the sensations were real, and his checking behavior was not repetitive. He avoided going to places that have no toilet facility. The author diagnosed him as a case of generalized anxiety disorder with panic disorder. The patient responded favorably with an SSRI (citalopram). He had no fear of death. This case may be an example of incomplete or partial Koro with anxiety/panic disorder. The author very rightly commented that "Koro is rarely observed in the western hemisphere, and the cases reported are usually associated with other major psychiatric disorders. The typical symptoms of Koro are rarely reported in Caucasians."

[37]. A. W. Shindel, M. M. Garcia, T. F. Lue: Penis panics: A brief history of koro, dhat, and related disorders.
The Journal of Urology, 2008, 179(4), 310–311.

It is a discussion paper based on the review of world literature on Koro and Dhat. They noted that Koro-like syndrome is mentioned in Chinese medical texts from 300 B.C. In India, ancient Ayurvedic texts stressed the value of semen and caution against indiscriminate ejaculation. The pathognomic role of sexual impropriety, masturbation, infidelity, and seminal nocturnal loss in both disorders is highlighted. In some instances, malign external influence like witchcraft is also implicated. They mentioned the Koro epidemic of Singapore and magical penis loss in Senegal. They concluded that:

> Phobic anxiety about damage to/ loss of the genitalia has been reported throughout history and in men from all corners of the world. On occasion, socio-cultural factors have led to widespread "penis panics" affecting entire populations. (p. 311)

[38]. F. Bures: mind dismembered- In search of the magical penis thieves. (Letter from Nigeria)
Harper's Magazine, 2008, June, 60–65.

This is an adventurous but ethnographic and emic study by the author who was deeply interested in the serial phenomena of penis theft in African countries and ultimately his keen interest pushed him to visit

Lagos, Nigeria, facing climatic hostility and narrowly escaped mass attack for his curiosity. He provided a detailed observation and literary account of his first hand experience of local culture and penis-loss incidents and activity of penis thieves on the streets of Lagos. This is a very interesting description, with academic references and a sense of satire, the author very minutely and in a psychological way unfolded the socio-cultural mystery behind the African phenomena of penis-thieving.

* * *

Box 8.1. Some African News Media report of Penis Theft

'Nigerian witch steals man's penis'

EISH! / 8 DECEMBER 2000, 10:03PM /

Lagos—Police in Lagos late on Friday detained a woman who had been stripped and beaten by a mob after a man accused her of "stealing" his penis.

A spokesperson at Ikoyi, the Onikan police station, declined to reveal the identity of the woman, who was beaten up and led down a busy road, half naked, by a mob of about 100 people.

Members of the crowd said that the woman was a witch who had magically 'stolen' the penis of a man in the crowd.

No-one in the crowd, who were insulting and hitting the woman and had torn off her shirt and bra, said they had actually seen any evidence (the man was holding tightly on to his trousers) but all appeared to believe his story.

The Onikan police station spokesperson refused to say on what grounds the woman was being held or whether the claims of the man that his member was missing had been verified.

Belief in the power of women to magically 'steal' mens' private parts by an incantation or simple handshake are widespread across Nigeria and much of west Africa. Sapa-AFP [https://www.iol.co.za/news/eish/nigerian-witch-steals-mans-penis-55656].

THE TELEGRAPH

Congo police arrest penis snatchers

Police in Congo have arrested suspected sorcerers accused of using black magic to steal or shrink men's private parts.

8:15AM BST 23 April 2008.

There has been a wave of panic and attempted lynchings triggered by the alleged witchcraft. Reports of so-called penis snatching are not uncommon in West Africa, where belief in traditional religions and witchcraft remains widespread, and where ritual killings to obtain blood or body parts still occur.

Rumours of the bizarre theft began circulating last week in the capital Kinshasa. They quickly dominated radio call-in shows, with listeners advised to beware of fellow passengers in communal taxis wearing gold rings, who were blamed for the devastating curse.

Purported victims, 14 of whom were detained by police, claimed that sorcerers simply touched them to make their genitals shrink or disappear.

But some residents said the "victims" were simply trying to extort cash by promising a cure, proved by the reappearance of their genitals.

"You just have to be accused of that, and people come after you. We've had a number of attempted lynchings. … You see them covered in marks after being beaten," said Jean-Dieudonne Oleko, Kinshasa's police chief. Police arrested the accused sorcerers and their victims in an effort to avoid the sort of bloodshed seen in Ghana a decade ago, when 12 suspected penis-snatchers were beaten to death by angry mobs.

"I'm tempted to say it's one huge joke," Mr Oleko said. "But when you try to tell the victims that their penises are still there, they tell you that it's become tiny or that they've become impotent. To that I tell them, 'How do you know if you haven't gone home and tried it'," he said. Some Kinshasa residents accuse a separatist sect from the nearby Bas-Congo province of being behind the witchcraft in revenge for a recent government crackdown on its members.

"It's real. Just yesterday here, there was a man who was a victim. We saw. What was left was tiny," said 29-year-old Alain Kalala. [https://www.telegraph.co.uk/news/1898902/Congo-police-arrest-penis-snatchers.html].

* * *

[39]. N. Coull, T. O'Brien: Street urology: beyond the formulary.
BJU International, 2008, 103, 721–722.

This reporting is valuable for alerting all Koro researchers because of recent repotting of Koro or Koro-like symptoms associated with dependence or withdrawal of abusive substances. The authors cited different research data to show how other commonly abused drugs cause urogenital symptoms/side effects and sexual dysfunction. They described the drugs like Cocaine, Opioids, Ecstasy, Cannabis, Ketamine, and Steroids. They provided applicable mnemonic CHECKS to identify and check for the use of cocaine, heroin, ecstasy, cannabis, ketamine, and steroids for all young people presenting with sexual dysfunction.

2009

[40]. L. F. Charlotte, J. Bycroft: Street urology: beyond the formulary.
BJU International, 2009, 104, 5, 722. (L)

This is a letter in response to Coull and O'Brien's article in *BJU International, 2008, 103, 721–722* (review No 39 above). They identified that amphetamine was missed from the report. They reported that the vasoconstrictive effect of amphetamine in some patients and is known as "speed dick," "speed willy," or "whizz dick." Amphetamine is a psychostimulant and may cause shrinkage of the flaccid penis (third of normal size) for the duration of the drug's effect. They also cited Bloor's (2004) paper and also mentioned the cannabis-induced Koro in the literature.

[41]. L. Faccini: The incredible case of the shrinking penis: A Koro-like syndrome in a person with intellectual disability.
Sexuality & Disability, 2009, 27(3), 173–178.

This is a fascinating report on a 47-year-old male with a learning disability and fixated pedophilia. His intellectual disability was due to a brain injury at birth due to forceps delivery. There is a history of at least 25 children whom he rubbed and touched. He was also engaged in limited instances of public masturbation and obscene phone calling. His fixated pedophilia was a non-exclusionary type. He reported that a baby (internalized imagined companions -IIC), inside his head forced his compliance to engage in infant/child-like activities with the threat that it would shrink his penis if he did not comply. This experience was managed by focusing on him contending in his "new me" behavior of being an assertive leader, which helped a rapid restabilization. The author proposed that this Koro-like symptom may be an example of the depersonalization syndrome, where a dissociative mechanism affects the body image integrity. Individual therapy to highlight a "New me" as an assertive leader helped reduce his anxiety and distress concerning Koro-like symptoms.

[42]. L. Faccini, J. Tucker: The return of koro and the companions in a person with intellectual disability: Follow up assessment and dynamics.
Sexuality & Disability, 2009, 27(4), 239–248.

This is a follow up of the previous case reported by the author (Sexuality and Disability 27(3): 173–178). After a detailed assessment and therapy, the IIC of the baby was banished. But subsequent follow up showed that baby has returned and said that:

> the baby had taken over his body, … Usually, he reported that the baby "moves around" within his body on a near daily basis "going into my penis, playing with my butt", but with the preference of "staying more in my penis and stomach" (previously he reported that it only lived in his head).

The authors believed that this.

IICs were created to deal with his trauma, loss and loneliness. Two conditions that may have contributed to the formation of the IICs involve him having an exceptional creative imagination, and since having difficulties with interpersonal relationships and relating, the development of Schizoid Personality Traits. (p. 247)

[43]. F. Maner et al.: Secondary koro: A case report.
Klinik Psikofarmakoloji Bulteni, 2009, 19(Sup 1), S168–S170. [Article in Turkish]

The authors stressed the classification of Koro as primary and secondary. They discussed a Koro-like symptom in a male case of paranoid schizophrenia.

[44]. K. Marlowe: The cultural myth of Koro conceptualization: Time for a rethink.
Transcultural Psychiatry, 2009, 46(2), 375–376. (L)

This letter was written in response to Buckley et al.'s (2007) paper published in Transcultural Psychiatry (review no 26 above). The author challenged Koro's concept as a culture-bound Asian disorder, mainly because of Koro's widespread reporting from diverse regions, ethnicities and secondary to other diseases, ranging from substance abuse to psychosis. The author believes that the term "genital retraction syndrome" (Edwards, 1984) is a more useful descriptive term than Koro. The author tried to restrict the phenomenology of individual Koro from the epidemic Koro. In the former, a shared cultural idiom of distress may play a role. The latter is a collective expression of anxiety among the poorly educated population without knowledge of the "biomedical approach to distress." By referring to African genital theft epidemics, the author supports the sociological concept of collective behavior.

[45]. H. Yang, C. Tranulis, O. Freudenreich: Keeping culture-bound syndromes in cultural context: The case of Koro.

International Journal of Culture & Mental Health, 2009, 2(2), 86–91.

This is a discussion paper with a case report. The authors attempted to explain the difference between culture-bound syndrome Koro and Koro's sporadic cases associated with other psychopathology. They mentioned the justification of considering the differences between the "surface grammar" and "deep grammar" of clinical presentation. The case they presented was a 56-year-old, single, first-generation Italian American with a long history (15 years) of schizophrenia. In addition to his disorganized behavior with severe anhedonia and anxiety, he had multiple bodily delusions, including a sense that his penis has shrunken and continuing to shrink. The authors stressed that it is a Koro symptom that omits his severe psychopathology according to surface grammar. But according to deep grammar, his core presentation was schizophrenia with a Koro-like symptom, which guides the appropriate treatment intervention. The authors very nicely elaborated on the role of culture and their different dispositions in selecting the penile symptom choice- which they exemplified with Chinese culture and Western (American) culture. They stressed the importance of locating the deep grammar in the context of local culture (in this case) rather than labeling it with Koro by the rule of the presentation's surface grammar. They further elaborated that:

> It is not surprising that Koro, as a culture-bound syndrome, can share some presentations with non-culture specific syndromes or vise versa. Efforts should be made to look for a 'deep grammar' that can further understanding and guide interventions. In this case, we would argue that schizophrenia with its perceptual problems is the 'deep grammar' and that personal history, body shape and American cultural symbols related to sexuality not only colored and shaped the context of symptoms, but also played a contributing role in symptom genesis and maintenance (90).

Observation: This conceptual framework of surface and deep grammar is helpful in the understanding and diagnostic precision of primary and secondary Koro or Koro and Koro-like symptoms (KLS).

[46]. H. Evans, R. E. Bartholomew: Outbreak: The Encyclopedia of extraordinary social behavior.
Anomalist Books, 2009, San Antonio, TX

With a scholarly disposition, this book contains a detailed reporting of extraordinary social behaviors (outbreaks), spans more than two millennia, and provided a very insightful analysis of the events from the historical and cultural context. It covers many topics and incidents covering many facets of human behavior, viz., collective behavior, deviance, social and perceptual psychology, sociology, religious dimension, social anthropology, sociology, and mental health. It discusses Genital shrinking scares (pp. 194–203); Koro in different South-East Asian Countries; Epidemic koro, and Genital vanishing scares (pp. 203–206). It is an excellent reading to develop historical insight and current sociological affairs relating to mental ill-health and psychiatric epidemics.

2010

[47]. L. Faccini: From peter pan to a normal man: A happy ending.
Sexuality & Disability, 2010, 28(4), 297–299.

This is a summary paper of the follow-up of a patient with a learning disability, who initially showed Koro-like symptoms, imaginary companions, and sex offending behavior, reported earlier (2009). After treatment for eight months, the patient recovered.

[48]. L. Jie: Koro epidemic among school children in Guangdong, China.
World Cultural Psychiatric Research Review, 2010, 102–105.

This is a crucial Koro epidemic reporting from a school in Fuhu village, Yangxi County of Guangdong province, China. The author also provided some helpful information about Koro in China: it usually occurs in southeast China's coastal areas, especially when the community faces social stress. He reported one child Koro case from Sichuan province in central China.

Report of the epidemic: it involved 64 male students within three days in late May of 2004. The age range was 6–15 years. In the Fuhu village, a Koro epidemic had occurred in 1963, involving 50 adults for about ten days. Koro is called in this village as S*suo-yang* (shrink of yang organ, i.e., penis) and *kong-suo* (panic shrink). The author gave a very nice history of the epidemic background as follows:

1. On May 21, 2004—a third-grade boy student had an attack of Koro and ran home, subsequently treated by a local healer (80-year-old lady) by *aijiu* (moxibustion).
2. On May 23, the school principal summoned all the school children (393 boys and 287 girls). Using a microphone explained the incident and warned them to be cautious and take emergency measures if they experience such symptoms.
3. On that day, four boy students have a Koro attack.
4. Next day, 60 boy students had Koro attacks.
5. 63 students received *aijiu* treatment from the same lady healer.
6. Local administration by public health education mitigated the spreading panic in the locality.

The author reported two sets of research data from this area. One compares the Eysenck Personality Questionnaire (Chinese version) among the 64 Koro victims and 64 non-koro control groups. Koro subjects showed a lower E score (Extravert) than the non-koro subjects, meaning Koro students were less sociable with timid personalities. Interestingly, in a similar research design, Chowdhury (1991) found a high score of E and N (neuroticism) among the adult Koro victims of the 1982 Indian epidemic.

The research was done in 2009, and that was a survey using the Folk Belief Questionnaire among adults (n 61) and school children (n 36), which showed that 57.4% of adults and 59% of children believed that Suo-yang was a dangerous condition. A similar perception of "dangerousness" about Koro is reported by Koro patients and community in a social response study of the North Bengal Koro epidemic by Chowdhury (1992b, 2008) from India.

The healing lady's detailed account is fascinating; she told her professional experience about an adult Suo-yang epidemic in the village in 1963. Interestingly, no female student was affected. The author suggested that academic stress among male children may be an underlying factor.

[49]. M. R. Llompart, J. M. J. Llobera: A report on Koro syndrome.
*Formacion Medica Continuada en Atencion Primaria, 2010, **17** (5), 339–340.* [Article in Spanish]

[50]. D. Mitchell: Koro in Eastern Indonesia 1999–2010.
Asia–Pacific Psychiatry, 2010, 2 (3), A7

The author presented this short paper at the 14th Pacific Rim College of Psychiatrists Scientific Meeting, held at Brisbane, 28–30 October 2010. This is valuable research to our understanding of Koro because this report is from Indonesia, where the concept and the disorder were first reported in 1895!

From his fieldwork in Indonesia, the author presented the interview materials with three traditional healers who treat penis-retraction syndromes within three different ethnolinguistic groups in the Makassar region in Eastern Indonesia. He observed a surprising diversity in the names of the disorder, clinical presentation, and folk aetiologies.

The author provided some vital information.

1. In the west and central Flores, Koro is attributed to black magic known as "ru'u pota" (shrinking spell).
2. In eastern Sumba, koro is known as "hei lulu" (everything pulled inside), and the role of individual vulnerability and life stress is implicated.
3. In Makassar, the term "koroq" is used about black magic that wives use to punish their unfaithful husbands. In recent years, the fear of losing sexual function has replaced the fear of death from Koro.

The author also reported a Koro epidemic in Ende's town in 1999, where rumor and suggestibility played an important role. This is a very informative research presentation.

[51]. E. Ntouros, A. Ntoumanis, V. P. Bozikas, S. Donias, I. Giouzepas, G. Garyfalos: Koro-like symptoms in two Greek men. *BMJ Case Report, 2010, March 15.* https://doi.org/10.1136/bcr.08.2008.0679

This is a Koro-like case report from Greece. The authors presented two unusual cases of Koro-like symptoms reported in the background of psychiatric morbidity.

The first case was a 40-year-old fisherman who attended an emergency with complaints of radiating burning pain at the penis root and the penis's shrinking toward the abdomen, causing a persistent sensation of strain. He also has three months history of depressive symptoms. He believed that he contracted some kind of virus that lived in his penis for the last 18 years after intercourse with a prostitute. For the last 18 years, he had periods of relapse with symptoms lasting for months and consulted many urologists, neurologists and had different laboratory tests. He was diagnosed with major depressive disorder (? Psychotic) and treated with citalopram 20 mg and quetiapine 200 mg for two months. This has improved his depressive mood and pain symptoms, "but the penile discomfort persisted, and his belief in the "genital virus" remained unshaken.

The second case was a 24-year-old man who presented with irritability, auditory command hallucination, and aggressivity. He also complained of a sensation that his penis retracts into the abdomen and expressed fear that it will eventually be lost. A history of sexual assault at age 17 generated a sense of guilt and confusion about gender and sex. He also reported that currently, he has the feeling that he had breast. He has been treated with olanzapine 30 mg and supportive psychotherapy. At three weeks, his koro-like symptoms disappeared.

The authors discussed the importance of clinical examination of past sexuality, sexual identity, and primary diagnostic workup in each case with Koro-like symptoms. In both cases, this KLS may be viewed as a delusional symptom as a part of their primary psychopathology.

[52]. J. R. Bermudez, L. C. A. Venegas, D. C. Melendez, M. E. Nadurille, F. Nente, M. F. Mendez: Cotard syndrome in neurological and psychiatric patients.
Journal of Neuropsychiatry & Clinical Neuroscience, 2010, 22(4), 409–416.

It is an exciting clinical paper on Cotard syndrome among neurological and psychiatric patients from Mexico City, Mexico. The authors discussed the concept and definition of Cotard syndrome and then briefly discussed the proposed mechanism of Cotard syndrome. They did a retrospective review of all inpatients from the National Institute of Neurology, Mexico, from March 2007 to May 2009. Among 1321 inpatient consultations, 63% had a neurological disease, and one (0.11%) had viral encephalitis and Cotard syndrome. Of inpatients, 36.2% had pure psychiatric disorders, and three (0.62%) had Cotard syndrome, associated with psychotic depression, depersonalization, and penile retraction (Koro syndrome). They reported 4 cases, including a Koro case. It is probably the second case report in the literature on Cotard with Koro syndrome.

The case: A 55-year-old man was hospitalized for recurrent psychotic depression. In addition to depressive features with persecutory delusion, he had apprehension "that his penis had shortened until it disappeared but refused to verify this problem in front of others." During routine examinations, he continued to express nihilistic beliefs like "I have no eyes" or "have no heart" during routine inspections. He was also convinced that his left hand was dead, and he was already a dead man. At age 51, he had a major depressive episode with psychotic symptoms and was treated successfully as an inpatient. In current admission, he was treated with medication (citalopram and olanzapine) and ECT.

The authors provided a very good discussion on different neurological and psychiatric conditions associated with Cotard syndrome. They discussed the core clinical presentation in asomatognosis, cotard, and depersonalization/derealization. Asomatognosia is the neurological loss of awareness of parts of one's body, usually associated with right hemispheric lesions. Clinically they may complain of feeling that parts of the body are missing or stolen or have decayed. The information table on the "issues that may be denied" (personal space- body or self/extrapersonal space- aspects of the world) in Cotard syndrome is clinically very useful. In the end, they provided a tabular description of the possible psychological mechanism of nihilistic delusion in different clinical conditions. This is a very scholarly written paper with lots of clinically useful information.

KORO LITERATURE: From 2011 to 2020

Preamble: A total of 37 publications are reviewed in this section. Some are Koro case or related reports, and some are discussion papers. Egypt, Iran, and Australia are the new countries added to Koro geography. Some extraordinary psychiatric associations with Koro include few critical publications, like Cotard's syndrome, erectile dysfunction, another culture-bound syndrome, Dhat syndrome, Othello and Capgras syndrome, and Alzheimer's disease. Most importantly, after many years, one sporadic female Koro case is reported from England. Two exciting topics—restless genital syndrome and the penis's vulnerability—will help understand penile pathology from a different clinical and social perspective. The genital shrinkage/vanishing epidemic in Africa unfold an additional cultural dimension. Four precious books in the context of Koro and psychiatric epidemics are also mentioned.

2011

[1]. D. Roy, S. Hazarika, A. Bhattacharya, S. Das, K. Nath, S. Saddichha: Koro: Culture bound or mass hysteria?
Australian & New Zealand Journal of Psychiatry, 2011, 45(8), 683. (L)

This is a report of two male Koro cases in the background of Koro's ongoing epidemic in Assam, a north Indian state. Both patients had a typical clinical presentation. The first was a 30-year-old single carpenter whose symptoms were triggered after receiving a mobile phone call from his brother regarding an ongoing "strange penis shortening disease." In the second one, a 23-year-old man whose symptoms were triggered after observing a television report of "penis-retraction disease" and believed that this disorder could cause intestinal obstruction. Both the patients responded well with low dose benzodiazepine and supportive psychotherapy. The authors challenged the concept of culture-boundness to Koro and supported the idea of mass psychogenic illness.

[2]. P. Bandineli, M. Trevisi, G. D. Kotzalidis, G. Manfredi, C. Rapinesi, G. Ducci: Chronic koro-like syndrome (KLS) in recurrent depressive disorder as a variant of Cotard's delusion in an Italian male patient. A case report and historical review.
Rivista di Psychiatria, 2011, 46(3), 220–226. [Article in Italian]

This is an exciting clinical case report of a 58-year-old single Italian male who had a long history of recurrent depressive disorder over 30 years. He was diagnosed with the recurrent major depressive disorder at age 54. In each of the past four depressive episodes, he had this terrifying perception that his penis was shrinking, which subsided with remission of depression. In this last admission, he believes that the penis' shrinkage would lead to impotence and change his gender. He expressed his anxious and fearful concern that doctors would cut off his penis and change his body to a female. He developed a concern for his penis at the age of 18 and had very low masculine self-esteem. He responded favorably with a combination treatment of venlafaxine 150 mg and olanzapine 20 mg for a month.

The authors suggested that nihilistic or hypochondriacal delusions are associated with depersonalization experiences. The feature of KLS here is sharing annihilation delusion, which may be called a variant of Cotard's delusion. The paper has a good discussion of Cotard's syndrome and Koro (with details from Chinese medical texts).

[3]. O. Aina, O. MOrakinyo: Culture-bound syndromes and the neglect of cultural factors in psychopathologies among Africans. *African Journal of Psychiatry, 2011, 14, 278–285.*

This is a significant research paper on African Culture-bound Syndromes (CBS). The authors very reasonably pointed out the Eurocentric or Western academic dominance in the International Classification system. In many instances, they believe, neglected the regional psychopathologies outside the Western territory. The authors put Africa's case, where many CBS is still outside any "internationally accepted classificatory systems."

They did a thorough academic literature search in the West African region, which occupied about 20% of Africa and included 16 countries, including 5 Anglophone, 9 Franco-phone, and 3 Luos-phone nations. They were able to identify 4 CBS's reported from these West African cultural areas: The Brain Fag syndrome (BFS), Koro-like or Magical Penis Loss syndrome, Ode ori, and Ogun oru.

BFS was first reported by Raymond Prince (1960) and later elaborately by Morakinyo (1980). They devoted a lengthy discussion on Koro—its nosological status, variations in sporadic and epidemic form vis-a-vis culture dependence or non-cultural basis, and finally, its resemblance with African Magical Penis Loss syndrome. They described the sequence of symptom patterns in Penis-loss episodes and demarcated their difference with Koro (penis/breast vanishes—magically taken away from the body, not shrinking as in Koro). They described the different fanciful accounts of penis theft from the media reports and stressed the importance of these events' mental health and forensic implications. One fascinating piece of information struck my mind with astonishment: that is reported in Punch newspaper on 1 February 2008 with the headline: "Okada rider alleges theft of private part"—Okada is the name of a commercial motorcycle. He "alleged that a passenger he picked up used "spiritual" pigeon to steal his penis." An interesting observation is worthy of mention here: when I visited Tripura, a North-Eastern state of India, after the 2015 Koro epidemic there, I met a villager in Sobrum village in South Tripura district who said that there are extraordinary pigeons fly here and people can identify one with a "high magical power" and where the pigeon seats (on the thatched housetop) that house will be affected by Koro illness. So people used to run after the flocks of pigeons and scaring them in such a way so that they could not sit down on any housetop. Magical tales have so much similarity in different cultures across the globe!

The authors provided a detailed account of two CBS from Yoruba culture. *Ode ori* (literal meaning "hunter of the head"-a sensation of an organism crawling through the head or other body parts that cause different somatic symptoms) and *Ogun oru* (literal meaning is "nocturnal warfare"). It is a neuro-psychiatric condition where the patient is "attacked" at night while asleep, awakens, unable to sleep with agitation, and showed abnormal behavior like bleating like a goat. #Research showed that this is a type of parasomnias or a type of nocturnal sleep epilepsy. They also described some other culture-bound concepts and beliefs of Africa like *Abiku, Ogbanje, Nikubon* (related to the idea of reincarnation), *and spiritual or marine spouse* and their mental health significance. *Marine Spouse* or *Mammy Water* is a concept of river spirits that are very powerful, troublesome, and wicked. They can appear as a beautiful woman who entices and seduce a male for his complete sexual faithfulness. Interesting to note that in real-life situations, the beautiful ladies are nicknamed "mammy water." This cultural concept strongly resembles the belief in the fox spirit in Chinese and far eastern cultures.

The authors stressed the importance of a paradigm shift in the nosological classification system. African CBS's, with many others, should be judicially incorporated into the system. They stressed that this attempt would strengthen cultural psychiatry's transcultural roots and guide to study and treat such disorders in different cultures and communities. This is a beneficial paper and provides a good insight into CBS in African culture.

This reminds my field experience in a tribal village Garopara in the South district of Tripura, India, where I studied an atypical hysterical epidemic among a group of villagers (12 persons). They showed different abnormal behaviors and mimicking animal calls (dog, fox, horse, crow, monkey, and cow). Locally it was called "jungle madness" (Chowdhury et al., 1993).

[4]. S. Ceraldi: A comparison of primary and secondary koro.
Annual Review of Undergraduate Research, School of Humanities and Social Sciences, School of Languages, Cultures, and World Affairs, College of Charleston, 2011, 10, 19–26.

This is a lovely short discussion paper addressing the different dimensions of Primary and Secondary Koro. The author described the clinical presentation of Primary Koro, which is mainly seen in an epidemic setting and having a cultural explanation underneath. Most of this type occurred in the South-East Asian countries. The secondary Koro is sporadic and lacks the sudden and acute presentation like the Primary one and is usually associated with some mental or organic pathology. The author pointed out the cultural acceptance of Primary Koro in south-east Asian cultures, which is opposite or non-existent in Western cultures. In drawing the conceptual difference of masculinity and sexual morality between Eastern and Western cultures, the authors tried to substantiate Koro's clinical manifestation and its similarity with Anorexia. The author suggested a similarity of "depersonalization" among Han Chinese and Western Anorexic females. I think it is a very simplified explanation and may invite some differences in opinions.

[5]. S. D. Mendelson: The Great Singapore Penis Panic and the Future of American Mass Hysteria
Create Space Independent Publishing Platform, 2011.

Dr. Scott D. Mendelson, a consultant liaison psychiatrist at the Roseburg VA Medical Center in Roseburg, Oregon, USA, explored the Singapore Koro epidemic's historical perspective. By a very meticulous approach to document this psychiatric epidemic, he gave a very lively account of this much researched and discussed phenomena for the general public's understanding. His previous book, "*Metabolic Syndrome and Psychiatric Illness*" was also a masterpiece and was accepted graciously by the medical fraternity.

2012

[6]. D. M. Devis, A. M. Stever, J. M. Terwilliger, M. T. Williams: The relationship between the culture-bound syndrome Koro and obsessive–compulsive disorder.
In, Psychology of Culture, Eds. G. R. Hayes and M. H. Bryant, Nova Science Publisher Inc, 2012, 213–221.

It is a very useful academic paper for a clinical understanding of Koro. The authors proposed that Koro is a form of Obsessive-Compulsive Disorder (OCD). They described Koro and its history, types, causes, and defining features. While describing Koro as an OCD, they cited several clinical examples to show the similarity of many Koro symptoms with OCD, like the perception of retracting genital is the primary obsessional anxiety and genital pulling is the compulsion. Avoidance of anxiety-producing stimuli is present in OCD, and many Koro cases consciously avoid touching or looking at their genitalia. Even if Koro is viewed as a body dysmorphic disorder (BDD), BDD is also considered an OCD-spectrum disorder. The response with treatment with CBT and SSRI antidepressant medication supports the contention that Koro is a culturally specific form of OCD or related spectrum disorder.

[7]. P. Alvarez, V. M. Puente, M. J. Blasco, P. Salgada, A. Merino, A. Bulbena: Concurrent Koro and Cotard syndromes in a Spanish male patient with a psychotic depression and cerebrovascular disease.
Psychopathology, 2012, 45(2), 126–129.

This is a very interesting case report of Koro-like symptoms with Cotard syndrome in the background of psychotic depression and cerebrovascular disease. This is the third report of Koro and Cotard syndrome in the literature. The authors provided a very detailed clinical description of the case.

The case: A 62-year-old widowed Spanish male was presented with severe psychotic depression with multiple organic pathologies: controlled atrial hypertension, type 2 diabetes mellitus, 13-year history of ischemic heart disease, acute myocardial infarction 2 years ago, surgical treatment of a subdural hematoma 7 years ago and mild cognitive impairment and gait disturbances of central origin for a year. This is his third admission.

In addition to depressive symptoms, he had several negation-type delusions. He believed that he is dead, the anus was closed, he could not swallow or defecate, and 20 days after admission, he expressed his conviction that his "penis was disappearing as the abdominal heat made it melt." MRI showed multiple chronic hemorrhagic lesions with signs of diffuse cerebral atrophy. MMSE was 25. He responded favorably with treatment with venlafaxine XR 225 mg, mirtazapine 15 mg, and olanzapine 10 mg. His depression and the Cotard and Koro-like symptoms resolved ultimately within 50 days.

The authors diagnosed this case as incomplete Koro. They suggested a commonality construct between Cotard and Koro, viz., somatic delusion on a specific body part (penis). They concluded that: "Hence, in this case, the Koro syndrome may be considered a subtype of Cotard syndrome in which the delusion of negation is limited to the penis." The authors also provided an excellent discussion and related literature survey.

[8]. K. H. A. Abdullah, S. Wahab: Koro-like symptoms with associated erectile dysfunction in a Rohingya refugee.
ASEAN Journal of Psychiatry, 2012, 13(2), 221–223.

It is a Koro-like case report from Malaysia. The patient was a 37-year-old single Muslim male, a refugee from Myanmar. He had major depression with psychotic and anxiety symptoms, secondary to erectile dysfunction a year ago. He visited a traditional healer who said his sexual impotence is due to his sinful act of premarital sex, and his girlfriend's spirit is residing within his body. During his recent visit, he complained of sudden onset of burning sensation on his penis and felt that the penis was shrinking and retracting into his abdomen. He also believed that his girlfriend's spirit inside his body was pulling his genital into the stomach. An episode of burning feeling is associated with dizziness and difficulties in breathing, which he described as a near-death experience. He believed that sufficient water intake would lessen the symptoms (otherwise, he will die). Thus, he used to drink a copious amount of water during this burning attack, which usually stays for 1–2 minutes. He responded partially with treatment with antidepressants and benzodiazepine. The authors explained his Koro symptoms in terms of a cumulative effect of migration stress, strong religious belief, the guilt of premarital sex, and resultant depression and erectile hypoarousal. If the authors elaborated a bit more on "religious guilt" and the "girlfriend's spirit," the paper would be more informative.

[9]. I. Crozier: Making up koro: Multiplicity, psychiatry, culture, and penis-shrinking anxieties.
Journal of the History of Medicine & Allied Sciences, 2012, 67(1), 36–70.

It is an extensive and scholarly discussion paper on the issue of Koro. The author very methodically analyses Koro's different dimensions as an illness- from its inception by Dutch physicians and its subsequent explanation in the ambit of Western psychiatry. Culture and anthropology's role shapes its perception as a culture-bound illness, further strengthened by the 1967 Singapore Koro epidemic. The consequent publications of Koro-like symptoms from diverse ethnicities and regions, including the genital-theft epidemic of sub-Saharan Africa, highlighted culture's critical role in culture-bound syndromes. He also pointed out the differences in clinical presentation between Eastern and Western Koro. The only link is being the core symptom of "penis-shrinking anxiety." By raising the issues of cultural artifacts to promote penis enlargement, the author questioned the underlying psychodynamics of Western Koro and thus commented:

> To understand koro, we have to look more closely as masculinities in various cultures, and question why these cultural contexts of masculine and corporeal anxieties are not raised in western cases in ways that they are in nonwestern cases. (p. 51)

There is a good deal of discussion on genital-theft panics of Africa with some comparison with Koro and very insightful analysis of African culture's role in transcultural psychiatry. The last part of the article discussed Koro's definition and inclusion in DSM IV, including Koro's universal definition as a genital retraction taxon as suggested by Simons and Hughes (1985).

This is a very insightful analysis of Koro phenomena over centuries. The author picks up appropriate social, anthropological, and global (migration) issues that influence genital retraction or Koro's perception and concept among the professionals. This is a must-read paper for all Koro researchers.

2013

[10]. P. Afonso, S. Saravia, Z. Gameiro: Schizophrenia presenting with Koro-like symptoms.
Journal of Neuropsychiatry & Clinical Neurosciences, 2013, 25 (Supl 1), E32. (L)

This is a case report of Koro-like symptoms in a 41-year-old Caucasian single man with schizophrenia from Lisbon, Portugal. The patient had a 15-year history of cannabis abuse and a 3-year history of heroin dependence, though he was entirely abstinent for the last two years. He was presented with intense anxiety secondary to a fear that his penis was getting smaller and retracting into his body and third-person auditory hallucination. Laboratory tests, including CT, ECG, and toxicology, were normal. He responded favorably with olanzapine 15 mg/day and diazepam 15 mg/day for two weeks. Six months follow-up was uneventful except for some negative symptoms. The authors suggested that the abnormalities of body perception may have some neurological links with KLS.

2014

[11]. M. Kimmel, C. Milrod, A. Kennedy (Eds): Cultural Encyclopedia of the Penis.
Rowman & Littlefield, Maryland, 2014.

It is a comprehensive account of the concept and constructs of the penis from the viewpoint of wide-ranging issues like cultural meanings, penis in antiquity, in art, in religion, in politics, in media, in music, and in the artistic imagination and different rituals concerning penis by people and communities over time. It contains a discussion on Koro (pp. 104–105). This is an excellent information source regarding the socio-cultural perception of the penis in different societies, cultures at different time period.

[12]. S. Zilavy: Culture-Bound Syndromes: Malaysia.

https://prezi.Com/ghfjoa7zypgg/culture-Bound-Syndromes-Malaysia
November 7, 2014

It is a report of Koro from Malaysia. The author said that Koro is still common in Malaysia. Two short cases from 2005 are reported. The first case was a 30-year-old unmarried male who had the Koro symptoms for the last 12 years and explained that it was due to "sinful and anti-religious acts dealing with his sexuality." The second one was an unmarried male who had a long history of Koro, for the last 15 years. He blamed his past prostitute visits during his adolescent years. No other information was available. It seems that both subjects had chronic Koro.

2015

[13]. J. G. Marques: Koro, Othello and capgras syndromes in one patient with drug-induced psychosis.
Psychiatrica Danubina, 2015, 27(4), 429–430. (L)

It is a case report of a 28-year-old married male with Koro-like symptoms from Lisbon, Portugal, at the background of multiple substance abuse, including alcohol. The clinical picture is of delusion of infidelity to his wife and the belief that she was replaced by a double. Along with other symptoms of drug-induced psychosis, he also had a "penis-shrinking sensation." He responded favorably with oral olanzapine 30 mg initially and paliperidone 9 mg daily subsequently. The author believes that right frontotemporal impairment may be responsible for the Koro-like perception. In this case, the clinical description favors a diagnosis of Koro-like symptoms (KLS) rather than Koro (as there was no fear of death and the complaint is of chronic duration). Given his delusional predisposition, the penile symptom may be labeled as a somatic delusion as well.

[14]. A. N. Chowdhury: Koro.
In, The Encyclopedia of Clinical Psychology, First Edition. Edited by R. L. Cautin and, S. O. Lilienfeld. 2015, pp. 1626–1629. John Wiley & Sons Inc.

It is a comprehensive account of Koro covering Koro's definition and concept or Genital Retraction Syndrome (GRS), the historical background of the term "Koro" and its corresponding orthography in the Chinese language, and its different names in different Southeast Asian cultures. There is a short discussion on Koro's culture-boundness, a timeline of several Koro epidemics, and a debate over its psychiatric nosology. The author tried to substantiate the differences among classical Koro, Koro-like symptoms (KLS), and other Koro-variants like the "penis vanishing or genital theft" epidemic in Africa. There is a short description of reported psychopathologies in Koro and its treatment and future research directions.

[15]. A. de-G. Aikins, V. A. Dzokoto, E. Yevak: Mass media constructions of 'socio-psychological epidemics' in sub-Saharan Africa: The case of genital shrinking in 11 countries.
Public Understanding of Science, 2015, 24(8), 988–1006.

It is precious research on the genital theft epidemic in 11 countries of Sub-Saharan Africa. The authors stated that the individual experiences ranged from "vanished, shrunk, disappeared, and stolen genitals or genital retraction" among 180 cases from 1992 to 2008, as reported in media. There is some confusion about psychopathology's exact nature—whether it is genital theft or vanishing or retraction or shrunken genitals—because these two sets of perceived symptoms indicate somewhat different psychopathology. The first one is typical of the African penis theft epidemic, and the second one is closer to the Koro epidemic. But unfortunately, this distinction is not made in this paper.

Apart from this, there is a much crucial sociological analysis that enriched this research. They tried to explain these episodes in individual psychopathology and extreme somatized anxiety with collective symptom expressions like Mass Psychogenic Illness (MPI). They also mentioned the pathoplastic role of social tension. They elaborated on the local cultural context, which provided a positive model for infectivity, further facilitated by mass media reporting. There is an in-depth analysis of mass media handling of the incidents. They analyzed the theme of the media reports as: "Eight causal theories emerged from the media reports on GS: witchcraft/sorcery, power of suggestion, social tension, psychiatric disorder, monetary gain, revenge, juju, and neurosis".

They provided a significant clinical presentation of the episodes as follows:

> The sites of GS accusation were usually public: markets, lorry parks and public lavatories. Onset was sudden, and descriptions of what had happened to the genitals included 'vanished, shrunk, disappeared, and stolen' for male cases and 'shrunk and sealed' for female cases. In most reports, the accused perpetrator was typically assumed to be a 'stranger' from another African country (e.g. Nigerians were the blamed for the Ghanaian cases; other West Africans were blamed for Sudanese cases). However, analysis of published names suggested that the 'strangers' were actually local. The perpetrators were both male and female. (p. 9)

They also described the mode of spread as well:

> The mode of transmission in all countries occurred after interactions with strangers in public spaces (e.g. being asked the time or for directions) that usually involved physical contact with the stranger (e.g. shaking of hands, being tapped on the shoulder) as illustrated in the Ghanaian, Sudanese and Congolese cases" .... " In one Zimbabwean case, the GS occurred after the male victim had sexual intercourse with the female perpetrator". (p. 10)

This is valuable research to understand the socio-cultural aspect and mass media coverage of the widespread penis theft/shrinking episodes epidemic in African nations.

[16]. C. T. Braun, M. E. Ricklin, A. Pauli, D. Ott, A. K. Exadaktylos, C. A. Pfortmuller: Death after sexual intercourse.
Case Reports in Emergency Medicine, 2015, Article ID 646438, 4 pages, Hindawi Publishing Corporation.

This is not a Koro paper. It is a very useful clinical paper that highlights death after sexual intercourse. Koro researchers may recall that death was referred to as a serious outcome of "improper sexual intercourse" in traditional Chinese medical texts. The authors reported a case of a 22-year-old female who presented to the emergency room with the complaint of seizure followed by unconsciousness while having sexual intercourse. CT scan showed an extensive subarachnoid hemorrhage with a breach in the fourth ventricle. She died after 48 hours in the intensive care unit. The published research data showed that 14.5% of all subarachnoid bleeding is precipitated by sexual activity. Studies showed male predominance; explosive coital headache is a common presentation. Death due to sexual intercourse is rare: 0.6% incidence among 5559 autopsy studies.

[17]. H. Chiang: Translating culture and psychiatry across the Pacific: How koro became culture-bound.
History of Science, 2015, 53(1), 102–119.

This is an excellent discussion paper on the emergence of Chinese Koro from Sinophone culture to Culture-bound Koro in the Anglophone psychiatric concept. As an expert historian from the Department of History, University of Warwick, UK, the author very elegantly analyses minutely how the idea of Koro emerged as a Chinese disease from the reportings of Dr. A.L. Gwee from Singapore and Dr. H. Rin from Taipae, both in the '60s. Then gradually, how Dr. P. M.Yap from Hong Kong termed it a Culture-bound illness opened the door for Koro's acceptance to the Anglophone academia. He showed how Gwee stressed Koro's long legendry Chinese medical heritage, beliefs, and practices. Gwee rediscovered all relevant Chinese medical texts and established the Chinese root of Koro very convincingly. Rin tried to introject Western psychodynamic concepts in his Koro patients blended with Chinese culture issues. Thus, " koro emerged as a clinical entity on the overlapping geocultural margins of Chineseness and Anglophone psychiatric medicine." He then discussed Dr. P. M. Yap's attempt to offer a rational logic and conceptual framework for Koro, acceptable to Western academia. He coined Koro's diagnostic term as "culture-bound depersonalization syndrome." So by the mid-1960s, it is generally believed that "koro had become a distinctively mental illness, no longer resembling pure somatoform disorder; as depicted in Chinese medical texts." In the 1970s, Koro earned more global reporting with more diverse psychiatric associations, which helped it unshackle its Chinese cultural bond and paved the way for new thoughts and propositions for its befitting inclusion in the upcoming classificatory scheme for DSM.

Observation: This is a must-read paper for all Koro researchers to understand Koro's early history clearly. Two critical pieces of information are valuable: 1. The most initial documentation of female Koro is in the reference of the Chinese medical text: New Compilation of Tested Prescriptions by Bao Xiang'ao, published in the nineteenth century. 2. Dr. Rin wrote an entire chapter on Koro in his textbook on Transcultural Psychiatry (In Chinese, 2007).#

This book is now reprinted with the name "Gift of Cultural Psychiatry: From Taiwan to Japan" Author: Lin Xian, Original author: Rin Hsien, Translator: Wang Jueying, Publisher Mind Workshop, 2007.

2016

[18]. A. Vrntriglio, O. Ayonrinde, D. Bhugra: Relevance of culture-bound syndromes in twenty-first century.
Psychiatry & Clinical Neurosciences, 2016, 70, 3–6.

This is a good commentary on the relevance of the nosology of "culture-bound syndromes" in the background of recent globalization and industrialization. The authors gave a short historical review of the use of the term and concept of "culture-bound" by Yap's work in 1962, which was subsequently used widely in psychiatric nosology. ICD- 10 (1992) of WHO used the term "culture specific disorders," and DSM-5 in 2013 abandoned this term and preferred the term "cultural concepts of distress." They argued about the validity and reasonability of the concept and the term culture-boundness as follows:

> What does 'culture-bound' really mean? We believe that the concept of boundness and whether certain illness are really bound to certain cultures is problematic. In particular, old traditional boundaries across cultures are becomimg more porous, with rapid globalization, cultural factors are becoming perhaps more diffuse and more accessible. The rapid increase in the use of social media and connectedness through increased and rapid access to media, including the internet, has added another complicating and complex dimension. (p. 4)

They provided five-point general guidance for a "culture-bound" presentation: 1. indigenous labeling as an illness; 2. Local names, 3. Symptoms have local EMI and local social response, 4. They are limited to a specific community or cultural area, and 5. Symptoms are localized, not global. They discussed how the concept of Dhat or Semen-Loss Anxiety Syndrome has changed over the years in different cultures.

[19]. L. Silva, C. Rapso-Lima, C. Soares, J. J. Cerqueira, P. Morgado: Koro syndrome in an obsessive compulsive disorder.
European Psychiatry, 2016, 33, Suppl. S618.

It is a case report of a Koro-like symptom, chronic in nature, in a 27-year-old single man who, from his age 23, harbored the anxiety related to his perception that his penis was shrinking and retracting into the abdomen. He described these thoughts were repetitive, intrusive, and ridiculous. Initially, the ideas were not very disturbing, but gradually he developed a solid obsessive doubt about his penile condition and was forced to verify his penis length several times a day. To mitigate his obsessive doubts and anxiety, he started to have mental images of sexual intercourse, compulsive viewing of pornography, and increased masturbatory behavior. He responded favorably with fluvoxamine 200 mg/day with CBT. The Y-BOCS score decreased from an initial 30 to 18 after three month's treatment.

[20]. K. G. C. L. Kapugama, L. N. Obadaarchchi, B. V. S. Ruwanpriya, K. A. L. A. Kuruppuarachchi: Depression presenting with genital symptoms—A series of unusual case histories.
Sri Lanka Journal of Psychiatry, 2016, 7(2), 23–25.

It is a significant clinical paper where the authors reported three depression cases, and all of them have very unusual genital symptoms. Every Koro researcher should be aware of these associations as often Koro with depression may present such symptoms and complicate the Koro presentation. Two cases are important in this regard.

Case 1: A 52-year-old lady of two children presented with depression features of one month's duration. Besides, she experienced a sensation in her vagina as if she was having sexual intercourse with a man. This sensation lasted for a day and made her very distressed. She also believed that her vagina is not working correctly. She has high guilt about a past relationship with a married man and has a girl from that relationship. She had a good recovery from combination therapy of imipramine and risperidone, and ECT.

Case 2: A 40-year-old single man developed depression with suicidal ideation and excessive alcohol consumption for three weeks and started to believe that his penis was getting smaller like a pre-pubertal boy. He blamed his frequent masturbation for this symptom. He visited a prostitute to check his penile size, and she positively endorsed his small penis. Being too distressed and concerned, he started comparing his penis size with others in the public lavatories. There was no fear of death. He responded poorly with fluoxetine, and thus a course of ECT was given, and he recovered from depression and penis symptoms. Interesting to note that in the next five years' follow-up, he had several episodes of depression. With each episode, he redeveloped the same beliefs regarding the shortening of his penis.

Both the case histories are essential to remember that similar penile concerns in Koro associated with depression are reported in the literature.

[21]. E. C. Serefoglu: Restless genital syndrome in a 38-year-old man- A case report.

Journal of Sexual Medicine, 2016, 13(5), 2, S210.

This is not a Koro paper. This is a fascinating report from Istanbul, Turkey, on Restless Genital Syndrome (RGS), a somatosensory disorder characterized by an unpleasant sensation in the genital area and pelvis. This is a case of a 38-year-old male who presented in a urology clinic with the complaint of "persistent unwanted genital arousal and tingling, stinging, and retraction feeling in his genitalia. He had a continuous impulse to grab genitals." His symptoms are worse in a sitting position and would alleviate in a standing position or on walking. He reported that this symptom vanishes in the setting of sexual thoughts or desires but is aggravated by masturbation. He is also having a persistent feeling of impending ejaculation all day. His symptoms significantly reduced after two months of treatment with 100 mg sertraline and 0.5 mg clonazepam daily.

The author concluded that:

> RGS has been defined as spontaneous intrusive and unwanted genital arousal (e.g., tingling, throbbing, pulsating) that occurs in the absence of sexual interest and desire. It occurs in about 1 percent of women and, so far, has only been diagnosed in a handful of men. RGS is a rare clinical entity among men and these patients are commonly misdiagnosed with chronic prostatitis. (p. 220)

2017

[22]. A. M. M. A. El-Tantawy: Chronic Koro-Like Syndrome co-morbid with schizophrenia and history of cannabis abuse in an Egyptian patient: Case report.
Arab Journal of Psychiatry, 2017, 28(1), 92–96.

This is the first sporadic case report from Egypt. The author presented a case of an Egyptian male of 27-year-old single, who has a long history of cannabis, tramadol, and alcohol abuse. Subsequently, he developed drug-induced psychotic florid symptoms like auditory hallucination, ideas of reference and delusion of persecution, loss of control, and thought disorder. During this episode, the author mentioned that "He experienced nihilistic delusions, which manifest as a belief that his penis would disappear." He was admitted and treated with ECT and antipsychotic medication. Still, his belief about the penis remained for three years.

He was on several medications. In the present episode:

> Psychiatric examination revealed the following positive findings: intense anxiety attacks secondary to a fear that his penis was getting smaller and retracting into his body. He felt compelled to extract it himself and in the process believed he might die. The complaint was more frequent and more severe when in the gym, public places and on public transportation. He stayed home most of the time where the attacks were less frequent. The worrying thoughts associated with the belief about his penis led to him performing religious rituals. There were no other psychiatric manifestations apart from depressed mood. (p. 93)

Observation: The authors mentioned the chronicity of penile perception in this case. Because of his ongoing drug-induced psychotic presentation, whether this Koro-like symptom is the delusional somatic features or not is a clinical question. One clinical issue remains to be answered whether the *probability* of the penis' disappearance is justifiably termed as "nihilistic delusion" because the organ is still there (not negated). The apprehension of loss is very close to obsessive rumination (anxiety) than nihilism, probably.

[23]. P. Garlipp: Koro- A Genital retraction Syndrome.
In, Unusual and Rare Psychological Disorders—A Handbook for clinical practice and research. Ed. B.A. Sharpless. 2017, pp. 167–176. Oxford University Press, New York.

It is a valuable collection of unusual human behavior that needs every Koro researchers' attention. All entries are well narrated with a case vignette and a note of historical and cultural contexts for the disorder. In Section IV, the five critical culture-bound conditions are described:

1. Koro —A Genital Retraction Syndrome—It is a comprehensive account of Koro. The author described classical Koro in South Asia and Koro-like (KLS) symptoms in Western countries. Some reference to historical records of Koro in the 1865 Chinese medical records is made.

By other authors: 2. Taijin Kyofusho; 3. Brain Fag Syndrome, 4. Jerusalem Syndrome and Paris Syndrome: Two Extraordinary Disorders, 5. Dhat Syndrome, and 6. Ataques de Nervios .

[24]. A. P. Romero, E. G. de Mergelina, L. B. Belda, J. F. P. Prieto: A systematic review and case report of the Koro syndrome in an intellectually disabled Caucasian patient.
European Psychiatry, 2017, 41, Suppl, S229–230.

It is a report from Valencia, Spain. The authors presented a case study and a systematic review. They described Koro's case in a Spanish male with intellectual disability at an acute psychotic background. They also did a systematic review of articles published in Pubmed following the PRISMA guidelines. They found 117 studies, of which only 29 met the inclusion criteria. They found:

> Data were analysed on several epidemiological and clinical characteristics. ….Koro syndrome is more often presented as a result of intoxication or as a part of a previous known psychotic disorder. Cases involving patients sharing their delusion have been only reported in Asia….. Pharmacotherapy and social support may be effective in ameliorating the symptoms. (p. 230)

[25]. M. Haghshenas, F. Malekpour, E. Yousefi, M. Shalbafan, N. Behtash, E. Shirazi: Koro-like syndrome in an Iranian 50 years old man; is it a variant caused by cultural issues?
Journal of Neurology & Psychology, 2017, 5(1), 3.

This is a Koro-like case report from Iran. The authors described a case of a 50-year-old married man with a three-month complaint of the gradual shrinking of the penis and fear about its total loss. There is a history of benign prostatic hyperplasia (BPH) and diabetes mellitus. He has advised tamsulosin for his BPH, but he refused because he thought this would enhance urination and cause the penis' shrinkage. He also has a host of anxiety symptoms and obsessional thoughts about losing his penis, decreased libido, and dysphoric mood. He was treated as an inpatient and with fluvoxamine (100mg BD), perphenazine (4 mg BD), and amantadine (100 mg BD). He was reviewed by a urologist, who firmly reassured him about his standard penis size. After a month, his symptoms reduced significantly, especially after the urologist's reassurance.

Observation: This case may also be called chronic Koro-like, but the symptom of OCD is noteworthy. It is entirely unclear why the authors brought the issue of Dhat syndrome when there was no clinical symptom suggestive of this disorder.

[26]. K. M. Griffith, E. A. Eichel, N. C. Brahm: Genital somatic complaints in a woman with schizoaffective disorder.
Psychiatric Annals, 2017, 47(2), 69–71.

This is a very useful clinical report that helps us widen our knowledge of genital psychopathology. Different types of genital somatic concerns and complaints are reported from female Koro cases. In this research, the authors described very unusual genital somatic complaints from a 32-year-old woman with schizoaffective disorder and mild intellectual disability background. There is a history of multiple genital concerns/complaints with numerous gynecological consultations. Her complaints were different types of pain in vagina with perception that a "membrane" on her vagina or a "piece of meat" is hanging from the vagina. She also displayed hypersexual behavior and believed that she was a man. She was not satisfied with the opinions of multiple examinations that her genitalia was normal. She is on a long list of medications: 15 mg haloperidol orally; 200 mg haloperidol decanoate IM injection two weekly; 30 mg olanzapine orally; 300 mg trazodone orally and 75 mg venlafaxine extended-release by mouth daily. Out of clinical suspicion, the doses of trazodone were reduced and stopped. She then showed a reduction of her symptom of genital pain and preoccupation with abnormal genitalia. She was diagnosed with Trazadone induced clitoral priapism. An uncommon side effect of trazodone is priapism- a persistent painful erection that lasts for 6 hours or more with sexual arousal.

The authors described clitoral priapism's mechanism with other research references. He pointed out trazodone's role because of its effects on serotonin 5-HT2A/C and alpha-1 adrenergic receptors. Some clinicians use alpha-agonist like phenylephrine or pseudoephedrine for its treatment. The authors commented that the incidence of priapism in males is 1.5/1000.000 man years. Literature showed six reports in females, including vulvar pain symptoms, restless genital syndrome, sexual tactile hallucinations, and persistent genital arousal.

[27]. F. Bures: The Geography of Madness: Penis thieves, voodoo death, and the search for the meaning of the world's strangest syndromes.

Melville House, 2017.

Like a cultural anthropologist, Frank Bures, an American writer, and journalist tried to understand the root of exotic "culture-bound" syndromes in their respective culture and community. He traveled from Singapore to Nigeria to Hainan Island in China and tried to discover the meaning of extraordinary mental disorders. In doing this, traveling across the cultures, he documented a lively account of illness/disease symptoms, their cultural significance, and communities' perception and reaction to these "abnormal"; behavior. He has unfolded the unique cultural stories like fiction from the lively account of people and organizations and thus provided a fascinating *emic* account of *Koro, Mamhepo, Ode Ori, and Running Amok*. This is a delightful travel book of different cultures with a different lens to understand culture-bound disorders.

[28]. J. N. Clark: The vulnerability of the penis: Sexual violence against men in conflict and security.
Men and Masculinities (2017). Pages 1–29. https://doi.org/10.1177/1097184X17724487

This is not a Koro paper. It is fascinating research in a new framework where the author explores sexual violence in men in armed conflicts. While dealing with the theme, two critical pieces of information were noted. This may be of interest to any Koro researchers.

The first one is an anthropologist Helliwell's (2000) work, whose fieldwork was with the *Gerai* community of Indonesian Borneo. The author stated about penis vulnerability as an "outside organ" that:

> Among the Gerai, the penis and male genitalia, far from being seen as threatening and potentially harmful to women, are viewed instead as vulnerable – and more vulnerable than women's genitalia – because they are outside the body. According to Helliwell (2000: 808–809), 'This reflects Gerai understandings of "inside" as representing safety and belonging, while "outside" is a place of strangers and danger, and it is linked to the notion of men as braver than women'. The externality of the penis, moreover, means that in some cultures, it is viewed as vulnerable to 'theft'. During a Koro epidemic in southern China in the 1980s, for example, Mattelaer and Jilek (2007: 1511) – a urologist and clinical psychiatrist respectively – were told that 'genital-robbing female fox spirits had been seen roaming the area'. This information sowed widespread fear among local people, causing the epidemic to 'spread' from village to village (Mattelaer and Jilek (2007: 1511). (p. 6).

The second important piece of information concerns penis disappearance episodes in Africa. It shows the local cultural perception that the penis can be vanished by magic or spell. The author cited the work of Goebel (2002) as follows:

> In rural Zimbabwe, wives can purchase 'husband-taming' herbs designed to control their spouses' behaviour—and in particular infidelity (Goebel, 2002: 463). If these herbs are misused, they can effectively emasculate a man. According to one healer, '…the penis will disappear with all the

testicles. Everything will go inside, no penis plain, and the husband will become very fat that same day'. (Goebel, 2002, 481)

2018

[29]. P. Sean, M. S. Madden, M. Patrick, M. S. Einhorn: Cannabis-induced depersonalization-derealization disorder.
The American Journal of Psychiatry Residents' Journal, 2018, February 3–5.

It is not a Koro report. It is a good account of cannabis-induced Depersonalization—Derealization disorder. A few articles in the literature reported an association of cannabis smoking in Koro patients, even Koro's attack immediately after cannabis smoking (Chowdhury & Bera, 1994). So this paper may be helpful to develop an insight into the depersonalization-derealization spectrum after cannabis use.

[30]. C. A. Romero, H. I. Garcia, I. A. Zabelta, C. S. Munoz, J. Klotz: What a fright (Koro syndrome). A case report.
European Psychiatry 48S, 2018, EV0233; page S405.

This is a short case report of a Koro-like symptom in a 26-year-old Spanish man. He has presented at the emergency room with a panic attack and the worry that his penis was smaller than usual and concerned about his genital retraction in the context of an acute dermatological reaction. Initially, he was diagnosed with acute and transient psychosis necessitating hospitalization and antipsychotics, but he was diagnosed with Koro after careful review. The authors stressed the need for clinical knowledge of health professionals on Koro to avoid diagnostic confusion and injudicious use of antipsychotic medications.

[31]. M. H. Connors, F. Lehmann-Waldau: Koro and denial of genital ownership.
Australian & New Zealand J Psychiatry, 2018, 52(11), 1097.

This is a fascinating case report from Australia. A 36-year-old single Caucasian man presented at the emergency department with high distress from "the belief that his penis had been stolen# and replaced with someone else's. The patient cited significantly reduced penile length as evidence for his claim. He has no urological issues, neither and changes in sexual function or gender dysphoria. A week ago, he cut his penis and poured boiling water, which was quite painful, and he was astonished at how he could feel pain if he has a "foreign penis." He failed to explain this penis transfer process and said that it was like magic. He was not sure who was responsible or the motives or where his real penis was kept. He requested staff members to locate his lost penis and return it to him. He showed his penis preoccupation during his two and half month hospital admission. He did not show any other psychotic symptoms. He had a history of schizoaffective disorder with prominent auditory hallucinations and depression. A urine drug test on admission was positive for cannabis. He attempted to get penis enlargement surgery through urology clinics. The trial with various antipsychotics failed, and eventually, he responded to clozapine treatment. The family's collateral history showed that he had longstanding body dysmorphic concerns and feelings of insecurity with women.

The author discussed how this selective penis misidentification differs from Koro and penis theft and commented that how the denial of genital ownership is clinically manifested with body dysmorphic concerns and psychotic vulnerabilities.

[# This clinical presentation reminds me of a similar display in a 47-year-old single male seen in West Bengal, India. One night, he presented himself to the hospital emergency with acute pain and distension in the lower abdomen. While examining, he disclosed that his penis and scrotum are stolen by a man he knew, and currently, there is no genital organ. There were moderate clinical depression and regular cannabis smoking.]

[32]. F. Elghazouani, M. Barrimi: When culture interacts with psychopatholoy.

Revue Medicale dr Bruxelles, 2018, 39(2), 108–110.

This is a Koro case report in a 43-year-old Moroccan male who presented with persistent anxiety, avoidance behavior, and a chronic belief that his genital organ may shrink or disappear and causing his death. This belief seriously impacted his professional and family life. He was diagnosed with the culture-bound syndrome as a sporadic case and chronic in nature. The authors tried to explain his perception as per the influence of Moroccan culture, which attributes great importance to male sexuality.

[33]. L. Silva, P. Morgado: Koro syndrome associated with obsessive–compulsive disorder: clinical case and brief review.
Brazilian Journal of Psychiatry, 2018, 67(2), January–June.
Print version ISSN 0047-2085 *On-line version.*

This is a case report of Koro with OCD from Portugal, previously reported in the European Journal of Psychiatry in 2016. In addition to the detailed case writing, the authors also do a short literature review on Koro.

[34]. M. Everest-Phillips: Anxiety politics in Singapore: The "Koro Crisis" of 1967.
Asian Journal of Public Affairs, 2018, 10(2), 53–66.

This is a very valuable analysis of the 1967 Singapore Koro epidemic from a geopolitical perspective. The author categorically traced the timeline of the pre-and post-outbreak scenario regarding the swine-fever epidemic, emergency public health steps of the government, media reportings, and Singapore Medical Association's involvement at the domestic backdrop racial and international political tension of the newly born nation-state of Singapore. He discussed in a very lively and analytical manner the dynamics of "Cultural Politics" (historical review of the concept and manifestation of Koro) and "Politics of Modernity" (interactions of local and regional political climate) in the genesis of the Koro epidemic in Singapore. The author also summarized three vital lessons from this analysis. These are: 1. Coordination among different government departments (public health, swine fever vaccination program, veterinary department, medical involvement, government public advocacy to earn trust and mitigate rumor); 2. Public health administration and trust–distrust dynamics of the different social groups. The outcome of Policy effectiveness of government administration and public trust. He cited two examples in this regard- Severe Acute Respiratory Syndrome (SARs) in Singapore and "Mad Cow Disease" episodes in UK; 3. Role of public education, health literacy, and technological use of complementary health messages to mitigate public health crises and emergencies. He also analyzed the perspective of the national, regional, and international political environment of the time. He stressed the sociological dynamics at the background of the mass-psychogenic episode: "The *Koro* hysteria reflected potentially explosive racial aggravations and religious sensitivities at a politically difficult moment, both domestically and internationally." Given the socio-political and economic climate and the struggling financial position of a new state in 1967, he commented that:

> The cause of '*Koro* epidemics' is ultimately political – and serious. The disease reflects the worry that citizens of a country can feel at being powerless in the face of rapid social change and economic transformation. (p. 64)

2019

[35]. M. Hussain, A. Hirsch, H. Seens, E. Moghaddam: Koro syndrome displaced rostrally: Nasal retraction.
Biological Psychiatry, 2019, 85(10), S260–261.

This is a very interesting paper and a new addition to Koro literature. According to Chinese medical text, any protruding external organ of the body like ears, nose, and even the tongue is considered yang elements and may be subjected to internal retraction and is regarded as a Suo-yang (Koro) equivalent. We got the report of tongue retraction from Malaysia (Chin & S'ng, 1995) and inward pull of limbs and ear and genital retraction in India's epidemic setting (Ghosh et al., 2013). In this report, the authors present another variation of Koro, i.e., nose retraction, and that too from a 54-year-old female with bipolar mania with a host of paranoid ideas. She believed that her "nose was disintegrating and retracted in her face" and she lost her ability to smell. She also had grandeur delusional ideas, like she came from another planet and came to save the world. She had paranoid ideation that some "gang members are taking out organs and selling them." She has multiple organic findings, including Cranial nerve 1 test- alcohol sniff test 0 cm for anosmia; the presence of diffuse atavistic reflexes suggestive of bilateral damage of the cortex, presence of Jamais Vu indicates the possibility of temporal lobe epilepsy. The authors stressed the association of psychiatric presentation (mood disorder with nasal retraction) in neurologic disease. It seems that anosmia may be a triggering factor for nose retraction and may be a delusional symptom. In any case, this is a rare example of retraction perception of a body part in the mixed background of psychiatric and neurological pathology.

[36]. M. Colthert, R. Langdon: Somatic delusions as motivated beliefs?
Australian & New Zealand Journal of Psychiatry, 2019, 53(1), 83–84. (L)

It is not a Koro paper. This is a good theoretical paper regarding the cognitive process by which monothematic delusional belief develops. The authors suggested that two critical questions help understand the psychological process of the development of delusional belief and may help identify the causes and neuropsychological brain area for the delusion. The two questions are: What prompted the delusional idea at the beginning? Why is the idea adopted as a belief? They discussed this issue, particularly with six types of delusion, viz., Capgras delusion, Cotard delusion, Fregoli delusion, somatoparaphrenia, mirrored-self-identification, and delusion of alien control. They explained their proposition with a Koro-like case reporting (Connors & Lehmann-Waldau, 2018) and a case of somatic delusion (rotting gum) in a man. This paper is helpful in understanding a single somatic delusion development and may help identify Koro symptoms associated with the psychotic process.

2020

[37]. M. Tau, A. V. Masukar: Koro delusion in mild cognitive impairment due to Alzheimer's disease.
Journal of Neuropsychiatry & Clinical Neuroscience, 2020, 32(2), 204–206.

This is a Koro-like symptom in a 78-yea-older man at the background of mild cognitive impairment due to Alzheimer's disease reported from New York. The authors identified the sign as "koro delusion." In one of his follow-up visits to the Neurology clinic, he complained that he "heard his penis shrink" and that it had "retracted." This was a great concern and anxiety to him. There were some other delusional symptoms present. Physical examination found no penile pathology. MMSE score was 24/30, and brain MRI was suggestive of Alzheimer's disease. The authors discussed the role of cortical lesions in psychosis, delusion, body image, and dementia and concluded that it is unclear which brain area is associated with Koro delusion.

References

Chin, C. N., & S'ng, K. H. (1995). "Koro"—Like syndrome affecting the tongue—A case report. *Medical Journal of Malaysia, 50*(2), 175–177.

Chowdhury, A. N. (1991). Personality profile of Koro patients. *Journal of Personality & Clinical Studies, 7*, 117–118.

Chowdhury, A. N. (1992a). Mass hysteria with animal identification: Study from a tribal village in Tripura. *Journal of Indian Anthropological Society, 26*, 67–74.

Chowdhury, A. N. (1992b). Psychic infectivity: The role of positive illness cognition in psychiatric epidemic. *Journal of Personality & Clinical Studies, 8*, 125–128.

Chowdhury, A. N. (2008). Ethnomedical concept of heat and cold in Koro: Study from Indian patients. *World Cultural Psychiatry Research Review, 3*, 146–158.

Chowdhury, A. N., & Bera, N. K. (1994). Koro following cannabis smoking. *Addiction, 89*, 1017–1020.

Chowdhury, A. N., Nath, A. K., & Chakraborty, J. (1993). An atypical hysterical epidemic in Tripura, India. *Transcultural Psychiatric Research Review, 30*, 143–151.

Diagnostic and Statistical Manual of Mental Disorders. (2000). *Fourth edition: DSM-IV-TR*. American Psychiatric Association.

Diagnostic and Statistical Manual of Mental Disorder (2013). *Fifth Edition.* American Psychiatric Association.

Edwards, J. W. (1984). Indigenous Koro: A genital retraction syndrome of insular South East Asia: A critical review. *Culture, Medicine & Psychiatry, 8*, 1–24.

Ghosh, S., Nath, S., Brahma, A., & Chowdhury, A. N. (2013). Fifth Koro epidemic in India: A review report. *World Cultural Psychiatry Research Review, 8*(1), 8–20.

Goebel, A. (2002). "Men these Days: They are a Problem": Husband-Taming herbs and gender wars in rural Zimbabwe. *Canadian Journal of African Studies, 36* (3), 460–489.

Gwee, A. L. (1963). Koro—A cultural disease. *Singapore Medical Journal, 4*, 119–122.

Helliwell, C. (2000). "It's only a penis": Rape, feminism and difference. *Signs, 25*(3), 789–816.

ICD-10. (1992). *Classification of mental and behavioural disorders: Clinical description and diagnostic guidelines*. World Health Organization.

Illechukwu, S. T. C. (1992). Magical penis loss in Nigeria: Report of a recent epidemic. *Transcultural Psychiatric Research Review, 29*, 91–108.

Kirmayer, L. J., & Santhanam, R. (2001). The anthropology of hysteria. In P. W. Halligan, C. Bass, & J. C. Marshall (Eds.), *Contemporary approaches to the study of hysteria: Clinical and theoretical perspectives* (pp. 251–270). Oxford University Press.

Mattelaer, J. J., & Jilek, W. (2007). Koro—The psychological disappearance of the penis. *Journal of Sexual Medicine, 4*, 1509–1515.

Morakinyo, O. A. (1980). Psychophysiological theory of a psychiatric illness (The Brain Fag Syndrome) associated with study among Africans. *Journal of Nervous & Mental Diseases, 168*, 84–89.

Prince, R. H. (1960). The "Brain Fag" syndrome in Nigerian students. *Journal of Medical Science, 106*, 559–570.

Prinz, A. (1998). "Kaza bosolo"—A culture-bound syndrome among the Azande of northeast- Congo. Ethnotherapies. *Curare, 14*, 53–57.

Simons, R. C., & Hughes, C. (1985). *The culture-bound syndromes: Folk illnesses of psychiatric and anthropological interests* (R. C. Simons & C. Hughes, eds.). D. Reidel.

Yap, P. M. (1951). Mental disorders peculiar to certain culture: A survey of comparative psychiatry. *Journal of Mental Science, 97*, 313–327.

9

Indian Koro Research Publications: From 1943 to 2020

Preamble: This section reviewed Koro and related publications that appeared mainly from Indian research on Koro and were primarily published in Indian journals. A review of 100 publications during 78 years (1943–2020) is presented. There are several Koro case reports and the Koro epidemics report from West Bengal, Assam, Tripura, and Kerala. Some are discussion papers. There are two reports on Jhin Jhini epidemic. There are some contemporary newspaper reports on the Koro epidemic from West Bengal, Mumbai, and Assam. It seems that India is now becoming a Koro-prone country. It has seen at least eight epidemics involving many states since 1982. Koro is reported in association with substance abuse. The author presents a rare paper on "art in Koro" that sheds new light on Koro symptom formation's psychosexual dynamics. Some Indian Koro research has been published in overseas journals also.

The earliest reference of genital shrinkage as a clinical phenomenon is noted in the descriptive account of the dream conversations of an ascetic by Dr. Sarasi Lal Sarkar in 1943. Except for Dr. A. P. Pillay's publications in 1953 and of Dr. A. Venkoba Rao in 1978, there is virtually no

A. N. Chowdhury, *Koro*,
https://doi.org/10.1007/978-3-030-87962-4_9

mention of genital shrinkage/retraction or Koro or Koro-like symptoms in the literature published from India till 1980. From 1981, Koro started appearing by name in the Indian medical press with increasing frequency, especially after the 1982 Koro epidemic in India's Northeastern states. This review includes reports of four (1982, 2010, 2016) Koro epidemics (from West Bengal, Assam, Tripura, and Kerala state) and few sporadic cases. In some of my publications, I appended some additional input from my research work.

1943

[1]. S. L. Sakar: A study of the psychology of sexual abstinence from the dreams of an ascetic.

International Journal of Psychoanalysis, 1943, 24, 170–175.

The author reports a Koro-like feature in the dream conversations of an ascetic. The reference is related here to Sadhana's (meditation) preaching and consequent changes in sexual morphology. That reminds one of Koro symptoms, the difference being that it is the expression of distress in the latter, whereas, in the former, it is the desired goal of sexual restrainment of *Sadhana*. He stated:

> By the restraint of the sexual passion (produced by practicing Sadhana) the activities of the penis are destroyed. It then gradually shrinks and becomes small. Then it becomes inverted and draws itself within the body in such a way that its very root enters into the body. By this process its appearance becomes that of a female sexual organ, while really it is the disappearance of the sexual organ from outside the body. This is nothing more than the outward development of an ascetic. (p. 174)

Asceticism is an integral part of the Hindu religion. For details, one may see Zysk (1991).

1953

[2]. A. P. Pillay: Anatomical Problems of sex.
In, Sex Society and the individual. A. P. Pillay & A. Ellis (Eds), International Journal of Sexology, 1953, p. 488, Bombay.
Reviewed by U. G. Duff in *The Eugenics Review, 1953, 45*(3), 189–190.

A. P. Pillay, an eminent sexologist from Bombay, reports that preoccupation with genital morphology constitutes most of his patients' complaints. He describes one of his clinic cases, a 29-year-old unmarried man with a history of masturbation and passive-active homosexuality who complained of "poor erection, premature ejaculation and shrinkage of penis" and constant nocturnal emission, which started after first heterosexual contact at age 28. The patient took Unani medicine, which corrected his excessive seminal emissions but not the poor erection. This is probably one example of "attenuated Koro"—a term later used by Rao in 1978. Here, Koro's classical and dramatic clinical sequences are lacking in the context of complaints of genital morphological changes (smallness/shrinkage of the penis) by neurotic patients.

1956

[3]. G. M. Carstairs: Hinjra and Jiryan: Two derivatives of Hindu attitudes to sexuality.
British Journal of Medical Psychology, 1956, 29, 128–138.

This is the author's fieldwork in a village (Deoli) of Mewar district of Rajasthan in India. It elegantly described semen value's emic perspective and its relation to the Hindu community's sexual code and ethics. The local worldview of sexuality (heterosexual) about the preservation of semen has many similarities with the Chinese medical concept of semen as the reservoir of health and masculine strength. The author described a culture-bound neurosis, "Jiryan" now called Dhat syndrome. It is an excellent reading to develop an insight into the social aspect of somatization and its relation with the concept of "spoiling of semen" among

Hindu men. A similar description and social beliefs about semen anxiety in South Asian cultures is described by Edwards (1983).

1973

[4]. J. S. Neki: Psychiatry in Southeast Asia.
British Journal of Psychiatry, 1973, 123, 257–269.

It is a very informative discussion paper that highlights the affairs of mental health in India. He believes that there is no classical Koro (like Chinese) in India or Sri Lanka. He proposed "Ascetic Syndrome" for severe sexual abstinence, psychosocial withdrawal, and weight loss.

1978

[5]. A. Venkoba Rao: Some aspects of psychiatry in India.
Transcultural Psychiatric Research Review, 1978, 15, 7–27.

It is an excellent brief account of psychiatry in India with a culture-bound syndromes (CBS) selection in the Indian subcontinent. The CBS like possession syndrome, the Indian Dhat syndrome, the ascetic syndrome, malignant anxiety, and suchi-bai (obsessional neurosis) are included. The paper also discusses at length depression in the Indian context. The author asserts a strong cultural belief in the clinical expression of different sexual neurotic disorders like Dhat or Ascetic syndromes. He shows the similarity of semen cognition between Indian and Chinese culture, where "semen is held to bestow robust physical and mental vigor, longevity, and supernatural powers" in them both. The author describes a specific form of Indian sexual neurosis relating to penile morphological change, which he terms as an "attenuated form of Koro." He states:

> An attenuated form of Koro, a syndrome characterized by fear of retraction of the penis into the abdomen, is familiar to psychiatrists in India. Patients suffering from this disorder show impotence and hypochondriacal preoccupation with the size and shape of the penis and the quality and quantity of semen. This syndrome is invariably attributed to

masturbation. Improved literacy and socioeconomic standards, and sexual education on simple scientific lines help prevent the development of this disorder. (p. 9)

1981

[6]. G. D. Shukla, D. N. Mishra: Koro-like syndrome: A case report.
Indian Journal of Psychiatry, 1981, 23, 96–97.

This is the first Koro-like case report from Jhansi, India. The authors describe a 20-year-old Hindu single male who presented with one-year-old complaints of severe anxiety, a feeling of gradually diminishing size of the penis and scrotum. Others have noticed that he was restless and spending anxious nights with his hands in trouser pockets—holding or manipulating his genitals. For the last year, he also visited many types of healers. He responded well to anxiolytics and four sessions of narcosynthesis with pentothal sodium. It was revealed that he masturbated pretty frequently, and subsequently, after reading some books, he developed intense guilt over his urge and practice of masturbation. The authors believe that probably this anxiety and guilt were operatives in the background of his complaints. His anxiety and sleep showed some improvement, but his ideas about shrinking genitals persisted. After a month, he developed a florid psychotic state (aggressive, violent, and frank thought disorder). He repeatedly said that "he had no penis and no scrotum, although he was gripping these structures firmly with his right hand and become violent on being asked to leave them free." He became symptom-free with a course of eight ECTs along with neuroleptic medications.

Note: *J. McGilvray reviewed Shukla and Mishra's (1981) paper in the Transcultural Psychiatric Research Review, 1983, 20, 59–60.*

1982

[7]. P. K. Chakraborty: Koro: A peculiar anxiety neurosis (a case report).
Indian Journal of Psychiatry, 1982, 24 (2), 192–193.

This is the second Koro case report from Ahmadabad, India. The author describes a case of a 19-year-old college student with two-year complaints of generalized weakness, frequent nocturnal emission, and a feeling that his penis was getting smaller day by day. The patient made a hole in his right trouser pocket through which he used to hold the penis so that it would not disappear inside the abdomen. The patient attributed his habit of too frequent masturbation as the cause of this sickness. Anxiolytics and supportive psychotherapy failed to relieve his shrinking-penis conviction, but he showed remarkable improvement when added neuroleptics. The authors express that cultural belief of sexual physiology and pathology has a crucial role in Koro, which may aptly be designated as "culture-bound psychogenic disorder."

Observation: The symptom here very much befitting a notion of a chronic Koro-like state, as the symptom duration was two years, and there was no fear of death like that of classical Koro. Moreover, his multiple medical consultations and numerous somatic complaints raise a strong possibility of some hypochondriacal somatic (penile) concern. Premorbid schizoid personality and remarkable response to neuroleptic medication also invite suspicion of somatic delusion!

1982 Koro Epidemic in Northeast India

[8]. P. S. Sachdev, A. Shukla: Epidemic Koro syndrome in India. *Lancet, 1982, ii, 1161.* (L)

It is a brief report of a Koro epidemic from Northeast India. The authors reported a cohort of 60 Koro cases from a village near Guwahati (Assam) from 600 households. The report is a detailed analysis of 30 patients (17 male and 13 female). The majority of cases were from the age group of 20–40 years, and about 2/3rd of them were married and were mostly from lower economic class. The disease was locally termed "*Jhinjhinia bimari*," meaning a tingling illness as the onset symptom was a tingling sensation in the legs. The authors report different social modes of treatment, viz. cold water pouring, lime juice drinking, and manual holding of the "shrinking" penis.

[9]. A. Chakraborty, S. Das, A. Mukherjee: Koro makes an epidemic appearance in India.
Transcultural Newsletter, 1982, III, 3–4 December.

It is an abstracted review of the Koro epidemic of Northeastern India. It provides a very brief account of the epidemic scenario with evidence of extreme panic that the epidemic created in this region as follows:

> Parents who were convinced their sons' penises were shrinking had tied string thread to the foreskin and secured it to another thread tied around the waist. As a result, ulcers formed on the foreskin. In the hilly Darjeeling district, doctors had to measure boys' penises at intervals to show parents there was no shrinkage.

The authors suggest that mass fear and panic may relate to the previous "mysterious disease" epidemic involving death in this region, which turned out to be cerebral malaria. In some parts, Koro was termed "Kattao" meaning "cut off".

[10]. D. Dutta, H. R. Phookan, P. D. Das: The Koro epidemic in lower Assam.
Indian Journal of Psychiatry, 1982, 24, 370–374.

This is a report of the Koro epidemic of Assam, which took place from June to September 1982. Four districts (Goalpara, Kamrup, Darrang, and Nagaon) out of ten were affected mostly by this epidemic.

This is a well comprehensive report of the first Koro epidemic on Indian soil and provides detailed features of the outbreak from Indian culture and Assamese ethnicity. The authors describe 83 cases, 64 male and 19 female. The main findings are grouped under the following headings.

Demographic Characteristics: The age range was 4 to 40 years, where most cases (55.4%) were between 20 and 29 years. Marital status—59% of the patients were single and 41% married. Religion—83.1% were Hindus, 15.7% Muslims, and 1.2% Christians. Ethnicity—61.4% were Assamese (Hindu, Muslim, and Tribal), 24% were Bengalese, and 1.2% were Rajasthanis. Education—3.6% were students of some professional courses (Engineering, Law, and Chartered Accountancy), 9.6% were graduates, 44.6% were educated up to secondary level, and 19.3% were illiterate. Occupation—43% had no work, including two minor and twelve homemakers, 33.8% were workers, and 23.8% were students. Socio-Economic Status—61% from middle economic classes, 27% lower economic class, and 6% were from the upper level.

Clinical Characteristics:

1. Time and place of attack—74% started indoors while 24% were outdoors. In 10 cases, there was no record. 79.4% of attacks occurred between 6 p.m. and 6 a.m., with a maximum record between 7 a.m. and 1 p.m.
2. Presence of hearsay history or witnessing a Koro patient—72.3% of the cases had definite exposure to gossip, discussion, or seeing a Koro case on the day of their attack or within the previous 2–3 days. Most of the subjects showed great apprehension about the alleged infective nature of the illness.
3. Duration of attack—Koro attacks lasted from five minutes to five hours, with an average duration of 25 minutes.
4. Symptoms—
    - (a) Genital—shrinkage and the inward pull of the penis in males and shrinkage or inward pull of the breast in females were the main presenting feature. Out of the 19 females, only nine (47.3%) had Koro breast symptoms, and no one had genital complaints. The remaining female cases showed varieties of anxiety symptoms. Thirty-three males (70.1%) had shrinkage and the inward pull of the penis.
    - (b) Anxiety symptoms—Different psychosomatic expressions of anxiety were present. These are fear, apprehension, palpitation,

sweating, sinking feeling, air hunger, extreme retrosternal pain, excessive thirst, restlessness, and a sense of impending death.

(c) Disturbed Consciousness—A tingling sensation started from the toes with upward radiation in some cases. It was followed by a dizziness and fainting spell, which varied from a semiconscious state with abnormal movements to total dissociation of variable duration.

(d) Relapse—12% of cases had a history of relapse within 30 days of the first attack.

The author failed to trace any significant contribution of overt sexual perversions or overindulgence among the cases. The illness earned a local Assamese name—"Jhin-Jhinia" in the community. Mass-education initiatives by media and administration were instrumental in mitigating the epidemic's spread beyond September 11, 1982.

1983

[11]. Editor, TPRR: News and Views: Koro epidemic in India.
Transcultural Psychiatric Research Review, 1983, 20, 150–151.

It is a publication of the same report of Drs. A. Chakraborty, A. Das, and A. Mukherjee appeared in the *Transcultural Newsletter*, 1982, Vol. III, No. 3 & 4, December 1982.

[12]. D. Dutta: Koro epidemic in Assam.
British Journal of Psychiatry, 1983, 143, 309–310. (L)

It is a brief report on the Koro epidemic of lower Assam, India, reported in response to three epidemic psychosis (BJP, 1982, 141: 98–99) by Harrington. She mentioned some interesting observations on the Assam Koro epidemic (June 1982). The local name of the disorder was "Jinjina Bemar" (tingling illness—tingling sensation of the body). She mentioned the role of a local rumor to precipitate the epidemic—"a lethal disease had struck the people bringing instant death or making the person impotent." She mentioned different indigenous strategies to combat the disease as "pouring copious cold water, drinking gallons of lemon water, smearing of chalk paste or lime paste over the ear lobules and also over the private parts." Both sexes were affected.

[13]. D. N. Nandi, G. Banerjee, H. Saha, G. C. Boral: Epidemic Koro in West Bengal, India.
International Journal of Social Psychiatry, 1983, 29(4), 265–268.

This is a brief report of the West Bengal Koro epidemic with three case reports from rural areas. The first case was a 19-year-old Hindu single male resident of a village on Calcutta's outskirts. After hearing Koro's discussion while traveling on a train, he developed the illness on returning home. The second case, an 18-year-old single Muslim female of Beldanga, Murshidabad district, developed Koro breast symptoms (shrinkage of the breast followed by burning and trembling of the breast) during an attempt to see some male Koro cases of her village on that day. The third one, a Hindu unmarried female of 16-years of age from a village of Howrah district, developed breast symptoms. She had a history of anxiety neurosis a year back. The authors believe that Koro is an acute anxiety reaction where suggestion plays an important role.

[14]. A. Chakraborty: An epidemic of Koro in West Bengal (India).
Indian Journal of Psychiatry, 1983, 25, 138–139.

It is a brief report of the West Bengal Koro epidemic, with a special mention of the North Bengal region. The epidemic wave came from the adjoining part of Assam to the North Bengal region of West Bengal, further spreading to South Bengal. Koro's dramatic presentation and associated traditional healing rituals (cold water pouring), including prevention with lime paste marking and wearing black arum slices, have been reported. Koro, in a young boy with a frank psychotic attack, was also recorded. Various local names for the disease, e.g., *Kattao* in North Bengal, *Jhin-Jhini* in lower Bengal, and *Disco* in Calcutta, are reported. The author attempts to explain North Bengal's epidemic in terms of social stress, the existing tension between local inhabitants and immigrant refugees from Bangladesh.

1984

[15]. D. N. Nandi, G. Banerjee, S. Bera, S. Nandi: Mode of spread of epidemic Koro in a village of West Bengal.
Indian Journal of Psychiatry, 1984, 26, 331–334.

This is a report of the West Bengal Koro epidemic with an excellent psychoanalytical study of mass response to illness rumors in the community. It describes a case of a businessman of a village of Malda district, who acted as the key messenger of the illness news, which he dissipated among the villagers on his way back home. He first discussed the news of this terrifying penis disease in a shop where four persons fall victim to Koro instantaneously in a chain reaction. Some panicky customers carried this news into a nearby village where, upon hearing from them, two married women were struck by the malady. The businessman's younger brother underwent a Koro attack when the family listened to the man's news of this dangerous disease.

This is an excellent account of social contagion where a terrified businessman terrorized others and helped spread the illness in the community. This example illustrates the dynamics of group psychology in disseminating rumors by the process of ego identification among people with suggestible personalities. The age range of the affected five personas was 18 to 22 years. Both the female cases had a history of hysterical attack, and one male patient had a concurrent affective disorder (phase not mentioned). The authors describe a unique incident of mass fear where a group of people came with their little sons, whose penises were tightly tied with rope. The fathers, not the sons, made the complaint of penile shrinkage. The authors thus commented:

> Psychologically the fathers were the real victims of the epidemic. But the symptoms were not centered on their own organs (i.e., mutilation of the self). It spilled over the organs of those whom they hold as dear as the self. (p. 333)

[16]. R. Khubalkar, O. P. Gupta: Psychodynamics of Koro (a case report).
Indian Journal of Psychiatry, 1984, 26, 180–181.

This is a Koro case report of a 21-year-old unmarried male from Wardha, Maharashtra. The patient here lacked the classical presentation of Koro but complained of gradual diminishing of penis size at the background of existing erectile dysfunction and mixed anxiety-depressive complaints. The treatment compliance with psychotherapy and antidepressants was good. The psychosexual history of the case is important. He had a strained family relationship. Intense masturbatory guilt and exposure to pornographic literature were instrumental in the symptom choice. A previous psychological fear of penile pathology (he read in some books that excessive masturbation leads to reduced penis size) was a cue that hastened the Koro symptom expression.

1985

[17]. P. S. Sachdev: Koro epidemic in Northeast India.
Australian & New Zealand Journal of Psychiatry, 1985, 19, 433–438.

It is a comprehensive report of the Koro epidemic of Northeast India (Assam) with three case reports. It is an extended version of the author's earlier paper published in Lancet in 1982.

The first section of this paper contains a short phenomenological description of the Koro symptom with historical references. The second part describes the survey findings of the epidemic in four villages of the Kamrup (Chandrapur) and Nowgong (Goverdhanpur, Khatbashi, and Kajoli) districts of Assam. Together, the villages make up about 600 households and 4000 people, of whom 60 persons were affected by Koro.

A detailed analysis of 31 cases (18 male, 13 female) showed the following demographic features. Age—Highest frequency (41.9%) was in the age group of 20 to 30 years. Marital status—29% were single, and 71% were married. Education—41.9% were illiterate; 38.7% had 5–10 years of schooling; 16.1% had high school education, and 3.2% had a college education. Occupation—25.8% were student; 6.4% farmers;

9.7% fisherman; 38.7% housewives, and 19.6% had other jobs. Socio-Economic Statue—61.3% belonged to the low and 38.7% to the middle economic class. Religion—90.3% were Hindus, and 9.7% were Christians. Ethnicity—Non-tribal constituted 67.7% and tribal 32.2%.

The clinical features of the cases showed the following characteristics. Time of attack—67.5% of the attacks occurred in the evening, 6.4% in the afternoon, and 19.1% in the morning. The number of episodes: one attack was noted in 61.3% cases, two in 22.3%, and more than two in 16.1% cases. Residual symptoms were present in 51.6% of cases in the form of either anxiety symptoms (9 patients) or tingling (2); sleep disturbances (3); fear of recurrence (5); paraesthesia in genitalia (1); faintness (1); pain abdomen (1); or headache (2). Premorbid personality—in 58.1% of cases, abnormal personality trait was present as follows: anxiety (12 patients), dependence/passivity (10), emotional instability (2), and shyness (8). History of past psychiatric illness was present in 9.7% of cases. 38.7% of patients had a significant family history like major depression (2 cases), conversion disorder (1), sleep disturbance (1), physical illness (4), and Koro syndrome (4). Sexual history showed that excessive masturbation was present in one case; excessive nocturnal emission in 4; Dhat syndrome in one; marked ignorance of sexual matters in 5; and poor heterosexual relations in 4 cases. Five patients also had an additional psychiatric diagnosis, two with major depressive disorder, recurrent (in remission), two with conversion disorder, and one with schizophrenic disorder. A study of patients' attitudes toward Koro's causes evinced that 16.1% regarded Koro as a physical illness; 9.7% viewed it as entirely psychological, and 28.8% conjectured it as both. 48.4% were noncommittal. Heat and humidity were also attributed to be the primary physical causative factors. The author discusses the "hot and cold" model of the illness with passing reference from Indian Ayurvedic treatises viz. the Caraka Samhita. The author remarks that the complaints about the gradual reduction of penis size are common psychosexual problems encountered in patients with sexual disorders.

[18]. O. Somasundaram: The Malleus Maleficarum and its psychopathology of sex.
Indian Journal of Psychiatry, 1985, 27, 123–126.

This is an exciting discussion paper that compares sexual psychopathologies as depicted in the recent DSM-III and the old document of fifteenth-century descriptions, viz. the Malleus Maleficarum, or the Hammer of the Witches, written by Henry Kramer and James Sprenger.

The author points out that a phenomenon akin to Koro is described in Chapter 7, Part II, question 1 of the Malleus Maleficarum, as follows:

> Witches can take away the male organ not indeed by actually despoiling the human body of it, but by concealing it with some glamour.

An exceptional example of penis loss noted in this book is a man from Ratisbon, who recovered his member after threatening the witch. This penis-loss phenomenon has gained recent interest, especially after the Nigerian epidemic (Ilechukwu, 1992). These accounts reflect the Western tradition of penis-maleness-witch myth not very far in its content and form from that encountered in Tanzania, China, Malaysia, the Black American culture, or Ghana, so far as the male fear of castration from a female castrator is concerned. This last theme has been analyzed in-depth by Prince (1992) and Kirmayer (1992).

[Note: Sprenger and Kramer (1849), in their most infamous book "Malleus Maleficarum", described the transient disappearance of the penis (described as "glamour") by witchcraft. About 200 years earlier, Guazzo (1608), in his Compendium Maleficarum, provided a list of sexual disorders enacted by witch's spell. The seventh or last issue in the list was "narrowing of the female genitals" and "retraction, hiding or actual removal of the male genitals" (Durst & Rosca-Rebaundengo, 1991). These accounts helped to have a robust social belief in demonology-witchcraft in Europe and were instrumental in social gender exploitations and violence like witch haunting and killings.]

1986

[19]. D. N. Nandi, G. Banerjee: A psychoanalytical study of Koro. *Samiksa, Journal of the Indian Psychoanalytical Society, 1986, 40, 94–104.*

This is a discussion paper mainly devoted to Koro's psychological explanation in terms of castration fear with three case illustrations. The first section describes, in brief, the historical background of Koro about Chinese cultural beliefs with a short account of global Koro occurrences. The second part contains a short descriptive note of three Koro patients, a 22-year-old married woman from Jalpaiguri, a 17-year-old married man from Calcutta. The third one, a Hindu unmarried female of 16 years of age from a village of Howrah, developed breast symptoms. Interestingly, the first and the third cases developed depression after three years and one year of their Koro attacks, respectively.

The authors provide an excellent discussion on castration anxiety about the clinical phenomenon of genital retraction and fear of death in Koro. The authors assert that loss of potency emanating either from the loss of penis or breast has a crucial psychoanalytical significance to the person, viz. It represents the damage of the body image and injury to narcissism. They draw an example of symbolism in the male Koro situation as:

> The sensation of heat stands for the sign of sexual excitement and the effect to cool is to get rid of the excitement. Painful state associated with castration anxiety can be explained as punishment for sexual act and expiation for guilt sense. The fear of impending death arising out of punishment for expression of sexual wishes and guilt is well evident. (p. 101)

In females, the authors try to explain the Koro symptom choice as a phenomenon of "phallic passivity," passive oral striving, and phallic identity (breast). The situation of breast loss "gives her an opportunity to get rid of her obvious feminine identity and to satisfy her unconscious wish to be a man."

1988

[20]. A. N. Chowdhury, P. Pal, A. Chatterjee, M. Roy, B. B. Das Chowdhury: Analysis of North Bengal Koro epidemic with three years follow-up.
Indian Journal of Psychiatry, 1988, 30, 60–72.

It is the report of the North Bengal Koro epidemic of 1982, West Bengal state with three years follow-up. The authors formed a Koro Study Team who collected case data from the District/Sub-Divisional hospital of the four districts (Darjeeling, Jalpaiguri, Coochbihar (or Koch Behar), and West Dinajpur) of North Bengal region of West Bengal state, India. During the epidemic, they collected a total of 405 Koro cases [357 (88.15%) male and 48 (11.85%) female], and during the three years follow-up periods, they collected ten patients (all were male) from the same region. They discussed the district-wise epidemiology and epidemic nature of this comparatively lengthy (from July to December 1982) epidemic. They also discussed the nature of the epidemic spread from urban to rural or vice versa in the districts. Details of the demographic distribution of the cases are also reported. Interestingly in the follow-up years, no female patient was reported. Subsequently, different aspects of clinical features, including penis perception and social cognition of Koro illness research, were done. Figure 9.1 shows the district-wise distribution of cases.

1989

[21]. A. Chakraborty, D. C. Bag: Genesis of the Koro epidemic in West Bengal and Assam: Implication of Turtle Cults.
Human Science, 1989, 38, 142–149.

This is a brief research note on the theoretical postulation of the Koro epidemic's genesis. They stressed the symbolic theme of turtle-cult and Jungian psychology of the collective unconscious. The authors provide a short account of the Koro epidemic of Assam and West Bengal. They discussed the various hypotheses regarding the genesis of Koro illness and its epidemic form. They attempt to explain the Indian Koro epidemic in terms of social stress, refugee versus non-refugee (indigenous/permanent) community clash, and stresses.

The authors believe that the tortoise cult is a significant cultural theme related to possession of the land and having symbolically to do with the Koro illness and its outbreak. They believe that a fusion of self, sex, and soil, as seen in fertility cults, is operative at the root of the Koro epidemic because "the threat of displacement from the soil thus may

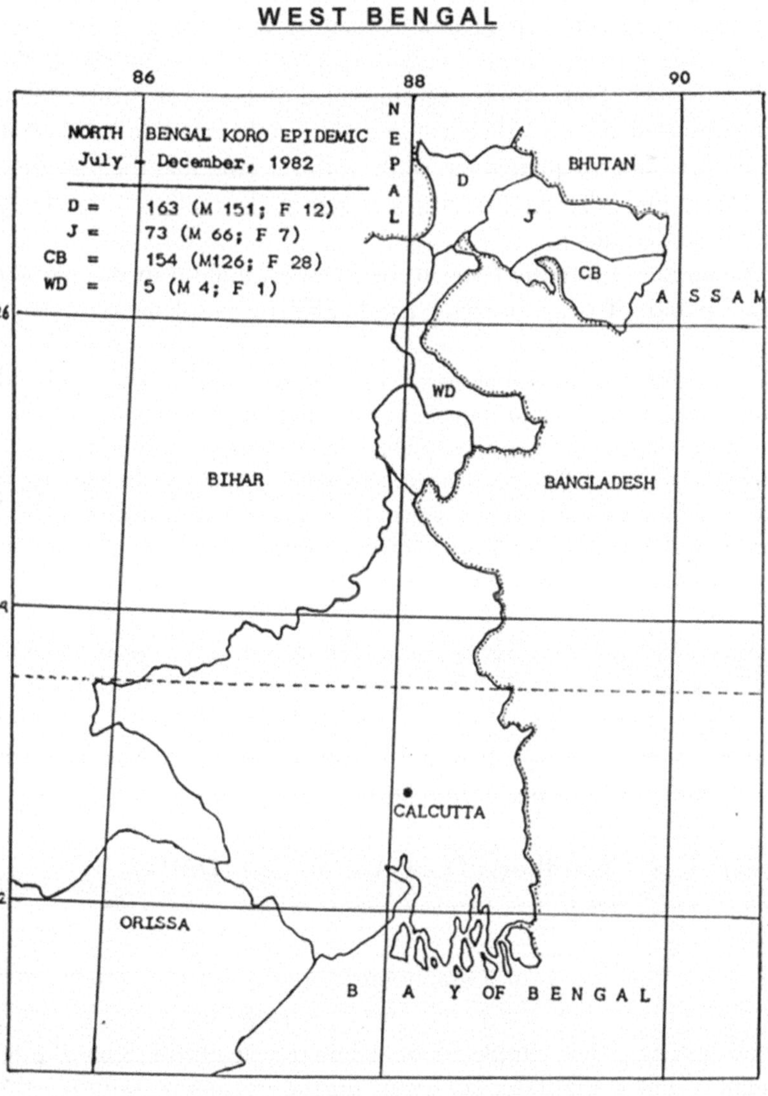

Fig. 9.1 District-wise distribution of Koro cases in North Bengal (D = Darjeeling; J = Jalpaiguri; CB = Cooch Behar; WD = West Dinajpur)

give rise to atavistic fear of loss of identity symbolized by the penis." They mention the mythical link with cultural customs and rituals about the tortoise, symbolically representing the dimensions of virility, stability, and immortality. Thus, they assume, "It is only where folk beliefs and Hindu mythology equate the tortoise with the land that the phenomena arose, and once the atavistic fear was activated, it affected the refugees and the settlers alike."

The authors apply the Jungian theory of symbolism in this particular situation and offer the following psychoanalytical explanation:

> We suggest that the symbiosis of the collective identity with land and the key sexual power to impregnate the land are all symbolized by the tortoise which is archetypally apprehended and incorporated in the collective unconscious. The threat of dispossession of land which amounts to unconscious violation of the archetype activates it with highly charged emotional reaction and a self-protective withdrawal as it were in the unconscious plane. (p. 148)

They conclude that the Koro phenomenon is an expression of identity problems related to land. In support of this contention, they cite the correlation between the ongoing ethnic clashes or tension or geopolitical stresses of human displacement in the areas of Southeast Asia from where the epidemic of Koro has been reported.

[22]. A. N. Chowdhury: Draw-A-Penis-Test (DAPT).
Journal of Personality & Clinical Studies, 1989, 5, 97–100.

This is the description of a graphomotor projective test, Draw-a-penis-test (DAPT) to elicit the penile perception of the drawer, devised by the author. DAPT attempts to elicit kinetics of morphological change of penis: Trait penis state, i.e., penis during normal condition without sexual arousal (flaccid penis) and State penis condition, i.e., penis during sexual arousal (extended penis). For perceptual comparison, the drawer is asked to draw a penis of an average person (without any genital disease) and his own penis during these two states. All the measurements are expressed in centimeters. The author recommended at least five dimensions of penile perception is elicited from these DAPT drawings: Penis length (PL); Nature of the penis root (close or open); Identifiable glans penis; Maximum width of the shaft and any Associated drawing. The author also provided some DAPT data on eight groups of subjects: Normal person; patients with anxiety neurosis; neurotic depression; psychogenic impotence; Dhat syndrome; hydrocele; scrotal filaria; and Koro (Table 9.1).

Clinical Utility of DAPT: DAPT drawings offer an overall penile perception of the drawer. DAPT scores project important factors of clinical significance for the psychodynamics of the patients and their illness. The perception of length and width of the penis may be related to the construct of masculinity or may reflect some psychosexual conflicts. The presence of glans or open and close roots may indicate perceptual integrity concerning the patient's organ image. Associated drawings are of crucial clinical significance in terms of conflict-laden body areas related to sexuality or their Explanatory Model of Illness (EMI). All these findings will help to map out the patient's cognition of body reactivity landmark (Fisher, 1959) or symptom localization (Cassel, 1965) or psychosexual symptom formation (Fisher & Cleveland, 1958) or any dysmorphophobic perceptual trend.

It should be remembered that the DAPT scores of any patient group should always be compared with those of a matched control of normal subjects. DAPT results may help to interpret the psychosomatic symptoms referable to the genital system. DAPT values of the penis length perception of different groups are presented in Table 9.1. Some DAPT drawings are shown in Figs. 9.2a–f.

[23]. A. N. Chowdhury: Neuroticism, extraversion and sex-guilt cognition in the genesis of Koro.
Samiksha. Journal of Indian Psychoanalytical Society, 1989, 43, 57–64.

It is valuable research on the psychometric assessment of personality and sex guilt of Koro patients of India's North Bengal Koro epidemic. On a large sample size (n 162) of male Koro patients with age-matched

Table. 9.1. DAPT Scores of penile length perception (n 484)

Group	No	Age (yrs)		Penile length perception in cm							
		Mean	SD	Normal Penis				Self Penis			
				Flaccid		Extended		Flaccid		Extended	
				Mean	SD	Mean	SD	Mean	SD	Mean	SD
Normal Subjects	164	27.2	8.8	7.6	1.5	9.4	2.2	8.1	1.2	9.7	1.4
Anxiety Disorder	84	30.7	9.7	5.6	1.3	8.1	1.8	5.4	1.3	8.1	1.6
Depression	36	24.1	6.4	6.2	1.7	7.3	1.0	5.8	0.9	6.4	1.1
Psychogenic Impotence	40	25.6	11.8	6.1	0.8	8.4	1.7	5.3	1.1	5.7	0.7
Dhat Synd	27	21.4	5.3	5.9	1.4	7.9	2.3	4.8	1.4	6.4	1.3
Hydrocele	43	29.5	8.8	6.8	1.1	8.2	1.4	7.5	1.9	8.6	1.3
Scrotal Filaria	33	31.3	7.2	6.9	1.4	8.1	1.3	7.6	1.5	8.4	1.5
Koro Patient	57	27.9	8.6	4.7	1.5	5.8	1.3	3.8	1.4	4.8	1.6

DAPT Drawings:

a

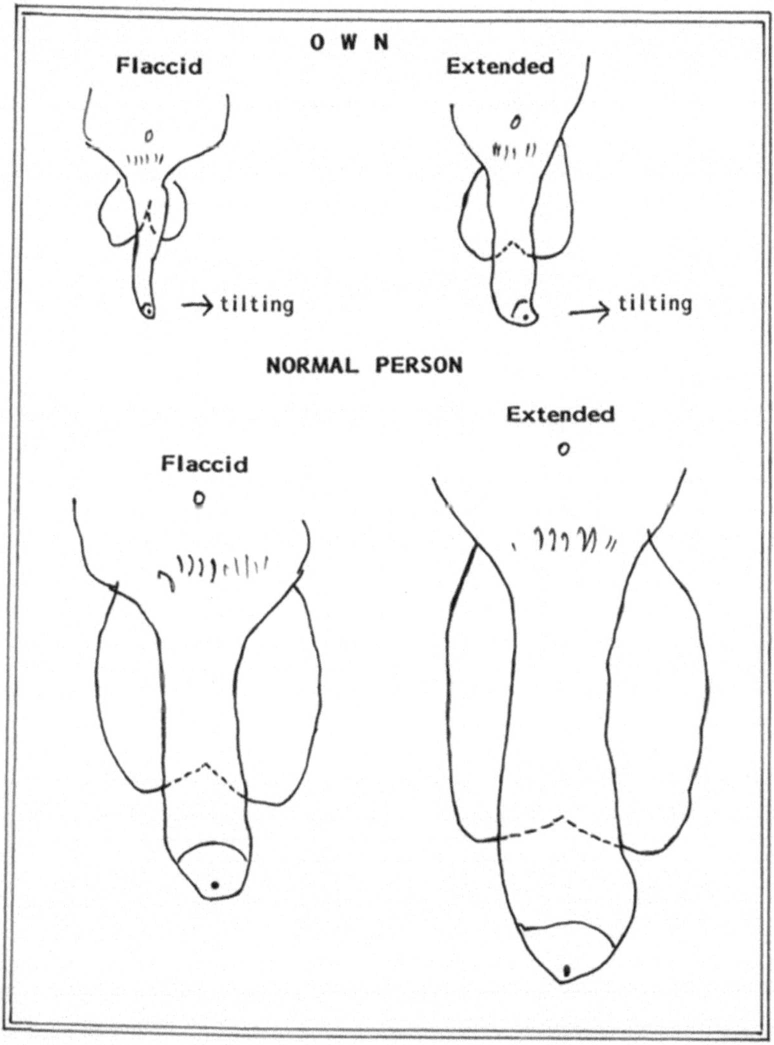

Fig. 9.2 (a) An urban Koro patient; (b) Two rural Koro patients; (c) A patient of Anxiety neurosis; (d) A patient of Dhat syndrome; (e) A Normal subject; and (f) Associated DAPT drawings. A. Patient of Dhat Syndrome. B. Patient with Scrotal Filaria

b

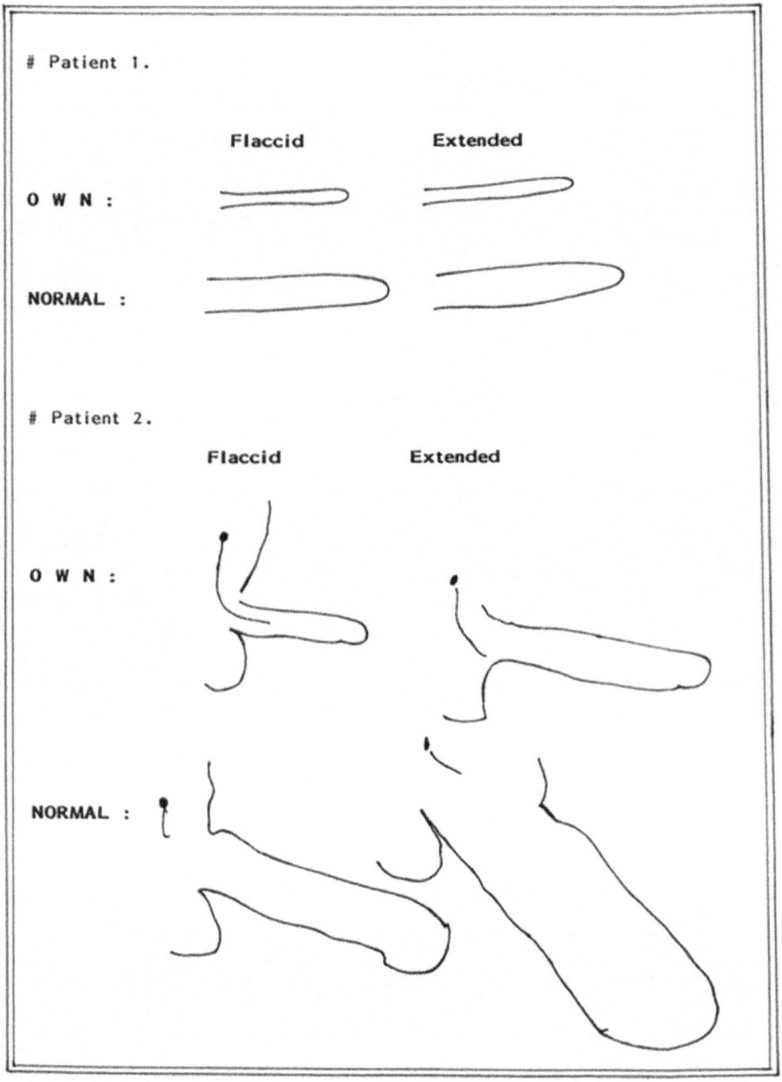

Fig. 9.2 (continued)

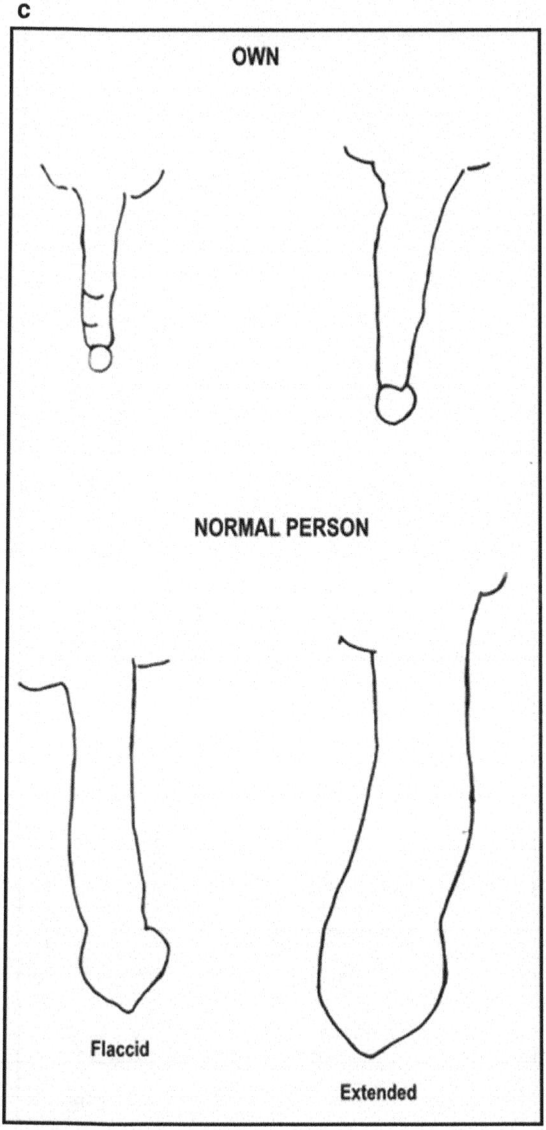

Fig. 9.2 (continued)

d

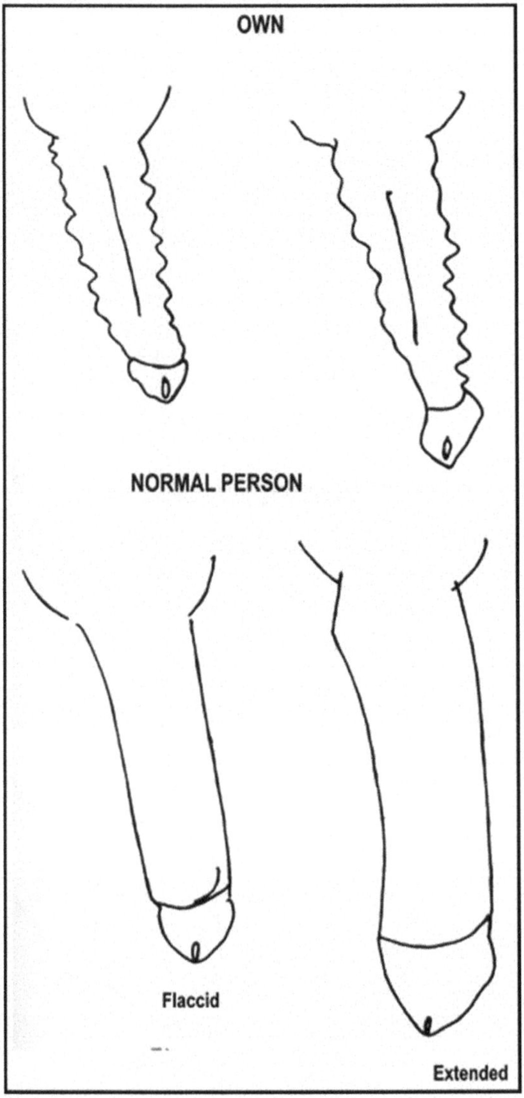

Fig. 9.2 (continued)

e

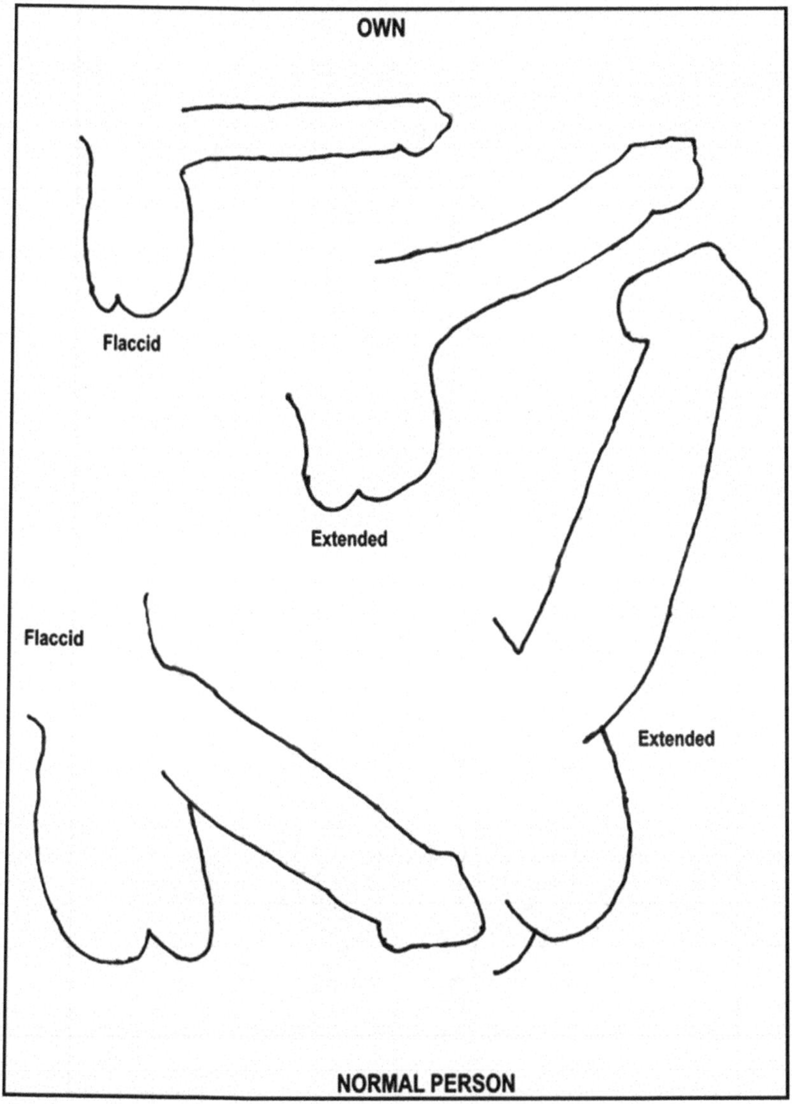

Fig. 9.2 (continued)

f

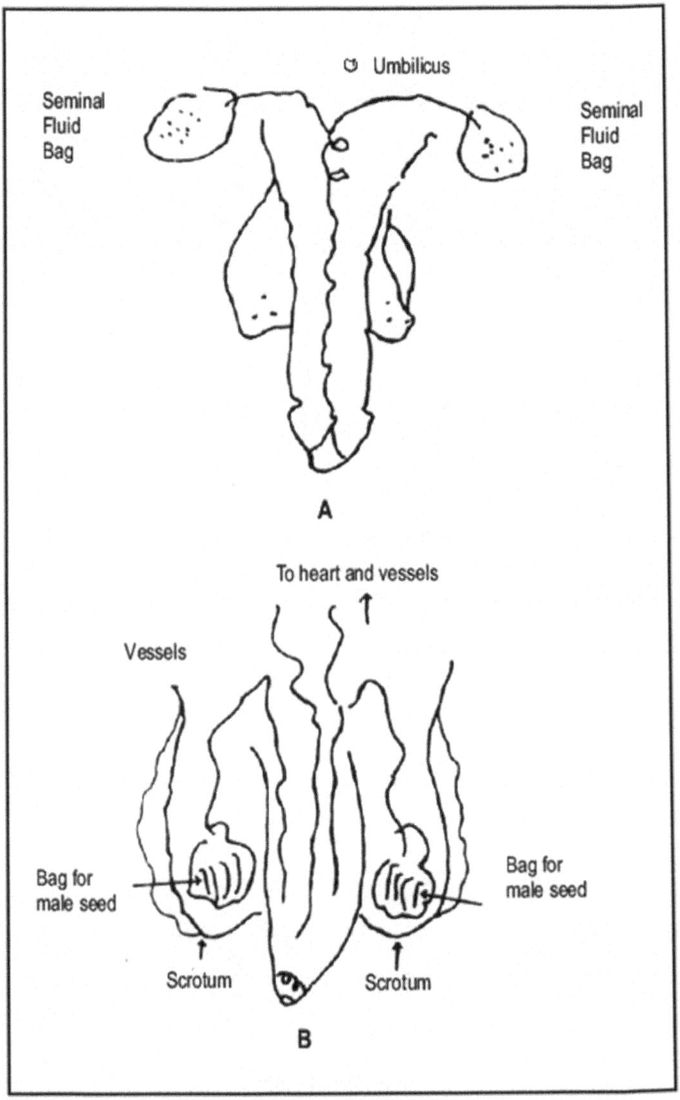

Fig. 9.2 (continued)

control, the author used Eysenck's Personality Questionnaire (EPQ) (Eysenck & Eysenck, 1975) (validated in Bengali—Chowdhury, 1989a), a Diagnostic questionnaire. A Questionnaire on sexual conflict and guilt was devised for the purpose of following guidelines from Mosher (1966), and Mosher and Cross (1971). The salient findings were:

1. Highly significant (p-value almost 0) excess of different psycho-sexual abnormalities in Koro patients than normal subjects. These abnormalities are: spermatorrhoea; impotence; ejaculatory difficulties; extramarital sexual relations; prostitute visit; incest; and sexual weakness.
2. Highly significant (p-value almost 0) sexual conflict and guilt.
3. Significant scores on Neuroticism ($p < 0.01$) in comparison to average and Extraversion ($p < 0.05$) in comparison to anxiety neurotics.
4. Highest percentage of Hysteria diagnosis (35%) followed by Anxiety Neurosis (21.7%).

The implications of these findings are discussed concerning the psychodynamics of Koro symptom formation.

[24]. A. N. Chowdhury: Koro among kinships.
Indian Journal of Social Psychiatry, 1989, 5, 24–26.

It is an interesting report of Koro affectivity among the same family during the Koro epidemic in North Bengal, India. A total of 21 cases from 9 families with five types of kinships are reported. The different types of kinships were: Brother–brother; Brother–sister; Father–son; Father–daughter; and Husband–wife. The author observed the time sequence of Koro attacks in detail with some relevant psycho-social histories of the cases. He cited one exciting incident of a marriage ceremony where the bride was first affected by Koro, and then her husband, followed by 16 males and five women, was involved in a chain reaction. The author discussed the Koro vulnerability in the same family members with sequential identification and modeling.

[25]. A. N. Chowdhury: Penile perception of Koro patients.
Acta Psychiatrica Scandinavica, 1989a, 80(2), 183–186.

This is the first psychometric study of the penis perception of Koro patients. All patients (single male, 20 each from the urban and rural background; age range 20–40 years, range 27.7 years) were taken from the 1982 North Bengal Koro epidemic, India. The author devised a graphomotor projective test—"Draw-a-penis-test (DAPT)" used to elicit penis image of the drawer—both his own penis and of an average person of his age. DAPT also evokes the changed penile conditions, i.e., flaccid and extended state. The data of the Koro patients were compared with four controlled groups (matched for age, marital status, education, and residence): average person, patients of scrotal filarial, hydrocele, and anxiety disorder. The time interval of Koro attack and DAPT administration was 8–21 days, a mean of 14.2. This controlled DAPT measurement (in cm) showed a perceptual abnormality of penis image in Koro patients. They perceived less penis length, both of their own and for a normal person, and failed to effectively perceive the morphological change of penile states in terms of length increase. In the perception of "normal" penis length—in flaccid state length perception, Koro patients differed ($p < 0.01$) from the normal, hydrocele, and scrotal filarial urban groups. In the extended state of penis image, Koro patient's length perception differed ($p < 0.01$) from all the controls. In the perception of "own" penis, Koro patients displayed the smallest penis length image than the controls ($p < 0.01$). This perceptual abnormality in organ image is discussed with Koro vulnerability and psychopathology.

[26]. A. N. Chowdhury: Dysmorphic penis-image perception: The root of Koro vulnerability.
Acta Psychiatrica Scandinavica, 1989b, 80(5), 518–520.

It is one of the extended studies of penis perception of Koro patients from the 1982 North Bengal Koro epidemic, India. In an earlier study, the author reported that, despite having an average length of the penis, Koro patients perceived smaller penis length, in both flaccid and extended states than normal subjects. To examine the influence of response bias, a longitudinal study was done. It records penis perception of the same patients (20 urban and 20 rural cases) serially over some time—three times over two years. The first DAPT was within three weeks of the Koro attack, the second DAPT was around six months, and the third DAPT was after two years. The penile perception was calculated by using the graphomotor projective test DAPT (Draw-a-penis-test). The study showed a remarkable constancy in their perception of penis length over time. This dysmorphic penile perception was discussed concerning their Koro vulnerability.

[27]. A. N. Chowdhury: Biomedical potential for symptom choice in Koro.
International Journal of Social Psychiatry, 1989c, 35, 329–332.

This is valuable research from the 1982 North Bengal Koro epidemic of India. The author analyzed different biomedical issues about Koro among 162 male Koro patients (mean age 25.86 ± 6.13 yrs) and compared them with age-matched controls (a normal person without Koro or mental illness). Among the five anatomic-sexual factors, venereal disease and scrotal filarial were significantly excess in Koro patients than normal controls. Similarly, among the six probable biomedical onset conditions, the highest frequency of extramarital intercourse (23.5%), exposure to cold water (19.1%), and a febrile episode (14.8%) were important findings. The implications of these biomedical factors concerning the hyperinvolution of the penis in Koro are discussed.

1990

[28]. A. N. Chowdhury: Diagnostic nosology of Koro.
Journal of Personality & Clinical Studies, 1990, 6, 207–209.

This is a research attempt to diagnose Koro as per psychiatric diagnostic terminology. 60 male Koro cases were taken randomly from a sample pool of 81 cases from Darjeeling district. The age mean of the sample was 22.78 ± 4.5 years. Multiphasic questionnaire (MPQ) of Murthy (1965), and Murthy and Lakshminarayan (1968) were used for diagnostic screening. MPQ has administrated at the first clinical contact with the cases and the range of the time interval between Koro attack and MPQ screening was from 6 hours to 3 days (mean two days). The patients were divided according to their severity, i.e., the number of Koro attacks, viz. single attack—mild ($n = 28$), two attack—moderate ($n = 15$), and more than two attacks—severe ($n = 17$).

Following was the diagnostic distribution of the Koro cases. In the mild category, neurosis showed higher frequency (60.7%) with higher percentages of hysteria diagnosis (46.4%). A similar picture was observed in the moderate variety. Though neurosis constituted a higher frequency (52.9%) in severe cases, psychosis also constituted 35.3% of diagnoses. 75% of the Koro cases were identified by MPQ diagnosis, of which neurosis was 56.7% and psychosis 18.3%. Individual diagnostic positions showed the highest percentage of hysteria (35%) followed by anxiety neurosis (21.7%), paranoid schizophrenia (11.7%), and schizophrenia (6.7%). The correlation between the MPQ diagnosis and Koro severity showed that: Anxiety neurosis and schizophrenia showed a positive correlation. In contrast, hysteria showed a negative trend, and paranoid schizophrenia did not reveal any such tendency. As a whole, neurosis displayed a negative correlation ($r = -0.81$), while psychosis showed a positive trend ($r = 4.40$). Only hysteria diagnosis showed significance with a 10% error.

The author suggested that pathological anxiety is the primary psychodynamic ingredient in Koro. This anxiety in its malignant form encroaches into the psychotic territory and is expressed as "depersonalization" (Yap, 1965), or; "hysterical delusion" (Gwee, 1968) or dysmorphic penile perception (Chowdhury, 1989b). This is probably related to the severity of Koro illness. The present finding is indicative of such a relationship. In the mild form, hysteria diagnosis occupies a major share, while in the severe form, this position is replaced by anxiety neurosis and schizophrenia. More research is needed to substantiate these diagnostic propositions.

[29]. A. N. Chowdhury: Trait anxiety profile of Koro patients.
Indian Journal of Psychiatry, 1990, 32, 330–333.

This is the first report on the psychometric assessment of Trait Anxiety (TA) among Koro patients. The author used Spielberger's State-Trait Anxiety Inventory, 1970 (Bengali adaptation, Chowdhury 1989c) in a large sample (n 186) of Koro male patients of the North Bengal Koro epidemic. Two groups (average person and patients of anxiety neurosis) of age-marital status-residence matched control were used as a comparison. The TA assessment time interval was within 48 hours (mean 28.5 $\pm$ 21.2) of the Koro attack. Koro cases showed a significantly higher TA score (45.6 $\pm$ 4.9) than the normal subjects (34.5 $\pm$ 5.2) and closer to the anxiety neurosis group (52.0 $\pm$ 5.5). The importance of a high level of trait anxiety in Koro vulnerability was discussed.

[30]. A. Chakraborty: Identity, Land, and Sex.
In, Psychiatry: A world Perspective. Ed. C. N. Stefanis, Vol. 4, 1990, Elsevier Science Publishers B.V. Holland, pp. 222–226.

This is a discussion paper where the author attempts to correlate the ever-increasing geopolitical tension with stress in recent times. These are resulting in a vast mass of "uprooted humanity" as refugees or voluntary migrants, with their loss of identity and the consequent displacement of this collective social anxiety into various somatizations, including Koro. She refers to a similar proposition made by Murphy (1982) in the context of Koro epidemics of Singapore and Thailand. She explains the Koro epidemic of Northeast India in light of the rising identity conflicts arising out of the rapid migration of people from Bangladesh to these regions. As a secondary explanation, she forward the Hindu beliefs and health practices, including the tortoise cult. She offered a socio-anthropological model. The fusion of self, sex, and soil form a fertility cult, which creates a group ego having "mystical identification" with the soil of the inhabited land and thus "the threat of displacement from the soil may give rise to atavistic fear of loss of identity symbolised by the penis."

The author refers to the anthropological significance attached to the turtle cult in the Northeastern Indian culture and shows the linguistic similarities between the Indonesian name for the turtle (Koro) with

"Kacchap or Kantha" in North Bengal. She speculates on Koro symptomatology's possible connection with turtle cult prevalent in geocultural areas along the equatorial line, where the animal is found in abundance.

1991

[31]. A. N. Chowdhury: Dysmorphic penis perception in Koro.
Indian Journal of Psychiatry, 1991, 32, 330–333.

This is one of the series of research done by the author on the penis perception of Koro patients. This study attempts to explore the penis perception of the Koro patients (Urban n 20 + Rural n 20 = 40) by using a graphomotor projective test—Draw-a-penis-test (DAPT) . This controlled DAPT investigation of flaccid self-penis length perception showed a perceptual abnormality in Koro patients' penis image. They perceived reduced flaccid penis length despite their identical or even longer real length of the penis than the average subjects (n 40) or other patients' controls (Hydrocele n 40; Scrotal filarial n 31; and Anxiety group n 40). Difference between the real and perceived flaccid penis length showed that the Koro group perceived significantly ($p < 0.01$) less penis length than their real or actual length. The urban anxiety group showed a similar perceptual trend, though to a lesser degree ($p < 0.05$). Normal and hydrocele groups did not reveal any differences. Scrotal filarial, on the other hand, is perceived more than their real penis length. The author postulated that this dysmorphic penis-image perception might be the cognitive element that enhanced their Koro vulnerability and psychopathology.

---

[32]. A. N. Chowdhury: Penis-root perception of Koro patients.
Acta Psychiatrica Scandinavica, 1991, 84(1), 12–13.

This is one of the research papers on the penile perception among Koro patients from the 1982 epidemic in India. This research showed that the Koro patients perceived the penis [using a graphomotor projective test—the Draw-a-penis-test (DAPT)] as a detached organ with root-boundary definiteness as evidenced by their close penis-root perception (Fig. 9.3). They also displayed a reduced volumetric perception of penis-root than the matched control of normal subjects. The author thinks that these perceptual deviations in the penis-root image might be a psychodynamic contributor to their Koro vulnerability.

* * *

[33]. A. N. Chowdhury: Personality profile of Koro patients.
Journal of Personality & Clinical Studies, 1991, 7, 117–118.

This is a research report on the personality profile of Koro patients. The personality dimension of 49 male Koro patients of the North Bengal Koro epidemic was assessed by Eysenck's Personality Questionnaire, 1975, EPQ (Bengali adaptation, Chowdhury, 1989a). Koro patients displayed the profile of a combination of high neuroticism and extraversion scores on EPQ (Table 9.2).

A combination of high E and N scores, as the Koro patients displayed here, constitutes the "Neurotic Extraverts" group (Eysenck & Claridge, 1962). This high E and N association in Koro is probably responsible for their psychosexual pathology with sexual conflict and guilt (Rin, 1965) and subsequent symptom formation. A clinically significant percentage of Koro patients showed various sexual behaviors resulting in conflict and guilt over such approaches (Chowdhury, 1989d). So the Koro cases could be defined as "Neurotic Extravert" within the Eysenckian dimensional frame of the personality model (Eysenck, 1970, 1972). This disposition also explains Koro's phenomenological similarities and dynamics with anxiety neurosis and hysterical somatization reaction.

[34]. A. N. Chowdhury: Penis-shaft perception of Koro patients.
Journal of Indian Academy of Applied Psychology, 1991, 17(1–2), 41–44.

This is a research report of one of the series of penile perception studies among Koro patients from the North Bengal Koro epidemic. The penis is a dynamic organ that experiences shrinkage (flaccid state) as well as expansions. This volumetric morphological change in penis

Supplementary data:

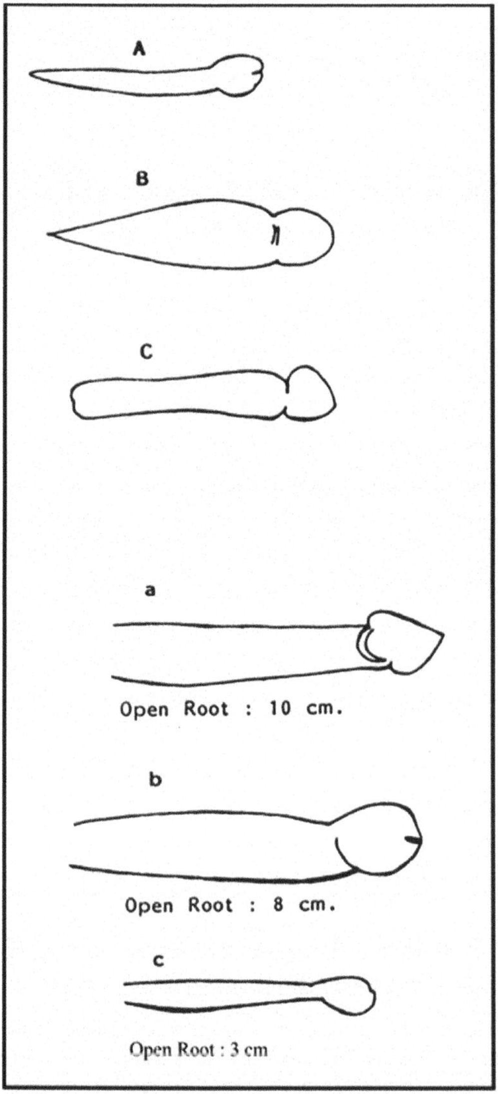

Fig. 9.3 DAPT Root Measurement (Own-Penis-Flaccid State) (A, B, C = Closed Root drawing of Koro, Hydrocele, and Anxiety neurosis cases. a, b, c = Open Root drawing of Scrotal filarial, Normal subject, and Koro cases)

Table 9.2 EPQ scores of the group

Group		P	E	N	df
Koro ($n = 49$)	X	4	14.86	16.27	
	SD	1.43	3.70	3.75	
Anxiety Neurosis ($n = 30$)	X	4.27	7.03	16.30	
	SD	0.91	1.52	1.33	
	t	0.215	1.393*	0.009	77
Normal ($n = 50$)	X	3.82	12.42	8.78	
	SD	1.04	2.16	1.45	
	t	0.144	0.808	2.645	97

*$p < 0.005$
P = Psychoticism; E = Extraversion; N = Neuroticism

size is a unique fact. The author examined the perception of penis-shaft volume, viz. the maximum shaft-width of the penis, both during flaccid and extended state among Koro patients. The study also examined the "extraneous" penis-shaft image (way of perceiving others) by the same Koro patients to explore the perceptual differences between their "own" and "normal" penis-shaft width perception. A graphomotor projective test DAPT (Draw-a-penis-test) was used to evaluate the perceptual dimensions of penis-shaft perception. This controlled DAPT investigation shows that Koro patients perceived reduced volumetric penis-shaft measurement, viz., less "maximum shaft-width" than the controls (a group of normal persons, patients of hydrocele, scrotal filaria, and anxiety neurosis). This perceptual deviation in the penis image was discussed concerning their Koro vulnerability and symptom formation.

[35]. A. N. Chowdhury: Role of medical cognition in psychiatric outbreaks: Study from North Bengal Koro epidemic.
Indian Journal of Behavioural Sciences, 1991, 1, 64–67.

This is a very important and first of its type of study where the author tried to elicit the region's health care providers' medical cognition during the 1982 North Bengal Koro epidemic. Research has shown that the "Illness perception" and "response" are mostly socially learned phenomena because the magnitudes of symptoms and disability are products of subjective experience and social definitions (Mechanic, 1977). The process of labeling involves the orientation of people about sick-role. The acceptance of sick-role is guided and reinforced by the opinion and attitude of the help-providing therapists in the community (Ramaan & Murphy, 1972). The "doctor" is essential because his opinion provides a scientific basis for social cognitions (Menzel, 1960). He thus helps in the adaptive response to deviant behavior. Otherwise, people accommodate illness perception through social cognitive constructs, such as searching for meaning, social attribution, and social comparison (Cobb, 1976; Mechanic, 1972, 1975). This investigation studied the local treatment people's cognitive responses—physicians, general practitioners, surgeons, and paramedical staff, to the massive Koro epidemic in the region concerning Koro's illness model.

[36]. A. N. Chowdhury: Medico-cultural cognition of Koro epidemic: An ethnographic study.
Journal of Indian Anthropological Society, 1991, 26, 155–170.

This is a report on Koro's social cognition (medical and community) during the North Bengal Koro epidemic, highlighting the reinforcing force of medical understanding (by local health care providers), which strengthens the community folk help-seeking behavior with its accompanying health hazards. Interestingly, the region's medical cognition was very similar to the community perception about Koro illness in terms of its disease nature, seriousness, risk, infective potential, and causation. Even in the treatment opinion, there were also quite identical assumptions and similar responses between the two groups. The folk or traditional treatment for Koro represents the general social cognition about its causes. The section on casualty from folk/conventional treatment of Koro is an important contribution of this paper as it showed the different serious health hazards of such therapies, including death. This is a significant issue because, in any future such epidemic, sufficient preventive precaution should be taken and advocated in the community through a mass-educative approach so that people would be sufficiently aware of the risk–benefits of the folk treatments.

1992

[37]. M. S. Bhatia, K. N. Thakur, R. Chadda, S. Shome: Koro in Dhat syndrome.
Indian Journal of Social Psychiatry, 1992, 8, 74–75.

This is an interesting case report of Koro in association with another culture-bound syndrome, viz. Dhat syndrome. The authors present a case of a 26-year-old married male. He was presented with complaints for a month of the gradual shrinking of the penis leading to the point of total disappearance (into the abdomen) at the background of a host of bodily distresses (weakness, fatigue, sleeplessness, worthlessness, and sad mood) due to passage of Dhat (semen) with urine for last three months. The patient responded entirely to the treatment with amitriptyline (75 mg OD) for a month.

[38]. A. N. Chowdhury: Koro social response (urban): A longitudinal study of North Bengal Koro epidemic.
Indian Journal of Psychiatry, 1992, 34, 46–52.

It is a report on Koro social response from an urban community of Darjeeling district during and after (longitudinal) the 1982 North Bengal Koro epidemic. To test the social cognition hypothesis on Koro, the author devised a protocol on "Koro positive illness paradigm," which tries to tap the cognitive responses from Koro-affected (n 58) and non-affected families (n 58) over some time. The paradigm addressed the following five assumptions or constructs: (1) Whether Koro was regarded as an illness?; (2) How serious was Koro illness?; (3) Cognitive assessment of the seriousness of Koro illness; (4) Cognitive evaluation of risk imposed by Koro; and (5) Consistency or differences in this social cognition of Koro over time. Koro social response rating was done on the same sample three times: First, at the height of the epidemic; Second, was at an interval from the first 29.5 ± 3.4 days; and the Third, was at the gap from the second 30.67 ± 4.5 days. The cognition intensity related to Koro vulnerability in all its cognitive dimensions has significantly diminished gradually with time. That was well corroborated with the gradual weaning of the incidence curve of the Koro illness in the region. The different aspects of the epidemic spread from a sociopsychological perspective were discussed.

[*This paper woned the "Marfatia Award" of the Indian Psychiatric Society at Its Annual Conference at Cuttack, Orissa, in 1988*]

[39]. A. N. Chowdhury: Psychic infectivity: The role of positive illness cognition in a Psychiatric Epidemic.
Journal of Personality & Clinical Studies, 1992, 8, 125–128.

Infectivity is a biological construct of Preventive and Social Medicine. In psychiatric epidemics, the nature of infectivity evolved from a psychological construct, i.e., a product of cultural cognition of the community's illness model. The author attempted to examine the nature and features of Koro's positive illness cognition from both affected and non-affected families in a rural community at the background of the ongoing Koro epidemic in the North Bengal region. The author devised a "Social Response Pattern" tool, which tries to elicit a cognitive assessment of Koro illness paradigm in terms of: illness type; estimated seriousness; risk to physical or sexual health or life; infective potential; and the chance of infectivity. It was found that Koro was perceived as a positive illness with high infective potential by both family groups. Thus a positive social environment with a cognitive model of high Koro vulnerability was created, facilitating the spread of the epidemic without any social resistance. Koro's credibility as a very contagious illness increased the construct of "infectivity", which strengthened the various cognitive cycles in the community and facilitated its spread.

[40]. A. N. Chowdhury: Koro in Schizophrenia with a case report from industrial set up.
Industrial Psychiatry Journal, 1992, 5(1), 47–59.

This is a case report of Koro at the background of florid schizophrenic illness in a 46-year-old single male from a milk factory. He expressed persecutory delusion, ideas of reference, and auditory hallucination. He believed that some of his workmates had cast some spell on him to make him impotent. Treatment with a course of haloperidol intramuscular injection controlled his excitement and delusion of penile retraction in a week.

[41]. A. N. Chowdhury: Clinical analysis of 101 Koro cases.
Indian Journal of Social Psychiatry, 1992, 7, 67–70.

This is a beneficial clinical report on the clinical features of 101 male Koro patients from the North Bengal Koro epidemic. The author provided the different components of Koro symptomatology in four primary categories, viz. Premonitory symptoms; Physical symptoms; Mental symptoms; and Genital symptoms. Interestingly, two other Koro genital symptoms were reported: complete loss of penile sensation and penile shortening without retraction. Fear of death, though, was the principal conceptual component of Koro anxiety. Still, other themes were also reported, i.e., fear of damage of sex organs, fear of physical ill-health, and feeling of being chased or talked about. This analysis reveals a wide range of symptoms associated with Koro illness.

[42]. A. N. Chowdhury: Koro in affective disorder with a case report from industrial setup.
Industrial Psychiatry Journal, 1992, 5(2), 71–83.

This is a report of Koro (seven cases) in association with the affective disorder (mainly depressive disorder) from the North Bengal Koro epidemic cases. The author presented an analysis of 20 case reports (all were male) from global Koro literature (1921–1992) who had associated depressive disorder with Koro. Except for two cases, all were sporadic cases. This analysis showed how depressive illness with somatization and or depersonalization is variously associated with the disturbed body (organ)-image perception in Koro. The author also presented a series of seven Koro cases (three males and four females) who had episodes of depression/bipolar affective disorder with some hypochondriacal/somatic symptoms.

[43]. A. N. Chowdhury: Psychopatho-sexuality in Koro patients.
Journal of Indian Academy of Applied Psychology, 1992, 5, 71–83.

This is an analysis of the sexual history and psychosexual behavioral profile of 162 male Koro patients (104 single, 58 married) of the North Bengal Koro epidemic. The age mean of the sample was: 25.9 ± 6.1 years. Sample selection was based on two criteria: (1) cases above the age of 15 and (2) patients interviewed during the first three weeks of the epidemic. A sample of normal subjects, marital status matched (100 single and 60 married) was taken for comparison. The age mean was 26.1 ± 5.6 years. All subjects were given "Sex-Guilt Questionnaire". This was devised for this purpose, in line with the construct of Mosher (1966) and Mosher and Cross (1971). The study reveals a definite positive history of aberrant sexual behavior (like incest, extramarital sex, and prostitute visit); psychosexual difficulties (orgasmic difficulties, spermatorrhoea, impotence, and weak sexual power); and mild to severe sex guilt in Koro patients compared to normal subjects. The present finding supports the earlier assumption regarding the role of abnormal sexuality (and concomitant guilt and anxiety) in Koro, thus providing transcultural support for the potential role of psychosexual pathology in Koro's genesis.

[44]. D. N. Nandi, G, Banerjee, H. Saha, B. Sen, A. Bhattacharjee: An epidemic of "Jhin-Jhini"—A strange contagious psychogenic disorder in a village in West Bengal.
Indian Journal of Psychiatry, 1992, 34(4), 366–369.

It is not a Koro research. The reason for its inclusion in this review is because the same name "Jhin-Jhini" was also used to designate Koro illness in the Assam epidemic, reported by Dutta et al. in 1982. To properly understand the local syntax of *Jhin-Jhini*, the reader should also be aware of this epidemic.

It is a retrospective study of an epidemic of Jhin-Jhini in a small village Arkhali, in the North 24 Parganas district of West Bengal, which took place in March 1982. The time is important as it coincides with the

Koro epidemic in the state as well. The presentation of Jhin-Jhini was as follows:

> The disease struck a person all of a sudden with a sensation of tingling and numbness in the legs which spread upward throughout the body. Within a few seconds the patient is seized with the horror of impending death and cries for help before he becomes speechless and motionless. Unless rescued, he would fall flat on the ground. (p. 366)

With emergency help and aid, they recovered after half to two hours. Eighteen people (9 male and nine female) were affected within two months. Most cases were married (13 out of 18 cases). The literal meaning of *Jhin-Jhini* is the sensation of tingling and numbness in limbs and body. The authors clarified this episode with Koro and stated that it was a rapid onset and disappearance of functional mental disorder. There was no concern for genitalia. The condition spreads very rapidly. Villagers believed that an evil spirit enacted it.

1993

[45]. A. N. Chowdhury: Jhin-Jhini—A hysterical contagion.
Indian Journal of Psychiatry, 1993, 35(2), 141. (L)

It is a response to Nandi et al. (1992) reporting on Jhin-Jhini epidemic (above). The author referred to a similar outbreak in Teliamura town in Tripura state, where more than 60 people were affected. It affected both men and women between the ages ranged from 9 to 48 years. The chief complaint was the sudden loss of power in the lower limbs so that the affected person cannot move or walk. Local people identify the cause as an insect bite. The epidemic persisted for nearly two weeks, and a common sight during these days was "the lame and immobile 'Jhin-Jhini' patients were carried to the hospital in cane-baskets." The author also reported two cases of Jhin-Jhini from a rural district of West Bengal. Both were sisters—the elder one (19 years) developed a loss of sensation in both the lower limbs with profuse crying for hours together. The younger sister (14 years) developed this Jhin-Jhini after six days, and it affected her upper limbs so that she was unable to write, which caused her excuse for not appearing in the final examination at her school. Her marriage date was postponed for this illness. The author discussed the diagnostic status of Jhin-Jhini as per ICD-10 as Dissociative motor disorder—Disorders of movement and sensation (F44.4). He also cited different examples of this symptom of Jhin-Jhini in other psychiatric presentations among cases from the Eastern Indian culture. The symptom of "Jhin-Jihni" may be present in some localized hysterical epidemics in rural areas of West Bengal (Chowdhury & Brahma, 2005).

[46]. A. N. Chowdhury, D. J. Bagchi: Koro in heroin withdrawal. *Journal of Psychoactive Drugs, 1993, 25(3), 257–258.*

It is a Koro case report of a 26-year-old single man who developed Koro symptoms during the heroin withdrawal phase. He was a regular user of heroin for four and a half years. He refused hospitalization and agreed to symptomatic home treatment with dextropropoxyphene, chlordiazepoxide, and nitrazepam. On the fifth night after the commencement of treatment, he developed Koro symptoms while using the toilet. The description of the onset is quite dramatic:

> … family members found him terribly excited, trembling with rolling eyeballs, holding his genitals with both hands and repeating the words, "this is the end, this is the end; free it, free it" with a peculiar intonation. When asked, he responded in a frightened voice that his penis had reduced into his abdomen and was 'locked' there and could not be taken out. (p. 257)

Important clinical findings are: features of mixed anxiety-depressive reaction, some elements of dissociation (trance-like state) during the episode of penile retraction, and he had no previous knowledge of Koro. The authors concluded that hyperaroused psychological state during heroin withdrawal, along with compensatory repeated self-stimulation by masturbation, may have a potential role in the genesis of sudden dysmorphophobic penile perception in this case.

[47]. A. N. Chowdhury: Glans penis perception of Koro patients.
Acta Psychiatrica Scandinavica, 1993, 87(5), 355–357.

This is one of the series of penis—perception research of Koro patients done by the author on patients of the Indian Koro epidemic of 1982. Using a graphomotor projective test—DAPT (Draw-a-penis-test) found that Koro patients have significantly less perception of glans penis than the controls (normal subjects, patients of Hydrocele, Scrotal filaria, and Anxiety neurosis)—Fig. 9.4. The author asserts that this perceptual deviation in the glans penis image influenced the penile perception and sexual-behavioral profile of the Koro victims (Koro patients who omit the glans in the DAPT had a significantly higher age to start masturbation) and probably facilitated their Koro vulnerability.

* * *

[48]. S. S. Damodaran, S. H. Nizamie: "Incomplete koro"—A forerunner for mood disorders: Two case reports.
Indian Journal of Psychiatry, 1993, 35, 60–62.

The authors report two interesting bipolar affective disorder cases where the Koro symptom appeared in association with the depressive features but disappeared during the phase of mania. Both the cases had sufficient neurotic sexual preoccupation with masturbatory guilt. The symptoms of moderate depression, suicidal ideas, and high level of anxiety with ideas of reference in the first case (20-year-old college student) showed favorable response to treatment with imipramine 150 mg/day and psychotherapy. Still, on the 10th day after discharge from the hospital, he developed manic symptoms when he claimed to possess a "very big penis." The second case (18-year-old college student) had a classical Koro presentation, i.e., "Penis becoming smaller and getting pulled into his stomach." Treatment with haloperidol, amitriptyline, and then ECT was not helpful because of the side effects. The patient eventually developed (3 days after the second ECT) florid symptoms of mania and "claimed to have a big penis." Treatment with sodium valproate showed promising

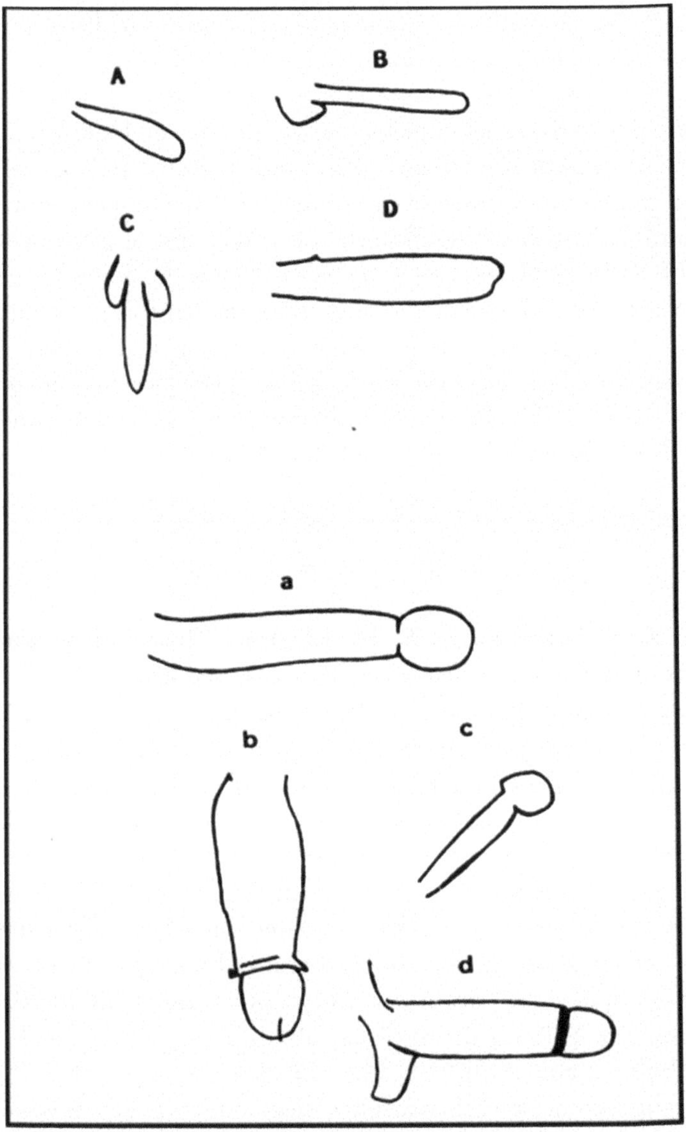

Fig. 9.4 DAPT—Glans Penis Identification (Own-Penis-Flaccid State drawing) (A, B, C, D = Penis without Glans—drawing of Koro, Hydrocele, Scrotal filaria, and Anxiety neurosis cases. a, b, c, d = Penis with identified Glans—drawing of Scrotal filarial, Normal person, Koro, and Hydrocele cases)

results, and all his sexual symptoms were gone by the end of a fortnight's treatment. The authors provided a detailed clinical history and development of the symptoms with some cultural explanation of penile perception with pathological mood states.

Observation: This report shows how the body (organ)-image distortion parallels with mood-congruent state in affective disorder.

[49]. A. N. Chowdhury: Age-specific trait anxiety in Koro patients. *Journal Personality & Clinical Studies, 1993, 9, 15–18.*

Many researchers have identified Koro as atypical hysteria (Lapierre, 1972) or psychological hysteria (Gwee, 1963). The central point of these nosological attempts is related to the clinical manifestation of anxiety in Koro. The author found a mid-position of Koro patients between normal subjects and patients with anxiety neurosis so far as the trait anxiety level is concerned. Moreover, it is an essential clinical impression, noted by many Koro researchers (Gwee, 1968; Ngui, 1969), that not all Koro patients exhibit acute anxiety reactions during their Koro attack. This overt or state anxiety projection is related to their covert or trait anxiety personality disposition. So it is a matter of clinical concern to see how many Koro patients have trait anxiety levels similar or dissimilar to those of anxiety neurotics, which being the standard referential psychopathology so far as the expression of both state and trait anxieties are concerned.

It was observed that not all Koro cases are presented with the typical symptom of acute anxiety. There are cases in which the genital retraction symptom probably sub-serves the purpose of hysterical attention-seeking without any overt anxiety reaction. This contention is supported by the present study's findings where single Koro patients in the age range of 26–30 years and married Koro patients of 21–30 years have an anxiety proneness personality disposition (trait anxiety) quite different from that of the anxiety neurotics. On the other hand, Koro patients of other age groups have identical trait anxiety profiles with that of the anxiety neurosis group. The proper delineation of the Koro symptom spectrum may indicate some confounding cases of hysterical or hypochondriacal cases in the epidemic cohort. But in the virtual scenario, these cases remain unidentified because of the epidemic rush and lack of formal clinical screening and study planning.

[50]. A. N. Chowdhury: Psychiatric morbidity and the Fox connection.
Transcultural Psychiatric Research Review, 1993, 30(4), 399–401. (L)

It is a letter in response to R. H. Prince's article: Koro and the Fox spirit on Hainan Island (China), *TPRR*, 1992, 29, 119–132. The author discussed Koro's culture-boundness so far as an example of the belief of an evil fox spirit in the Chinese Koro epidemic in Hainan Island. He also provided two additional examples of cultural faith in the fox spirit. A Japanese mental illness, Kitsunetsuki, is a possession by a fox spirit and Jackal's cult in Santal culture and folklore (a tribe in India). In Japanese folklore, the traditional belief is in the "soul replacement," i.e., the intrusion of an outside agent (possessed by a god or ancestors' spirit or animals) into the self (Wittkower & Rin, 1965). In Santal tradition, Jackal is called *Toyo*, who possesses a human voice and great supernatural power granted by the Sun god (*Chand*o) and the Moon god (*Ninda Chando*). A widely used Santal proverb on the wisdom of Jackel is the "wit of seven Jackals."

[51]. A. N. Chowdhury: Variations in the perception of the penis.
Journal of Sexual Health, 1993, 3, 156–160.

It is a theoretical paper on the perception of penis image regarding its morphology or functional capability. It discussed abnormal penis image viz. the apprehension of a "small" penis, which the patients may impute either to intra-abdominal pull (as in Koro) or to reasons other than abdominal pull (as in some cases of impotence or Dhat syndrome, or simply as dissatisfaction with a small size of the penis). The author tried to describe the problem related to the visual cognition of the penis by "Penis visibility and visual axis" and penile anatomic-physiological variation of penile morphology, viz. State (erected penis) and Trait (flaccid penis) penis condition and the impact of cultural cognition on them. The author described the visual scrutiny of the penis in the development of penis image or awareness and its role in alleged sexual dysfunction, both morphological and functional. Interesting to note that Yap (1965) mentioned this aspect of genital body image about depersonalization in Koro as:

> The genital portion of the total body-image is likely to be weakly structured and therefore more liable to catathymic distortion because the organ is toneless, beyond voluntary control. And its outlines dependent upon episodic emotional arousal. (p.48)

[52]. A. N. Chowdhury: Art in Koro.
Journal of Sexual Health, 1993, 3, 181.

This is a rare reporting from the 1982 North Bengal Koro epidemic. This is the only published report of any artwork by a Koro patient. The patient had a Koro attack during the sketching of this artwork during his schizophrenic episode. Analysis of the sketch shows a blending of cultural overtone, sexual morality with paranoid ideation. Analysis of this artwork highlighted some potential psychosexual dynamics befitting with the psychopathology of the subject.

* * *

"The case": AB. 24 years, unmarried Bengali Hindu male, educated up to class ten, worked as a helper in a small milk stall. He developed the schizophrenic illness at the age of 21 and was under psychiatric treatment with few relapses in between. His Koro attack occurred during such a relapse phase. He had some artistic abilities and used to draw sketches of the human figure and natural scenes. He experienced acute penile shrinkage one midnight while drawing such an illustration (Fig. 9.5).

This incomplete drawing shows probably a religious-philosophical theme with erotic references. The display of heterosexual union is in the center at the background of lotus petals intermixed with multiple geometrical lines resembling the tantric art in a mandala. The tantric art considers that the lotus is an archaic symbol—it is the first product of the creative principle (Mukherjee & Khanna, 1989). There are frequent uses of a definite number of lotus petals in tantric art, e.g., Srva-saparipukara

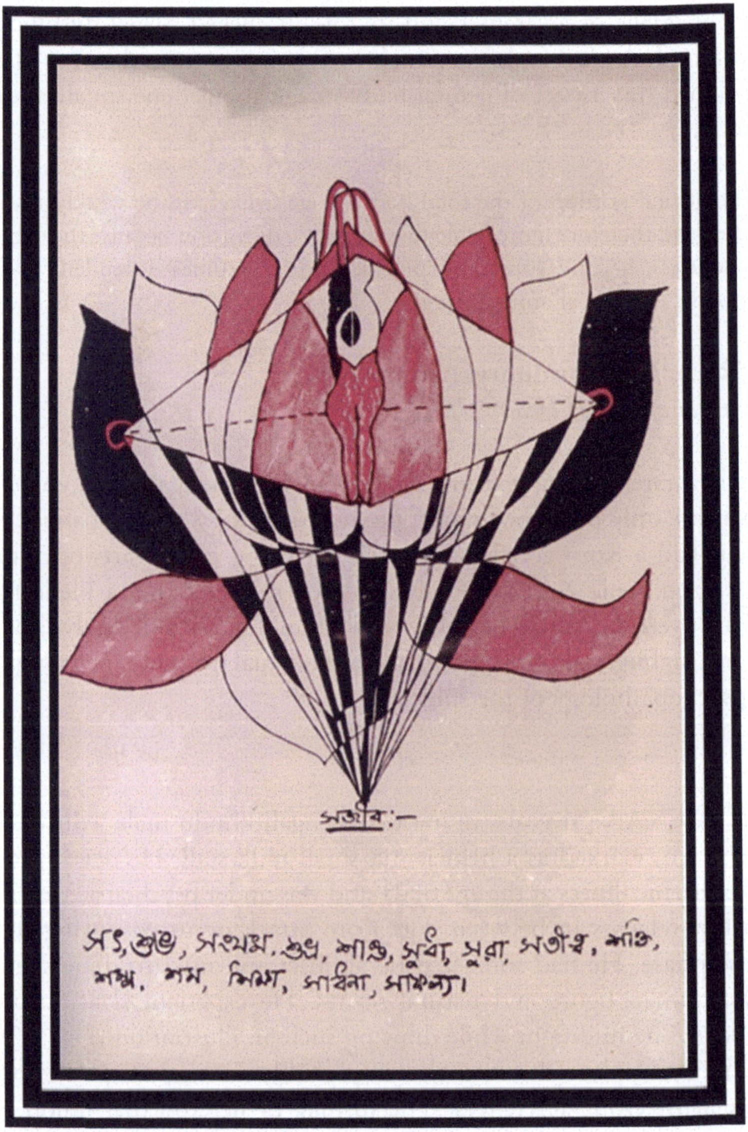

Fig. 9.5 Artwork by the subject. English translation of the Bengali words written at the bottom of the sketch: Honesty, Holy, Control, White, Calm, Nector, Alcohol, Virginity, Strength, Education, Meditation, Success (Written consent was taken for reproduction in an academic paper)

Chakra (ring of 16 petals) or Srva-saparipukara Chakra (8 petals)—both of which indicate the fulfillment of desire. The interwoven girdle of lotus petals usually symbolizes the "spiritual rebirth," and the center is the area of a cosmic zone representing the area of spiritual integration (Mukherjee, 1965).

The fifteen Bengali dialects written below the sketch are all beginning with the letter "S." They are as follows: The word at the pivotal point (below) from where the different threads originate is *Sajib,* meaning "animate." The word in the line written below from left to right are: *Sath* (honest), *Subba* (holy), **Sangjyam* (self-abnegation), *Subhra* (white), *Santa* (tranquil), *Sudha* (nectar), *Sura* (wine), **Swatittwa* (chastity), **Sakthi* (strength), *Sampa*—probably misspelled (lightning), **Sham* (restraint of passion), *Siksha* (learning), *Sadhana* (worship), and *Saphalya* (success). Word with asterixis are expressions of sexual principles of morality, with a bit of erotic flavor. The display and abstraction depicted by the interplay of white, black, and red color probably represent the conflicts concerning the spirituality and erotic instincts with a falling super-ego influence.

The patient displayed prominent schizophrenic symptoms like auditory hallucination, ideas of reference, persecutory delusion, and incongruent mood along with his Koro experience. The persecutory delusion was directed toward unidentified neighbors who were allegedly in constant search of an opportunity to inflict some harm to him. He said that, time and again, he expressed his sexual concern in the past. The concerns were mainly about his diminished "sexual energy," irrational fear, and anxiety of being impotent, though he gave no reason for this. Once, he blamed himself for the cause of the primary infertility of his elder brother's wife. He held the idea that an unknown magical force controls the "sexual energy and vitality" of the human race through cosmic rays. He explained the cause of the ongoing Koro epidemic as punishment by a "divine force" for the transgression of sexual morality by the people at large.

He said that he noticed this "moral deterioration" of people in their faces and eyes in recent times. He also explained his case as a punishment of "alert type" because, once, though for a little while, he looked toward his elder brother's wife with an "erotic look." He never masturbated as he firmly believes that loss of semen causes ill-health, and this vital fluid packed with "worldly force" should not be wasted for mere bodily pleasure. He recovered from his Koro experience within a week with the increment of doses of trifluoperazine, on which he was earlier put.

1994

[53]. A. N. Chowdhury, G. Banerjee, K. D. Sen, N. K. Bera, N. K. Sharma: Koro in West Bengal again: Report of nine cases.
Indian Journal of Social Psychiatry, 1994, 10, 27–30.

This report reports nine sporadic male Koro cases from four West Bengal districts between January and July 1993. Many of the patients reported a fascinating history of recurrent Koro attacks. One case (31-year-old, married, Nepali Hindu) was reported from Darjeeling Sadar hospital who had a typical symptom of Koro, and responded favorably with IM injection of B vitamin and oral diazepam.

Four cases were from the same village in the North Dinajpur district. All were of Ranbanshi ethnicity. Two cases (27-year, Single/26-year-old married) were from the same family, and they had Koro symptoms (penile retraction with fear of penis loss) after their first exposure to cannabis smoking. The third case had a history of recurrent Koro attacks (penile retraction with fear of death), 2–3 episodes a day, 3–4 times a week for five months. The fourth case had a solitary attack of classical Koro.

Two cases were from Taldi village under the Canning Police station of the South 24 Parganas district. This village experienced the 1982 Koro epidemic (9 males and two females were affected). The first case was a farmer and had a Koro attack in the background of fasting hypoglycemia. The second case occurred eleven days later in the same village and had a solitary episode. Both the cases were married. In the second case, there was a conflict with the next-door neighbor as the patient believes that they attacked him with some spell or black magic. Police were involved.

Two cases are reported from the Calcutta district. The first case was a single 28-year-old male who presented with recurrent penile indrawing complaints with mild pain accompanied by fear of sexual invalidism of three years. The inner pull increased whenever there was some friction of bare glans penis with wet clothing, which generated a burning sensation in the penis shaft. The problem started three years ago while he was rubbing the penis with a wet towel after a bath. He consulted a physician who prescribed a penicillin injection for his penile gonorrheal infection. Psychosexual history showed that he started masturbation at age 16, visited prostitutes over 23 times in the last four years. Mental state examination revealed an intense hypochondriacal bodily preoccupation with obsessive ideas and rumination.

The second case (28-year-old single) attended the hospital after reading a newspaper reporting on the reappearance of Koro cases. For the last ten months, he complained of episodic (once or twice weekly) partial penile indrawing without fear of death. He also complained of reduced sex drive and noticed the reduction of penis size by about 2 cm due to partial indrawing of the penis into the abdomen. This has added extreme anxiety to his already existing health-related preoccupations and compelled him to consult several health care persons, including astrologers, palmists, and folk healers. A mental state examination showed he had moderate depression with marked hypochondriacal concerns about alleged diverse bodily dysfunctions.

Observation: Analysis of these cases focused on four important clinical issues: (1) Fear of penis loss may well be an ideational component of Koro anxiety. (2) Over a considerable time, the stereotyped recurrent attacks provide the option for a newer nosology of "Chronic Koro". In such cases, the predominant features are the absence of acute anxiety, the presence of dominant fear of sexual invalidism (not death), and the lengthy-time course (weeks or months or years). (3) Two North Dinajpur district cases exemplify genital depersonalization as a psychological reaction following cannabis smoking. (4) The clinical importance of genital preoccupation in patients with strong hypochondriacal or obsessive health concerns.

---

[54]. S. M. Agarwal, P. G. Divakara, K. B. Pramanik: Koro in an industrial setting.

Indian Journal of Psychiatry, 1994, 36(1), 36–38.

This is a Koro case report from an industrial setup at Bokaro Steel City, Bihar, India. The patient is a 52-year-old married Hindu male who presented with complaints of poor penile erection, premature and retarded ejaculation, feeling that his penis was shrinking and drawn into his abdomen and might disappear if not held back. At other times he thought that his genitals had almost vanished. Also, he had palpitation, restlessness, sleep disturbances, vague pain in the chest, and other body parts. These symptoms intensify under work stress. He is having these symptoms for the last seven years and has consulted several doctors without any benefit. There is a history of masturbatory guilt and marital maladjustment due to poor erection and premature ejaculation. Rumination about family relations, sexual weakness, and work stress made him tense and anxious, and suddenly becoming overly worried about losing his sex organ and eventual death. He put his hands in the pocket to check the penis and scrotum, and for further reassurance, he frequently visited the toilet. He responded well with 30–60 mg of chlordiazepoxide and 25 mg of trimipramine daily and relaxation and dual sex therapy. He completely recovered in a month and showed no recurrence for five years follow-up. The authors suggested that chronic anxiety, multiple situational stressors, and sexual conflicts played a role in developing Koro-like symptomatology.

[55]. A. N. Chowdhury: Koro in females: An analysis of 48 cases. *Transcultural Psychiatry, 1994, 31(4), 369–380.*

This is a comprehensive report on female Koro, reported from the 1982 Indian Koro epidemic. It provided a detailed analysis of 48 female Koro cases' clinicopathological features. Breast symptoms were significantly more common (79.2%) than genital symptoms (12.5%). Fear of breast damage was the predominant ideational component in female Koro cases, followed by fear of death. Though the typical breast symptom reported in the literature is "nipple retraction." Still, in this study, some other breast symptoms were also noted, like breast pain, flattening of breast mass on the chest wall, pricking sensation in the breast, retraction of the whole breast into the chest cavity, and retraction of a single nipple. Labial retraction and vaginal pain were genital symptoms. Frequency analysis showed that patients with breast symptoms (79.2%) were significantly more prevalent than those with either genital symptoms alone (12.5%) or with both genital and breast symptoms (8.3%) – x2 = 64, df = 2, $p < 0.01$. The account also reported Koro's detailed breakdown and associated comorbidities like hysterical fainting, neurotic depression, psychotic depression, migraine, and lower limb arthritis.

The author also mentioned the scarcity of female Koro case report with international references. It is interesting to note that to date, female Koro cases were reported from epidemic settings mainly: 7 such reports showed a total of 146 (9.2%) female cases out of 1583 patients. The different psychosexual issues and local cultural contexts, and folk myths relating to female Koro are discussed.

[56]. A. N. Chowdhury, N. K. Bera: Koro following Cannabis smoking: Two case reports.
Addiction, 1994, 89(8), 1017–1020.

This is a report of two sporadic Koro cases from the rural area of West Bengal, India. In the first case (27-year-old single male), the Koro attack was followed by the first heavy smoking of cannabis with bodily dissociative symptoms and acute anxiety and fear of death. Traditional "water treatment" helped to have stopped the penis' retraction and subsequently showed complete remission with medical treatment. He also showed hypochondriacal traits. In the second case (26-year-old married male), a distant cousin of the first one, who knew his brother's Koro, developed penile retraction with acute anxiety and bodily dissociative feelings after heavy cannabis smoking. Interesting to note that both of them showed genital depersonalization only after cannabis smoking.

1995

[57]. A. N. Chowdhury: Koro and the Indian Psychiatrists.
Indian Journal of Social Psychiatry, 1995, 11, 78–80.

A discussion paper highlights that India is becoming a Koro-prone country since the massive Koro epidemic of 1982. It covers the report of the outbreaks from states like Assam, Tripura, Orissa, and West Bengal and sporadic cases from states like Gujarat, Uttar Pradesh, Bihar, and New Delhi. This opens up a new opportunity for the Indian Psychiatrists to observe and study this culture-bound syndrome from a close quarter. The paper also contains a gist of a global literature search on Koro.

[58]. A. N. Chowdhury, N. K. Bera: Koro in North Bengal A new: An unusual case.
Journal Personality & Clinical Studies, 1995, 11(1–2), 55–58.

It is a sporadic case report of a 35-year-old Indian male of Rajbanshi ethnicity (North Bengal region), who showed several episodes of a cluster of symptoms as: stereotyped episodes of abdominal pain, flushing, difficulty in breathing, feeling of cold extremities with penile retraction, and fear of imminent death for five months. The penile retraction component is typically a Koro-like attack but recurrent. During this period, he had at least a dozen episodes. Each attack was preceded by a cluster of autonomic symptoms, followed by a normal inter-attack interval, strongly suggestive of diencephalic or autonomic epilepsy. Mental state examination revealed a low mood with feelings of hopelessness, suicidal thoughts, and diminished libido, but the physical tests were standard. He showed some clinical improvement with anxiolytic and antidepressant drugs within 15 days but failed to report for follow-ups and EEG investigation.

Observation: Two critical clinical comments need attention: the scope of a newer nosology of recurrent or, more specifically, "Chronic Koro" and evaluating multiple, episodic, and stereotyped Koro symptoms in the light of possible epileptic phenomena.

[59]. A. N. Chowdhury: Yin-Yang dualism and sexuality in Chinese culture: A psycho-historical perspective.
Journal of Indian Anthropological Society, 1995, 30, 125–133.

This discussion paper focuses on the Taoist medical philosophy behind genital retraction in males from yin-yang dualism. The concept of Shook (Suk) Yang or Suo-yang or genital retraction as a grave sexual illness has its reference in the century-old Chinese Taoist medical doctrine.

The concept and the clinical presentation of genital retraction illness have been documented under various names. This paper deals with brief historical documentation of the yin-yang Taoist doctrine concerning sexuality in general and male genital retraction in particular.

[60]. A. N. Chowdhury, K. C. Rajbhandari: Koro with depression in Nepal.
Transcultural Psychiatry, 1995, 32, 87–90.

This is a sporadic case of Chronic Koro from Nepal. It describes the Koro symptoms in the background of depressive illness in a 27-year-old single Nepali male. He described his penile retraction as a slow process, "slow, snail-like indrawing" and took place over a few weeks. There was a history of sexual dysfunction, colored with intense sex guilt for the perceived transgression of cultural sex norms. The conceptual component of this morbidity was "penis loss," not death. He had no prior knowledge of Koro. He responded favorably with treatment with amitriptyline and nitrazepam.

1996

[61]. A. N. Chowdhury: The definition and classification of Koro.
Culture Medicine & Psychiatry, 1996, 20(1), 41–65.

This is a descriptive and extensive discussion paper on Koro. Here, the author attempts to analyze all the available data on Koro, especially the historical record of diagnostic nosology, its place in DSM-III and ICD-10, semantic confusion of Koro phenomenology, and the different cognitive ideational, physical, and psychological component of the clinical picture. He proposed a simplified classification as primary Koro (culture-bound expression) and secondary Koro (with other mental or physical or substance abuse disorders) of Koro—Table 9.3. There is a discussion on the age of onset, course, prevalence, family pattern, and folk treatment complications and directions of future research on Koro. A portion of the discussion was devoted to a recent study on body image vis-a-vis penis-image perception among Koro patients.

Table 9.3 Classification of Koro

1. Primary Koro: Culture-bound expression (Classical presentation)	1.0 Sporadic 1.1 Epidemic
2. Secondary Koro (may be a dual diagnosis)	2.0 With CNS disorders (neurology) 2.1 With alcohol and substance abuse disorder 2.2 With a psychiatric disorder (psychotic or nonpsychotic) 2.3 With other culture-bound disorders (Dhat syndrome) 3. With systemic disorders (medical/urological)

[62]. A. N. Chowdhury: Koro: A state of sexual panic or altered physiology?
Sexual & Marital Therapy, 1996, 11(2), 165–171.

This is a handy research paper addressing the biomedical context of the altered physiological state of the penis in the precipitation of Koro attacks in vulnerable individuals. The author surveyed the world Koro literature (up to 1992), including his research (Indian Koro epidemic), and substantiates physical factors' potential role in initiating or triggering the Koro perception. The central role of vasoconstriction in causing an acute hyperinvolution of the penis is already reported among sporadic and epidemic Koro cases. He described three factors as follows: (1) penile exposure to cold (water, wind)—119 cases of Koro have been reported after such exposure; (2) during excretory function as micturition or defecation (80 cases reported); and (3) an acute fear of Koro affliction (17 reported cases). It was concluded that "cultural beliefs do generate a background of cognitive sensitivity or proneness, based on which physiological or biomedical" conditions (cold, fright, genital-urinary activity or function) may facilitate or initiate the Koro perception. The author showed that the association between Koro perception on the one hand and cold, fright, sexual activity, or excretory functions on the other dose provides a reasonable probability that penile vasoconstriction is the real cause that may trigger Koro symptoms. The present analysis from various ethnicities and cultures across the globe shows that culture generates a background of cognitive sensitivity, based on which physiological or biomedical phenomenon initiates the morbid expression.

[63]. A. N. Chowdhury, G. Banerjee: Recurrent Koro in repeated Buprenorphine withdrawal.
Addiction, 1996, 91(1), 145–146. (L)

This is a case report of Koro in a 38-year-old single Indian (Assamese) male, who experienced 3 Koro attacks during repeated phases of Buprenorphine withdrawal. He took Buprenorphine for the last two years and was often injected into the dorsal vein of his penis several times due to the non-availability of other injecting sites. In his first attempt at stopping Buprenorphine due to fear of HIV/AIDS, he experienced severe opiate-like withdrawal symptoms, along with a strong intra-abdominal pull of the penis and scrotum. Buprenorphine injection helped regain a perceived normal state of genital morphology. About eight months later, in his second attempt (when he heard about the Koro illness by the local name of *Jhin-Jhini*), the Buprenorphine withdrawal led to a re-experience of genital retraction forced him to continue the drug habit. He made another attempt at cessation after being prescribed lorazepam by a general practitioner but had a severe Koro attack, and this time with a feeling of impending death. The symptoms diminished after Buprenorphine injection. This is the first report of Koro in Buprenorphine addiction.

[64]. A. N. Chowdhury: Cannabis: A note from Bengal.
Addiction, 1996, 91(6), 767. (L)

It is a letter in response to a discussion on the book "The health and Psychological Consequences of Cannabis use" by Hall et al. (1994), wherein describing the findings on cannabis abuse, the author mentioned about 3 cases of Koro with cannabis use in the context of body image disturbances. One patient had an episodic perception of reduced penile size (eight times in the last six months), coinciding with cannabis smoking. After stopping cannabis smoking, no such symptoms recurred at 2.5 years of follow-up.

[65]. A. N. Chowdhury: Sex guilt cognition in the genesis of Koro. *Archives of Indian Psychiatry, 1996, 3, 52–59.*

This is a paper on the "Sex Guilt" construct in Koro. A review of male Koro cases from the global literature and the author's research tried to endorses the hypothesis of sex-guilt cognition as an essential psychodynamic factor in Koro. Evidence from the literature survey has shown that at least three psychosexual abnormalities are noted in the male Koro cases irrespective of their origin, whether oriental or occidental. These are:

1. Conflict and guilt over sexual activities like masturbation, heterosexual relation with wife or prostitute or girlfriend, and conflict over sexual potency and sexual maladjustment.
2. Inadequate masculine self-image.
3. Hypersexual behavior and multiple sexual relations. It is also of clinical interest to note that most of the authors found a premorbid neurotic personality pattern or a history of frank attack of acute anxiety.

The present research among Koro cases of the North Bengal epidemic using Personality profile on EPQ (Eysenek & Eysenek, 1975) of Koro patients (n 49) found a significant score of Neuroticism (N) in comparison to normal and Extraversion (E) in comparison to anxiety neurotics. Assessment of trait anxiety level by STAI of Spielberger et al. (1970) showed a higher level of trait anxiety in Koro patients (n 186) than that of normal subjects. Based on these findings, a construct of "Sex-Guilt" theory is formulated as follows.

This high E and N association is probably responsible for varied psychosexual pathologies with resultant sexual conflict and guilt and subsequent symptom formation in Koro patients. Their high E disposition would make them react positively to sexual situations or encourage them to invite solitary or multiple sexual relations. In contrast, their coexisting high N personality component would make them react negatively to each situation. O'Neill and Kempler (1969) explain this situation by the "approach-avoidance conflict" concept: the N component helps raise the "avoidance" gradient above average. Correspondingly, the

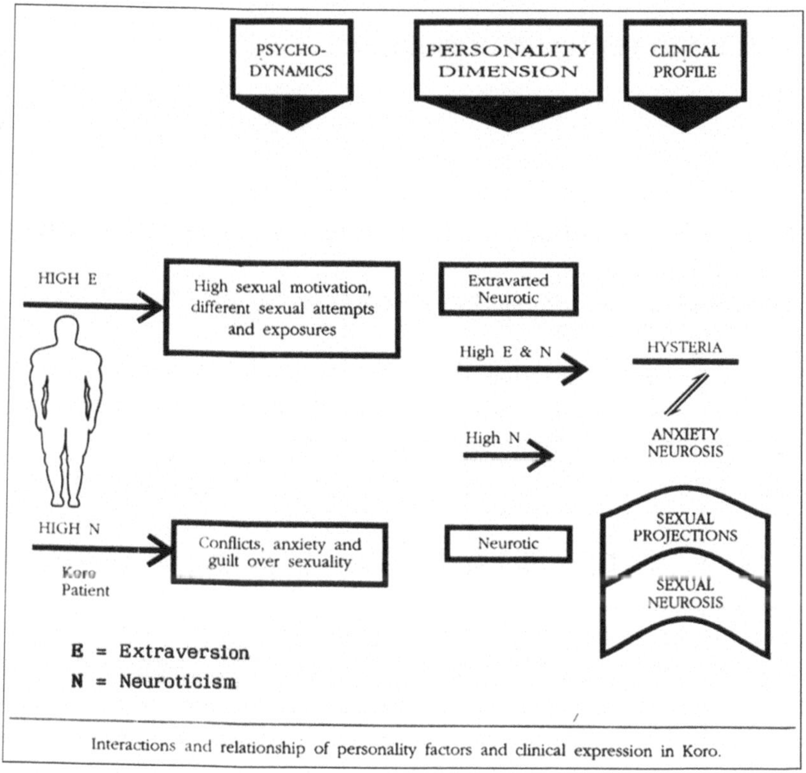

Fig. 9.6 Personality and sex guilt interaction in Koro

E component increases the "approaches" gradient above average. Psychodynamically, this is a critical paradox. Clinically a high percentage of subjects may show various sexual approaches resulting in cumulative conflict and guilt over each such "approach" behavior (Swensen, 1963; Wells, 1969). Koro patients display this interaction. Such interaction's clinical outcome depends on the E component's disposition over the N component and vice versa. Some may manifest a behavior akin to hysterical genital somatization, while some may exhibit acute anxiety neurosis with genital focus. Both, however, may be called sexual neurosis (Fig. 9.6).

1988 KORO EPIDEMIC IN TRIPURA

2000

[66]. A. N. Chowdhury: Animals with erotic symbolism: A transcultural account.
Journal of Indian Anthropological Society, 2000, 35, 171–177.

A brief discussion paper describes different animals representing erotic symbolism (including fecundity, masculine/feminine sexual power, and energy) in the world's mythology and cultures.

2003

[67]. A. N. Chowdhury: Tortoise: A psycho-anthropological perspective.
The Eastern Anthropologist, 2003, 56, 51–59.

This is a discussion paper that highlighted the psycho-anthropological aspect of the tortoise with a focus on its relationship with Koro semantic. "Koro" comes from the term for "tortoise" in Malay, Indonesian dialects (Wilkinson, 1932), and the imagery of genital retraction in Koro is linked with the turtle symbolism among the Chinese (Gwee, 1963). Different aspects of turtle symbolism in Chinese and Indian cultures are discussed.

2004

[68]. S. K. Praharaj: Koro and psychosis following steroid abuse.
German Journal of Psychiatry, 2004, 7(3), 49–50.

It is a case report of Koro in association with steroid abuse from New Delhi, India. The case was a 24-year-old single male taking dexamethasone 6 mg daily for the last six years to increase his health and vigor. The duration of current symptoms is two years. He was presented with hyperactivity, increased speech, emotional lability, persecutory and referential ideas, hearing of voices (arising from his body parts), fear, and observation of gradual retraction of penis size, which is becoming smaller by day. He checks and rechecks his genitals several times a day. He was diagnosed with steroid-induced Koro and psychosis. The steroid was stopped and treated with olanzapine 10 mg/day and lorazepam 2 mg at bedtime. By four weeks of treatment, he became asymptomatic.

Observation: Few things are worthy of mentioning here:

1. It seems from the clinical description that the person has a hypomanic state. There are some examples in the literature that during episodes of depression, people perceive shortness (or shrinking) of the penis, and in high or hypomanic (or manic) mood states, people perceive long or big penis. But unlike this here, the patient perceives retracting and smaller penis day by day. This is a new finding.
2. Is there a hypochondriacal spectrum that exists? Recourse to or abuse of steroids for health and vigor is indicative of body image concern. Does the scrutiny of penis size or hearing voices arise from the body parts (no specific mention of which body part) relates to heightened body concern?
3. It is more appropriate to identify this case as "Koro-like" as there is no acute onset, no fear of death from retraction. Instead, he had many worries about his penis condition, again pointing to genitally focused hypochondriacal health concerns.

[69]. A. N. Chowdhury, A. Brahma: Chronic Koro.
Eastern Journal of Psychiatry, 2004, 8, 57–59.

This is a sporadic male Koro case report from West Bengal. The subject presented with typical Koro symptoms spanning over three months. In each episode, he had multiple Koro attacks with fear of sexual dysfunction (not fear of death)—both functional and morphological (shortening of penile girth). He had previous knowledge of Koro illness. Given the chronic presentation over a lengthy period—the possibility of a "Chronic" course of Koro is suggested.

2005

[70]. N. Kar: Chronic Koro-like symptoms—Two case reports.
BMC Psychiatry, 2005, October, 12, 5, 34.

This is a case report of two Koro cases from Cuttack, Orissa, India. This paper reported a few interesting clinical facts about the Koro presentation.

The first case was a 30-year-old single male whose chief complaint was persistent fear for a gradual shrinking of the penis for the last 12 years. He believed that this sickness was due to his seminal nocturnal emissions and a couple of masturbatory acts during adolescence. He was highly religious and thought that the gradual shrinkage of the penis is an indication of his destruction and death. The author commented that he has overvalued ideas with an anxious mood. He consciously avoids seeing or touching his penis.

The second case was a 41-year-old single male, who complained of:

> gradual retraction of penis and scrotum into the abdomen. He had frequent panic attacks feeling that the end had come. The symptoms had persisted more than 15 years with a waxing and waning course. During exacerbations he spent most of his time measuring the penis by a scale and pulling it in order to bring it out of abdomen. He tied a string around it and attached it to a hook above to prevent its shrinkage during night.

He has a history of prostitute visits, contracted STD (gonorrhea and syphilis), and has a doctor shopping habit.

The author, given the period and repeated episodes, suggested the diagnostic label as Chronic Koro. The clinical description means some OCD traits in the first case and a strong hypochondriacal health concern in the second.

2008

[71]. A. N. Chowdhury: Koro social response during an epidemic: Study from India.
Scientific-Practical Reviewed Journal (Moscow), 2008, 3, 41–42.

It is a short publication on the author's study of social response to the Koro epidemic in North Bengal, India. The study explored responses from 366 people elicited by a predesigned "Social response pattern schedule" during the epidemic's height. 80.6% of the respondent viewed Koro as a form of physical illness, and 6% discarded its illness potentiality. 21.6% found no chance of infection from Koro-affected persons, and 43.7% considered it highly infectious. So far as the Koro health risk is concerned, 8.2% opined no risk; 32.2% perceived it as a life-threatening risk; and 38.5% viewed the loss of sexual power as the risk from Koro. The different aspects of community perception of Koro as an "illness" model were discussed.

2010

2010: KORO EPIDEMIC REPORTED from WEST BENGAL, ASSAM, TRIPURA, MUMBAI, and KERALA in INDIA

* * *

Box 9.1 News Paper Coverage of Kolkata Koro Epidemic in 2010 in STATESMAN

KMC move to treat Koro patients

10 November 2010

KOLKATA, 10 NOV: The Kolkata Municipal Corporation (KMC) has set up a special medical team to treat "Koro patients", member mayor-in-council (health), Mr Atin Ghosh, said today.

He said Koro is a culture-specific syndrome and a mental disorder. A Koro patient believes that his or her external genitals are retracting or shrinking, and fears that the organ will disappear.

Mr Ghosh said KMC has already conducted a study on the disease and found that 20 persons in several wards of the KMC are suffering from this syndrome. He said a section of astrologers, priests and exorcists is taking advantage of the situation selling amulets among the patients. A team of doctors of KMC will visit the places and meet the Koro patients for their treatment. If required KMC doctors will administer them a low-dose sleeping pill and a psychological counselling will be conducted, he said. Mr Ghosh said that the state health department should take the initiative for the treatment of the Koro patients. KMC health department will also urge state health department for the arrangement of the treatment of the Koro patients. Over the last few days a large number of people contacted the health officials regarding the disease. Educated people are no exceptions in this case, as those who believe themselves to be suffering from the disease are staying in the pond for a long time which they believe can help in curing the disease said a KMC health official. Sns

[http://www.thestatesman.net/index.php?option=com_content&view=article&id=348109&catid=73]

Box 9.2 News Paper Coverage of Assam Koro Epidemic in 2010

The Assam Tribune [India]

30 September 2010

It's a cultural syndrome, say doctors

Staff Reporter

GUWAHATI, Sept 29 – Doctors have discounted claims and apprehensions about the reported outbreak of a disease that affects males and females in peculiar ways. Senior doctors in Gauhati Medical College as well as those working in the rural interiors have rubbished reports which indicate that some males have seen their genital organs retract into their abdomen; while females have experienced the same with their breasts.

"There is absolutely no scientific evidence that such things have happened," said Dr MM Deka, Principal of Gauhati Medical College. He said that it could be traced to a cultural syndrome called Koro that is prevalent in Malay and Chinese population of Southeast Asia.

In countries like Malaysia, there is a belief that excessive sexual activity can lead to such conditions. But that cannot be called a disease, because no symptoms actually exist. "At best it is a cultural disease," Dr Deka remarked.

The senior doctor said that the syndrome has been reported mostly from the bordering areas of Assam, and could have spread via migration involving people and culture. "It is not a belief common to Assam, only once before was it reported in 1981–82", he noted.

Referring to the people who have reportedly fallen victims he said that, in almost all the cases they were from seriously disadvantaged background with no access to education. "Lack of awareness coupled to high stress levels made such people vulnerable to such beliefs," he observed.

Doctors, who have started receiving distress calls from people, believe that the media should refrain from sensationalism in this regard and play a responsible role.

Media persons and NGOs can play a positive role in sending a message of assurance to the masses, they add.

[http://www.assamtribune.com/scripts/detailsnew.asp?id=sep3010/city06].

2011

[72]. M. S. Bhatia, A. Jhanjee, P. Kumar: Culturebound syndromes—A cross-sectional study from India.
European Psychiatry, 19th European Congress of Psychiatry, EPA, 2011, (Suppl.1), 26.

It is a short report of a cross-sectional study on the prevalence of culture-bound syndromes presented at the outpatient department of a tertiary care hospital in Delhi, India's capital. Of 50 cases of culture-bound syndromes seen, Dhat syndrome was most common (80%), followed by Possession syndrome (14%), Ascetic syndrome (2%), Gilhari syndrome (2%), and Koro (2%). Depression was the most common associated psychiatric disorder.

[73]. S. Chakraborty, D. Sanyal: An outbreak of Koro among 19 workers in a Jute Mill in South Bengal.
Industrial Psychiatry Journal, 2011, 20(1), 58–60.

This is a valuable paper so far as the Koro demography in an epidemic setting is concerned. The authors provided many vital details of 19 jute mill workers, all male, from southern West Bengal. No timeline of the epidemic is reported. They also provide details of two case reports. Essential points the authors provided are: (1) 84.2% were single. (2) 63.2% not completed secondary education. (3) 12.5% had premorbid substance abuse. (4) 12.5% had a premorbid psychotic illness. (5) 15.8% admitted homosexual activity. (6) 12.5% had commercial sex worker exposure. (7) Majority of the cases believed that the disease was caused by overindulgence to masturbatory practices or nocturnal emission. (8) In 57.9% of the case, the primary health-seeking behavior was water immersion. (9) 5.26% of cases attempted mechanical penile traction resulting in abrasive injury on the glans penis. (10) None of the cases did meet any Axis I diagnosis of DSM-IV. (11) All cases believed that the disease occurred due to increased heat accumulated within the body that needed to be cooled down. (12) 26.3% of cases said "mobile phone as the initial information tool."

[74]. A. K. Nath, B. K.Bhowmic, J. M. Ghosh: A socio-cultural study of "Koro" epidemic in certain villages of Tripura.
Brochure of Conference of Indian Psychiatric Society, East Zone, 2011, 29–30.

This is a short report of Koro from two villages of Kamalpur district of Tripura, in the background of a Koro epidemic in the adjacent villages. They reported eight male Koro cases that happened within twelve days. Five cases belonged to tribal ethnicity, and three were from the Bengali community. The two adjacent small villages were Laijury north and west and Sashipal para, about 8 km away from this spot. Three of the victims were married, and five were single. The age range was from 12 to 38 years. Five victims were students, and three were cultivators. After the sunset, most of the attacks began with shivering for 2–3 minutes and then a tingling sensation in the penis and inward pull with heightened anxiety and fear of death. Local faith healers like *Tantrik* and *Ojha* were consulted, and they provided traditional treatment. Each episode lasted for 2–4 minutes, with an average of 3–5 times during 4–5 days.

From the description, it appears that all of them had recurrent Koro attacks within a specified time of 4–5 days. The authors also mentioned: "The people of the state still vividly remember the episode of Koro in 1998 when hundreds of young males and females were affected …restricted to about 20 km radius around Agartala, Capital of Tripura."

[75]. M. Sinha: Resurgence of Koro: Perception of mankind.
Asian Journal of Psychiatry, 2011, 4(2), 153–154.

This is a descriptive account of the 2010 Koro epidemic in West Bengal, India. The author provided a firsthand account of the clinical symptoms, the demography of the affected persons, the epidemic spread, and the community's preventive measures. Koro was known as "Disco" in the city. A significant female (breast symptoms only) population was also affected. Some presented with a tingling sensation all over the body associated with the penis' retraction; few complained of heat emanating from the body with a rise of body temperature. The age range was from 7 to 70 years. In rural areas, this illness news provoked some overvalued ideas bordering on a shared delusion. Folk treatment of water pouring and wearing of amulets contains charmed seeds of bottle-gourd was widely prevalent. In some communities:

> They have perceived it as a miraculous phenomenon created by 'Allah' or 'The Almighty' which has occurred due to some wrongdoings or misgivings in their daily life. To prevent further recurrences, the village leaders urged the folks to pray and read the holy 'Koran'. (p. 153)

2012

[76]. D. Bandyopadhaya, O. P. Singh, G. Saha: Mass Psychogenic Illness—Temporal spread and containment—A Southeast Asian story.
International Journal of Neuropsychopharmacology, 2012, 1, 243.

It is a poster presentation. The authors cited two recent examples of Mass Psychogenic Illness (MPI) . One is from India's Jharkhand state, where a rumor of henna or mehandi poisoning (a coloring agent used in body decoration, extracted from a plant *Lawsonia inermis*) was attributed to the death of a guest of the bride in a wedding ceremony. This triggered an epidemic of alleged Mehandi poisoning in the locality, involving 500 young women for two weeks. The second example was the 2010 Koro epidemic in West Bengal. The authors addressed the issues that affect the origin and spread of these Mass Psychogenic Illnesses and their containment.

[77]. G. S. Kalra, A. Bansod, N. B. Shah: A case report of Dhat and Koro: A double Jeopardy.
ASEAN Journal of Psychiatry, 2012, 13(1), 91–95.

This is an interesting case report where two culture-bound syndromes, Koro and Dhat expressed in a 32-year-old married male from Mumbai, India. From the clinical description, it appears that he was suffering from chronic Koro as the perception was very chronic in nature—extending for five years with a combination of different clinical features. "Stretching sensation" at the base of the penis was for five years, feeling that the penis is "getting buried" for one year, etc. His anxiety was more intensified by the positive endorsement from an alternative medicine practitioner who treated him. Subsequently, he developed Dhat syndrome, which led to sexual weakness, unsatisfying intercourse, and low mood. He was responsive to treatment with clonazepam (0.25 mg BID), relaxation, and psychoeducation. The authors described the role of culture, health care providers' faulty explanation, and ignorance of sexual physiology as the critical etiological risk factors for this "double jeopardy."

[78]. K. Promodu, K. R. Nair, S. Pushparajan: Koro syndrome: Mass epidemic in Kerala, India.
Indian Journal of Clinical Psychology, 2012, 39, 152–156.

It is a brief report on the Koro epidemic during August–September 2010 at three labor camps in Kochi, Kerala. Kochi is a rapidly developing metropolis in Kerala, and for huge construction work, thousands of migrant workers were hired from North Indian states like Bihar, Orissa,

West Bengal, and Assam. The laborers are usually live in temporary labor camps. The Koro epidemic struck the floating migrant labor population in some camps. In two weeks, about 100 subjects in three labor camps were affected. All were male. Most of the affected persons fled away to their respective native states. The authors surveyed one such base where they found 21 Koro victims, age range between 20 and 50 years, and education from illiteracy to 8th standard schooling. They also traced the index case. The symptom was first observed from a laborer from West Bengal (who had previous knowledge of the Koro epidemic in his native village) and subsequently affected a few co-laborer from West Bengal. Then it gradually spreads among the other migrant workers at a rapid speed and also affected Keralites.

Fear of panic prevailed, people started puja and worshipping rituals, TV channels and newspapers reported the epidemic as a significant event, construction work in many sites was stopped. One Keralite was hospitalized. Manual traction of the penis and cold water pouring was commonly used. They had a typical Koro attack with heightened anxiety and somatic symptoms like palpitation, breathlessness, sweating, and tremors. The attack spanned from 30 minutes to one hour. It is interesting to note that local people did not allow North Indian workers to mingle with them in the aftermath and disallowed them to enter local hotels and shops (for fear of contamination). They found three of the victims were having histrionic personality traits. They did not mention the ideational component of anxiety specifically. The authors suggested the following risk factors for Koro's development: illiteracy, poor living conditions, economic problems, occupational stress, and separation from home and family for a long time.

[79]. M. Panigrahi, S. K. Padhy, P. B. Behere: Understanding and managing complete from Sporadic Koro syndrome associated with depression.

Journal of Postgraduate Medicine, Education & Research, 2012, 46(2), 104–105.

This is a good clinical paper. The authors discussed the complete and incomplete forms of Koro and believe that this is considered a forerunner of mood disorder and to be understood in the context of psychosexual conflicts, personality patterns, and culture in some clinical situations. A comprehensive, holistic intervention model they espoused for treating the disorder.

The authors presented a 37-year-old married male. He had multiple premorbid pathologies like sexual conflicts, masturbatory guilt, sexual inadequacy, and situational stresses like strained relation with his father on whom he was dependent, rejection by the wife, and psychosocial stressors (nil income, no job, no permanent shelter). All these probably created a fertile ground for the emergence of a strong sense of loss of masculinity with eventual penile symptoms and reactive depression. He developed the complaints of:

> his penis had shortened and was retracting into abdomen, associated with severe anxiety and fear that this would ultimately cause death. These were occurring in episodes of 5 to 15 hours, daily. (p. 105)

A month later, severe depression sets in with attempted suicide and hospitalization. A comprehensive intervention involving antidepressant medication, psychoeducation, psychotherapy, biofeedback and relaxation therapy, family meetings to mitigate relational issues, and job opportunity helped the patient recover entirely by a couple of months.

2013

* * *

Box 9.3 News Paper Coverage of Assam Koro Epidemic in 2013 in INDIA TODAY

[https://www.indiatoday.in/magazine/living/story/19821015-koro-scare-a-rare-culture-bound-psychiatric-disorder-strikes-lower-bramhaputra-valley-772278-2013-10-09]

Koro scare, a rare culture-bound psychiatric disorder, strikes lower Bramhaputra Valley

October 9, 2013

UPDATED: September 4, 2014 10:48 IST

It was not a sight the orthodox Marwari owners of Gauhati's crowded Fancy Bazar would have fancied. A Bihari rickshaw-puller lay semi-conscious in the middle of the main market square, surrounded by over 100 men. Many more watched shyly from a distance and women scampered away giggling as two men stripped him and pulled desperately at his testicles.Face contorted in pain, he begged them to let go of him. But while everyone looked on sympathetically, the effort continued, until some young men standing by insisted that he be rushed to the hospital. The doctors at the nearby Gauhati Medical College Hospital immediately ruled that his problem was epilepsy and that a few more minutes of "pulling" could have killed him.

The scare in the lower Bramhaputra valley today is such that anyone suffering from the faintest form of numbness or unconsciousness is immediately diagnosed as having Koro, the rare culture-bound psychiatric disorder that makes a man feel that his testicles are sinking back into his abdomen.

The bizarre public torture that the rickshaw-puller survived on that September 13 afternoon was not the result of a sudden revival of some long-lost sadistic ritual. The men who seemed to be his tormentors were, in their own view, trying their best to save his life by preventing his testicles "from sinking back into his abdomen".

The scare in the lower Bramhaputra valley today is such that anyone suffering from the faintest form of numbness or unconsciousness is immediately diagnosed as having Koro, the rare culture-bound psychiatric disorder that makes a man feel that his testicles are sinking back into his abdomen.

Initially, no one really bothered when a few such cases were reported from the Garo Hills in Meghalaya in the first week of August. But the hysteria soon spread as more and more cases were reported from primary health centres, district and sub-divisional hospitals and private practitioners all over the lower Assam and Garo Hills area. Every week, hundreds of distraught men clutching at their genitals arrived at the hospitals, accompanied by wailing relatives pouring cold water over their heads. As the scare spread, someone theorised that only cold water could delay the "sinking".

Real Problem: Dr Deepali Dutta, professor of psychiatry, Gauhati Medical College, was the first person to tell a totally demoralised populace what the real problem was. She likened Koro to a disorder which until now was considered culture-bound with no history of breaking out anywhere outside the Malayan peninsula. Every since the outbreak of Koro in the area, she has been spearheading a campaign to inform people that Koro is neither a killing nor a disabling disease and that it is just an illusion which lasts for an hour or two. All India Radio shed its prudery to broadcast her informative talk and interview on the subject. The *Assam Tribune* too placed her reassuring article on Koro on its usually tepid edit page.

But such simplistic, modern theories do not find many buyers among the frightened and superstitious people of the area, as is evident from the way the scare has continued to spread. There are three home remedies touted wisely all over: applying lime to the earlobes and four other places on the body: drinking copious amounts of lemon juice; and pouring cold water over the head if the symptoms have already set in.

As a result of these lime and lemon "remedies", by mid-September the price of lemons in Gauhati had shot up from 20 paise a piece to 80 paise. And an increasing number of labourers and rickshaw-pullers went to work with lime marks on their earlobes. Even some of the officers of the state Government secretariat could be seen shyly carrying large flasks of cold lime juice around with them. In fact until these "remedies" became widely known, almost half of the rickshaws in Greater Gauhati were off the roads.

Thanks to the psychiatrists' campaign, the intensity of fear among new Koro victims has marginally decreased. But in spite of this, there is a steady rise in the number of cases and psychiatrists are unsure as to whether it is a "wave" phenomenon or a more persistent problem.

Few Details: Nobody has been able to give a scientific explanation for the "epidemic" yet. Dutta, who has only "some academic acquaintance" with the disorder, can give no more than its history in Malaysia. Encyclopedia Britannica, Americana and Asiatica are all silent on the subject. Even most medical books have no mention of it. The local psychiatrists are so starved of details on the disorder that they have rushed an SOS to senior psychiatrists at the University of Malaysia, Kuala Lumpur, where some research is reported to have been done.

According to doctors, the intensity of the current scare is so great because the outbreak of this neurotic "epidemic" has come close on the heels of a strange strain of malaria in the Siliguri area, in which the victims' genitals suffer atrophy, resulting in permanent damage. The Calcutta press has been full of stories on this. In fact in the beginning, some general practitioners mistook Koro as this dreaded malarial disease and advised their patients wrongly.

While the Siliguri malaria affected men and women alike, Koro understandably showed an almost exclusive preference for men. But according to Dutta's article there are cases known of women afflicted by this strange disorder. She says that in the case of women there may be a feeling of the breasts shrinking and an awkward feeling in the genitals.

Anthropological Aspect: What began as a joke and continues as a terror has become a medical and an anthropological riddle. While psychiatrists have no more than a few references from old journals and are trying to conduct fresh research on Koro, anthropologists are wondering if the outbreak in Assam is perhaps linked to the fact that the Ahoms originated farther east, not too far from the Malayan peninsula. According to an anthropologist, if the reasons for the outbreak are basically anthropological, then at least the frightening disorder will not spread anywhere else in the country.

Apart from Dutta and her department, most psychiatrists and anthropologists are disinclined to talk about the dreaded disorder in detail - a case of prudery combined with ignorance. As one psychiatrist rightly observed: "The hush has only helped quacks, some of whom charge up to Rs 500 for curing the disease - with nothing more than ground *multi-vitamin* tablets." And there seem to be no visible signs of the business slackening. Evidently, emotional turbulence comes naturally to the Brahmaputra valley. Only this time it is of a more formidable variety with no end in sight.

[80]. R. Kumar, H. R. Phookun, A. Datta: Koro: A culture-bound syndrome: An anxiety disorder.
Indian Journal of Psychiatry, 2013, 55 (SUPPL.1), S131–S132 (Poster 18.17).

A study report of 20 Koro patients attended the hospital in the background of an ongoing epidemic in Assam, India. Most of the patients were young single males of lower socio-economic strata. The three most prominent symptoms were: (1) Tingling sensation originated from the thigh and spread to the abdomen or other parts of the body. (2) Shortening of the penis. (3) Severe degrees of anxiety with increased worrying about genitalia, restlessness, increased sweating, and fear of death. This episode is of very severe intensity and short-lived. The authors commented that this presentation is well befitting an acute anxiety state, and most responded positively with psychoeducation and benzodiazepine.

[81]. S. Ghosh, S. Nath, A. Brahma, A. N. Chowdhury: Fifth Koro epidemic in India: A review report.
World Cultural Psychiatry Research Review, 2013, 8(1), 8–20.

This is a comprehensive report of India's 2010 Koro epidemic, which touched four states of India, viz. Mumbai, Assam, West Bengal, and Tripura. At least 4000 people were affected in Darjeeling and West Dinajpur districts. The present paper is a comprehensive report from the study of cases from Kolkata and adjoining districts (Howrah, North, and South 24 Parganas). Analysis of 55 patients (52 male and three female), who attended a tertiary hospital in Kolkata, was done. The authors provided very details of the clinical presentation with some new findings:

1. All male patients had presented with acute penile shrinkage and retraction symptoms and pain and pulling sensation in the penile region.
2. A "Flu-like" syndrome with fever (described as "Disco fever"), tremor, headache, burning sensation all over body with increased temperature

over the lower part of the body below the waist, sweating, and dryness of throat has been reported by 80% of the cases.

3. The acute penile pull was felt as sudden retraction with pain in the lower abdomen that lasted for 10–15 minutes with resultant shortening of the penis (in 7.7% cases, shortening or reduction of the scrotum also).
4. 95% of cases reported one attack, and 5% had several attacks (2–3) on the same day.
5. One male patient also reported a shrinking feeling of both arms, legs, and ears (as if there is a pull from inside) along with penile symptoms.
6. Fear of impending death was reported in 43.6% of cases. The remaining patients feared "dissolution or damage" (loss) of their male organs.
7. 15.4% of male patients' complaints of frequent loss of semen through urine (Dhat syndrome).
8. Two female cases had symptoms of retraction of nipples and fear of their body's disfiguration, and fear of some severe future health disorder (unspecified).

Most patients were treated with SSRI antidepressants (fluoxetine 60 mg or citalopram 60 mg daily) and benzodiazepine (clonazepam 500 mcg twice/thrice or alprazolam 0.25/0.50 mg twice or thrice daily) with supportive psychotherapy.

They provided valuable findings on the patients' explanatory model: 42.3% attributed their penile retraction and associated bodily symptoms to "bodily weaknesses." They also related this "weakness" with "body heat" as its consequence. They provided community or folk preventive methods, two water cooling treatment photographs, and lime paste smearing. The discussion highlighted Koro news's migration route from Mumbai to West Bengal (via mobile phone message), different associated sexual and psychiatric morbidities, prevention through carrying a copy of the chanted paper, and a page containing lines from the holy Koran, and the role of media.

* * *

Box 9.4 Media Report in Mumbai on 26.10.10
[https://archive.mid-day.com/news/2010/oct/261010-labour-camp-Goregaon-Aarey-Colony-Koro-mumbai.htm].

MID DAY

The curious case of shrinking genitalia

Mass panic at labour camp in Goregaon as twenty five men suffer from 'retracting' genitalia

2010-10-26
Mumbai

Mass panic at labour camp in Goregaon as twenty five men suffer from 'retracting' genitalia

Several labourers living in a work camp near Aarey Colony in Goregaon have been spending sleepless nights since Saturday after they found that the size of their genitals have been gradually reducing and getting inside the lower abdomen (Koro: see box). The panicked sit in a bathtub and family members pour water on them to cure them.

The relatives of the afflicted told MiD DAY that the workers have been suffering from Koro since Saturday. Govind Rai, a recent victim of Koro, said, "On Sunday night I experienced extreme heat emanating from my body.

My genitalia were retracting and I was really worried. Later, on my friends' advice, I jumped into a tub of iced water and sat there for three to four hours."

Rai added that the treatment worked and he was cured of the deadly disease by yesterday evening. Further investigations revealed that at least 25 people were suffering from the same ailment.

"We all are from Orissa, Bengal, Kolkata, but I have noticed that men from Orissa and Bengal are suffering the most," said Rai.

The construction site manager said, "We called the doctor last night but he, too, was unaware of the reason for the ailment."

One of the victims of Koro said, "I am shivering because of the cold and the heat that is emanating from my body. But, I will sit in the water only. I am unaware why I am suffering from this disorder. My relatives in Assam guided me on the disease and now I am feeling better."

Police officials from Aarey Colony came to the labour camp around 1 am and started questioning the labourers. They also took down the statements of the victims and other camp workers.

Inspector Girish Ahvankar said, "We will record the statement of the victims. However, this is not a police case."

Initial enquiry ruled out infection to be the cause of the epidemic, as no chemicals or detergents were present at the site.

A representative from the PR agency that looks after the publicity of the builder for whom the labourers work, said, "We were not aware that the workers were suffering from such an ailment.

A doctor was sent and we will look into the matter."

* * *

[82]. M. Srivastava, B. Pandit: Koro: A case report and review. *International Journal of Physiology, 2013, 1(1), 37–40.*

This is a sporadic Koro case report on a female from Varanasi, India. The patient was a 21-year-old single female who complained of sudden feelings of shrinking breasts and genitalia associated with fear of loss of womanhood and death. She was also showing some anxiety symptoms, along with a low mood. She repeatedly requested her parents to get her married as she believes that active sexual life may cure her condition. Her Hamilton Depression rating score was 14, and the Body Dysmorphic Disorder score was relatively high—87. She was treated with clonazepam (0.25 mg), and escitalopram (10 mg) with psychoeducation, and later olanzapine (10 mg) was added. After a month, she showed complete recovery.

The authors discussed this episode in terms of perceptual distortion as a part of body dysmorphic disorder. No triggering or precipitating factors are reported. The paper contains a useful literature review. This paper has the credit that it is the only sporadic female case report in the literature for the last eighty years.

2014

[83]. J. Noel, R. Krishnadas, R. Gopalakrishnan, A. Kuruvilla: Delusional disorder: An unusual presentation.
Indian Journal of Psychological Medicine, 2014, 36(4), 444–446.

This is not a Koro report but an interesting case report of a 19-year-old single college student who has 18 months history of firm belief and perception that whenever he assumed an upright position, he attained penile erection every time. He thinks that other people would notice this and ridicule him with derogatory comments. He tried to mask his alleged erection by changing his dressing pattern. In addition to that, he was socially withdrawn and absent from class with academic decline. To mitigate this problem, he changed his college to avoid the perceived ridicule and avoided the situations where he required standing upright like crowded buses, elevators, and shops. He attempted self-harm a year ago by cutting his wrist. He was on fluvoxamine and risperidone for seven months. All laboratory tests and andrological examinations were standard. He was diagnosed with delusional disorder. He responded well with risperidone and extensive CBT. Solitary bodily delusion, the strength of conviction, and the time, in the absence of first-rank symptoms of schizophrenia or affective disorders, he was diagnosed with psychosis. Similar situations and cases of Koro also warrant detailed clinical scrutiny for diagnostic precision.

[84]. R. Kumar, H. R. Phookun, A. Datta: Epidemic of Koro in North East India: An observational cross-sectional study.
Asian Journal of Psychiatry, 2014, 12, 113–117.

This is a 2010 Koro epidemic report from India. It is a comprehensive and detailed reporting of the Koro epidemic (70 cases, including two females), as observed in the Gauhati city, Assam.

The description of Koro demography is essential:

61.4% were within the age group of 21–30 years, and 70% were single. 68.5% presented at the hospital casualty department. 64.2% were from the Hindu religion, 34.3% were of Islamic faith, and 1.4% were Sikh. 62.8% were from lower socio-economic status 71.4% had education above high school. The authors provided a detailed clinical description as follows: 82.8% of cases had prior knowledge of Koro; 30% witnessed Koro attacks in the community; 85.7% of attacks occurred at home; and 72.8% of attacks were at night.

A host of anxiety symptoms accompanied the Koro attack: Tingling sensation (90%), restlessness (85.7%), sweating (75.7%), and palpitation (70%). The episode itself was comprised of (1) feeling of retraction or shortening of the penis; (2) tingling sensation originated from the thigh and radiating to the body; and (3) severe anxiety about genitalia and fear of death. Two female patients complained about the shortening and retraction of the nipple and female genitals inward with fear of death. The local name was "Jhinjhinia Bemar," and people believed that "bad air" or "bad spirit" was the cause of the illness. Patients were successfully treated with pharmacotherapy, psychotherapy, and mass education program. The photograph of traditional treatment (victim carried in a giant water bucket) is unique and enriched the presentation. The presentation is very standard and touched all the relevant issues of clinical significance. This is a fair reporting of the 2010 Assam Koro epidemic.

Observation: One crucial point is that the authors excluded some cases (numbers not mentioned) who have coexisting "schizophrenia, delusional disorder, other psychosis, or some significant medical or surgical genital's illness." Information on these patients may offer precious insight into the clinical diversity of secondary Koro cases.

[85]. P. Ramamourty, V. Menon: Koro presenting as acute and transient psychosis: Implications for classification.
Asian Journal of Psychiatry, 2014, 10, 116–117.

This is a fascinating Koro case report from Puducherry, India. The authors presented a sporadic case, which may be termed as "chronic Koro" in a 32-year-old married male with the complaints of "penis is shrinking for three days" with fear of death. His conviction became more intense when his wife inspected his genital and commented, "it looked smaller than normal." This reminded a case of folie a deux reported in a Homong refugee in the USA by Westermyer (1989). The authors labeled this as solitary somatic delusion and reported symptom remission after a prolonged sleep with antipsychotic (parental and then oral) medications.

The authors raised a nosological debate regarding Koro's classification. They proposed a clinically meaningful evaluation, which should be based on phenomenology, symptom sequence, and nature of dysfunction for its proper diagnostic labeling.

Observation: Some more information in the report would be helpful, like whether the episode of "penis shrinking" was episodic or continuous over the 72 hours? Some descriptions of any precipitating factor or previous acquaintance with similar symptoms or the patient's "Explanatory model" would help measure the psychotic or neurotic predisposition. The diagnosis of "acute and transient psychosis" also invites the question why it was not a hypochondriacal delusion or body dysmorphic perception?

2015

2015 KORO EPIDEMIC IN TRIPURA

[86]. P. Kanwar, R. Kumar, R. C. Sharma: Cannabis-induced Koro: A case report.
Indian Journal of Psychiatry, 2015, 57 Suppl. (1): S134. (Poster)

This is a report of Koro case triggered by cannabis smoking. A 30-year-old married male from Nepal presented with a history of first smoking 4–5 deep puffs of cannabis. After that, he experienced an episode of retraction of the penis into the abdomen associated with shortness of breath, fearfulness, hot flashes, chills, headache, and a sensation of impending death. For three months since the patient had smoked cannabis, he experienced similar episodes daily, which lasted 15–30 minutes. The patient had sought treatment from faith healers but did not improve. A diagnosis of cannabis-induced Koro was made. He was treated with paroxetine 25 mg/day and risperidone 1 mg/day, which worsened his symptoms. The medications then changed to escitalopram 10 mg/day, olanzapine 5 mg/day, and clonazepam 0.75 mg/day, and he became asymptomatic after four months. The authors commented that this case illustrates Koro's de novo onset after cannabis smoking and thus points toward the need for further research into the psychological and behavioral effects of cannabis.

[87]. J. Aneja, S. Grover, A. Avasthi, S. Mahajan, P. Pokhrel, D. Triveni: Can masturbatory guilt lead to severe psychopathology: A case series.
Indian Journal of Psychological Medicine, 2015, 37(1), 81–86.

The authors presented one case of a 25-year-old single male who had three years of delusional belief that his penis had started retracting into his abdomen, at the background of masturbatory guilt and onset of a depressive episode. Subsequently, he developed the firm conviction that he is passing semen through urine. He responded favorably with 150 mg of amisulpride but discontinued it. Within six months of stopping amisulpride, he developed the perception that his body shape changed into the feminine type and started to think that his penis and testicles would completely disappear into the abdomen and be expelled through stools. He will be ill due to the accumulation of urine inside the abdomen. He was diagnosed with undifferentiated schizophrenia with severe depressive disorder with Koro and Dhat syndrome. He responded well with a course of olanzapine, escitalopram, and modified bitemporal ECTs.

2016

[88]. A. Dan, T. Mondal, K. Chakraborty, A. Chaudhuri, A. Biswas: Clinical profile and outcome of Koro: A follow-up study from a Koro epidemic in West Bengal, India.
Indian Journal of Psychiatry, 2016, 58(Suppl 1), 571.

This is an important reporting of 92 Koro cases from the West Bengal 2010 Koro epidemic. The authors analyze 64 patients who attended different tertiary care hospital clinical departments and consented to the study over three months. The most critical clinico-demographic features are:

> (1) 81.2% of cases were single, and 76.6% were male. (2) 42.1% had education up to primary level. (3) 42.2% were agricultural workers. (4) 57.8% were of Hindu religion. (5) 95.3% were from a rural background. (6) 53.1% of cases were from joint families. (7) Past and family history of Koro was present in 27% (male 31%, female 13%) and 11% (male 6%, female 27%) of the subjects, respectively. (8) Psychiatric and physical comorbidities were present in 47% (male 41%, female 60%) and 23% (male 20%, female 33%) of the subjects, respectively. (9) 20% of the subjects needed indoor treatment, and 31% of the subjects received specific pharmacological and psychosocial treatment. (10) A new modality of psychosexual intervention, "sex education in vivo" was applied to patients of Koro with favorable result.

[89]. S. Debbarma, S. K. Das, A. Kumar, D. Debbarma, A. Das, T. Reang: Koro epidemic: A descriptive study.
Journal of Evolution of Medical & Dental Sciences, 2016, 5(76), 5634–5638.

This is a relatively comprehensive report of the March–July 2015 Koro epidemic of Tripura. The authors reported detailed psycho-social demography of 57 cases (49 male and eight female) from the Karbook (Gomti district) subdivision, Tripura. The epidemic was also documented from other areas like Shantir Bazar, Belonia (South district) subdivision, and villages of the Bishalgarh subdivision under Sepahijala district.

The salient findings of Koro demography are as follows: (1) Age group—50.9% in 17–30 yrs; (2) 78.6% married; (3) 50% with primary education; (4) 78.6% Hindu/21.4% Buddhist; and (5) 49.1% Day-laborer/35.1% unemployed.

Reported symptoms: Shrinking of the penis was the predominant clinical presentation among the 49 male cases and retraction of the breast (no vaginal symptom) among the 8 female cases; all had a fear of impending death. Besides, 20% of cases complained of “feeling cold,” and 45% of “reduced sexual function.” Traditional folk treatment was preferred by Ojhas, Tantric, local quacks, and priests. The predominant beliefs were that the illness was due to black magic, witchcraft, or spells of “mantra.” Very few cases turned to the hospital. Many of the victims offered “poojas” and religious worship rituals for a cure. The hospitalized patients responded well with small doses of benzodiazepine (clonazepam 0.5 mg or alprazolam 0.25 mg twice or thrice daily). The vast majority of the affected villages believed that the disease might infect them if they come closer to the affected person. So avoidance behavior and restricted movement of persons of the community were practiced. People also used traditional prophylactic measures to prevent affliction—herbal amulets or chanted paper containing “mantras” from the priest inserted in their armlets were used by many and were of high demand in the community. One important incident was reported that some people in the neighborhood were charged that they are causing this malady by casting black magic, and they were physically assaulted. The authors believe that these are due to some past familial hostility in the community.

2017

[90]. N. Bidani: A case of Koro syndrome.
Homeopathy 360. 2017. https://homeopathy360.com/2017/03/24/a-case-of-koro-syndrome/.

This is a case report of Koro in a 32-year married male from Hisar, Haryana, India. One night on an attempt of micturation, he “suddenly felt a loss of feeling in the genital region, and straightaway, the thought occurred to him that he would get a penile retraction.” He noticed that the penis was getting shorter, and his limbs are becoming cold and numb. This episode lasted for half an hour. He had a similar second attack, consulted a general physician, and recovered from his treatment within a week. A month later, while doing intercourse with his wife at night, he again noticed that his penis became flaccid and started retraction, along with some penile and scrotal pain. The following day he consulted a Homeopathy specialist. He disclosed that at age 24, he had sexual relations with a prostitute and was infected with gonorrhea, which generated high guilt in his mind. He was treated with homeopathic medicines and CBT and recovered. No further attack was reported at the one-year follow-up. Diagnostically this may be a case of chronic or recurrent Koro.

[91]. A. Dan, T. Mondal, K. Chakraborty, A. Chaudhuri, A. Biswas: Clinical course and treatment outcome of Koro: A follow-up study from a Koro epidemic reported from West Bengal, India.
Asian Journal of Psychiatry, 2017, 26, 14–20.

It is a valuable research paper on the 2010 Koro epidemic in West Bengal, India. The authors reported quite impressively the details of a large cohort of 90 Koro cases and followed up with 46 patients over three months. The paper provides many vital data like socio-demographic profile and intervention and outcome. The detailed tabulation of treatment modalities used is quite valuable. They stated:

> A typical subject was a young single male, educated up to primary standard, agricultural worker by occupation and belonged to Hindu rural joint family. Among the whole sample 23% were female. Majority were referred from either private doctors or hospitals or government hospitals and reported first at non-psychiatric OPD. Dropout and recovery rates were 28% (male 33%, female 13%) and 89% (male 89%, female 92%) respectively. 20%, 75%, 9%, 31%, 19% of patients needed indoor admission, oral anxiolytics, injectable tranquilizers, specific pharmacological and psychosocial treatment, supportive medical treatment respectively. (p. 16)

This paper is good reporting on the recent Koro epidemic in West Bengal. The authors reported a novel treatment modality—"sex education in vivo" to increase "sexual arousal" in some cases. This is a new treatment approach for Koro patients. But the question remains that whether sexual hypo-arousal is the aftermath or squeal of the Koro attack? It is a new research area to investigate. The authors got the opportunity to see so many Koro cases, but they haven't presented any patients' explanatory model—which would have been a rich contribution to Koro phenomenology.

Observation: Though they reported 15 female Koro cases, no female presentation details were reported (whether breast symptom or genital symptom or both). Female Koro is comparatively rare and usually found only in epidemics. So female clinical data is crucial. They also reported 12 excluded patients from their study sample because they "refused" or "having physical/ surgical complications." This is a critical piece of information and, unfortunately, was excluded. The reported "physical/surgical complications" from what? Was it due to the manual or mechanical traction applied to the penis? If it was so, this should be highlighted as a health hazard of folk treatment in Koro (Forensic issue). Information on these patients may also offer valuable insight into the clinical diversity of secondary Koro cases.

[92]. K. Garg, C. N. Kumar, C. Sharadhi: Koro: Much more than just a culture-bound syndrome.
Asian Journal of Psychiatry, 2017, 29, 146–147. (L)

It is a good discussion paper with a case report from Bangaluru, India. The authors presented a sporadic case in a 24 year old. It may be called "secondary or chronic Koro", who had three penile retraction episodes in three years. The average symptom duration was 5–6 weeks each, along with psychomotor retardation and social withdrawal symptoms. During the current episode, the mental state showed hypochondriacal delusional conviction. The patient relates his penile pathology with daily physical activities such as cycling, walking, and lifting, which he avoided. Based on the presence of delusion, negative symptoms, affective blunting, and significant psychosocial impairment and consideration of history, he was diagnosed with undifferentiated schizophrenia. He responded well with quetiapine 800 mg daily, along with vocational and recreational therapy sessions. The authors provided useful details of his treatment, both for past and present episodes. The authors discussed the confusion in Koro diagnostic label as culture-bound. They questioned Koro's culture-boundness, mainly when it occurs outside the traditional ethnic population or as secondary Koro associated with schizophrenia or other

CNS disorders. With more and more Koro reporting from diverse ethnic populations and different psychiatric or medical comorbidities, the term Secondary Koro or Koro-like symptom (KLS) is gaining more support. It is observed that in these cases, the culture has no pathognomonic role.

2018

[93]. A. P. Megha, J. T. Antony, K. S. Beevi, G. G. Chakkalakkudy, P. Kuttichira: A case of sporadic Koro from Kerala.
Indian Journal of Social Psychiatry, 2018, 34, 90–91.

This is a Koro case report in a 32-year-old divorced male from Thrissur, Kerala, India. The patient had difficulty in passing urine for the previous two weeks, and penis retraction was of 1-week duration. He presented to the hospital emergency at midnight. He was hospitalized and treated with clonazepam 12 mg/day and propranolol 20 mg/day, along with supportive psychotherapy. He responded favorably. He had no prior knowledge about Koro. The Koro attack started a week before the scheduled date to see the prospective bride for his remarriage. It is not clear from the account whether impotence was the cause of the first marriage's breakdown as his wife left him after two weeks of marriage. If it was the cause, then sexual anxiety may play a role in his Koro perception!

[94]. K. Garg, N. Das, C. N. Kumar: Koro in panic disorder: Beyond a culture-bound phenomena.
Asian Journal of Psychiatry, 2018, 31, 73–74.

The authors presented a fascinating case of recurrent Koro-like symptoms paired with episodes of panic attacks in a 25-year-old male from Bengaluru, India. Since the last two months before the clinical contact, he had ten episodes of typical panic attacks. During each episode, he developed intense fear that his penis has started to retract into the abdomen, and he would die when it abandons completely. He was utterly asymptomatic during the inter-episodic period. He responded favorably with treatment with paroxetine and clonazepam, titrated over four weeks. The authors questioned the concept of culture-boundness in Koro.

Observation: It seems from the case's behavioral description that some obsessive-compulsive elements were present. A more detailed analysis of the time sequence of Koro perception and panic attacks (which one is first to occur?) would help indicate the penile pathology's causal trigger. That may have some bearings on the primary diagnosis.

[95]. P. Kanwar, R. Kumar, R. C. Sharma: Cannabis-induced Koro in a Nepali migrant.
Asian Journal of Psychiatry, 2018, 31, 56–87. (L)

It is a Koro report in a 30-year-old married male, Nepali migrant laborer in Himachal Pradesh, India. This paper is a valuable addition to world Koro literature so far as the role of cannabis in body dysmorphic perception, viz. Koro perception.

This malady started three months ago, triggered by four deep puffs of cannabis. The patient's chief complaint was episodes of retraction of the penis into the abdomen with pain in the genital area and associated anxiety features. The authors described this Koro episode as recurrent: "Thereafter, similar symptoms started occurring daily more in the evening hours." The patient responded well with escitalopram (10 mg daily), olanzapine (5 mg daily), and clonazepam (0.75 mg daily), which was titrated over two month follow-up period. He also had psychoeducation.

Observation: It would have been more precise if they mentioned the number of episodes, i.e., frequency, because repeated Koro is almost a rare phenomenon. This frequency figure would have shed some new light on the recurrence pattern of Koro perception (even without cannabis)! I presume from the account that the patient has a history of three months, and in that case, he had roughly 90 episodes of Koro perception. If so, then it should have invited more diagnostic options (?OCD or hypochondriacal fear) and the "Chronic Koro" diagnostic label. Another information is missing that whether he smoked cannabis further.

[96]. A. Kapoor, R. Juneja, D. C. Singh: Cultural-specific syndromes in India—An overview.
International Journal of Current Research & Review, 2018, 10(11), 2–6.

It is a review paper on different culture-bound syndromes (CBS) seen in India. The authors pointed out the fact that CBSs are not included in any conventional classificatory system. The term and the concept were first incorporated in DSM-IV, and also in DSM-5 they are grouped as CBS without any definite category of disorders. To date, CBS is seen or considered based on the following shared characteristics:

1. Categorized as a disease in a particular culture,
2. Recognized as a disease in a specific culture but not in other cultures,
3. No definite or specific biochemical or organ abnormality present,
4. Usually treated by medicine and or conventional healers.

The authors discussed the clinical profile, probable nosological status, and treatment of different CBSs of the Indian subcontinent. They described: Possession syndrome; Dhat syndrome; Koro (mainly reported from Northeastern Indian states); Bhanmati syndrome (mainly in South India); Gilhary syndrome (mainly in Western Rajasthan); Culture-bound Suicide (Sati, Johuar, and Santhra)—largely historical; Jhin-jhinia; Suudu (mainly in Tamil culture); Ascetic syndrome (seen primarily on teenagers); different types of mass hysteria; Suchi-bai syndrome (obsessional neurosis of cleaning to avoid pollution, mainly seen in Bengal); and Gas syndrome. The authors stressed understanding the attribution pattern of a particular culture and patient's explanatory models about the distress in the evaluation and treatment of CBS's.

2019

[97]. A. N. Chowdhury, M. Chawla: Koro in female: A case report and a mini review.
European Journal of Psychiatry, 2019, 33(4), 182–185.

It is a Koro-like case report in a Caucasian female from England at the background of reactive depression (ICD-10 Code: F32). It is also the first Koro reporting in a Caucasian female. The subject was a 27-year-old single woman who developed Koro-like symptoms during an episode of reactive depression after the breakup of 7 years relationship. She anxiously reported that for one week, she felt as if her genital organ (vagina) was shrinking ("becoming flat") and as if receding into her abdomen. She also reported that her breasts were shrinking and getting smaller in size. These "thoughts were so recurring and disturbing" that she "checked the genitals and her breast in front of the mirror" quite a few times. Treatment with an antidepressant (citalopram) and supportive counseling resolve her depression and genital symptoms and concerns. The authors also did a mini review of world literature on female Koro.

2020

[98]. A. N. Chowdhury, A. Brahma: Update on Koro research methodology.
Indian Journal of Psychiatry, 2020, 62(1), 102–104.

It is a short discussion paper focusing on research methodology involving recent Koro researches. Given quite a handful of publications on the Koro epidemic (and some sporadic cases) in recent years, authors tried to focus on some of the essential clinical standards that should be addressed in the research to make the study more comprehensive and sound. They discussed the clinical distinction with definite criteria between Koro (classical form) and Koro-like symptoms (KLS). They stressed the importance of documentation of detailed demography and associated comorbidities if present. Culture-boundness in Koro is now questioned, and with the publication of DSM-5 in 2013, the cultural tag of Koro is abandoned. But until then, in some cultures, especially in Southeast Asian countries, culture does play an essential role in Koro. They also urged for the need for tracing the details of epidemic specificity in epidemic reporting. They discussed the importance of studying the explanatory model of illness (EMI) from the patients to understand its psychodynamics better. Treatment should record details of the drug name, dosage, and duration of treatment. This short commentary may be helpful to all Koro researchers.

[99]. S. Ghosh, A. N. Chowdhury: A case of two culture-bound syndromes (Koro and Dhat syndrome) coexisting with obsessive–compulsive disorder.
Indian Journal of Psychiatry, 2020, 62(2), 221–222.

It is a Koro case report of an 18-year-old Muslim single male (at the Koro epidemic background) from rural West Bengal. The subject also has another culture-bound syndrome Dhat Syndrome and subsequently showed symptoms of obsessive-compulsive disorder. The history showed different traditional help-seeking behaviors. He responded considerably with sertraline 150 mg and clonazepam 0.5 mg TDS with cognitive behavior therapy.

[100]. D. Banerjee, S. Sharma, S. Antony: Koro and migration: observational study of an outbreak of Koro in a migrant population working in South India.
Journal of Psychosexual Health, 2020, 2(2), 174–178.

This is a very interesting study of Koro in a migrant labor population, at the background of an epidemic, from Bangalore, South India. They came from the Eastern and Middle parts of India. It was a study of a cohort of 13 migrant workers (8 Male and 5 Female) from a population of 52, who attended the hospital within two weeks. The index case was a 29-year-old single mason who was having typical Koro symptoms. He believed that he had contracted this illness from a fellow worker who had this illness and with whom he shared a meal. There was no fear of imminent death, but fear of being infertile was there. He poured cold water on the penis several times a day. He disclosed that 5 of his fellow laborer also had the penis-shrinking illness, but they kept secret out of fear, shame, and stigma. Subsequently, 12 more patients (7 male and five female) attended the hospital clinic with Koro symptoms. Males complained of penile and scrotal retraction, while females felt that their breasts and vagina were shortening and disappearing within the body. Females fear that they may be losing the ability to bear children or lose the capacity for breast-feeding. All the patients showed good recovery with treatment with fluoxetine 20 mg and clonazepam 0.5 mg. Ten patients were treated with a single one-hour session of CBT.

The authors provided a few important clinical details as follows:

(1) 84.6% had previous knowledge of Koro; (2) Nature of genital shrinking belief: Delusional—61.5%; Ideas—23.1%; and Doubts—15.4%; (3) 76.9% had fear of death; (4) 69.2% belief the illness is contagious. The authors identified the stress of migration, social isolation, and stigma are the environmental risk factor for this epidemic in a closed migrant colony.

References

Cassel, W. A. (1965). Body perception and symptom localization. *Psychosomatic Medicine, 27*, 171–176.

Chowdhury, A. N. (1989a). Bengali adaptation of Eysenck's Personality Questionnaire. *Indian Journal of Clinical Psychology, 16*, 71–73.

Chowdhury, A. N. (1989b). Dysmorphic penis image perception—The root of Koro vulnerability. *Acta Psychiatrica Scandinavica, 80*, 518–520.

Chowdhury, A. N. (1989c). Bengali adaptation of Spielberger's STATI, From X. *Journal of Personality & Clinical Studies, 5*, 257–260.

Chowdhury, A. N. (1989d). Neuroticism, extraversion and sex-guilt cognition in the genesis of Koro. *Journal of Indian Psychoanalytical Society, 43*, 57–64.

Chowdhury, A. N., & Brahma, A. (2005). An epidemic of mass hysteria in a village in West Bengal. *Indian Journal of Psychiatry, 47*, 106–108.

Cobb, S. (1976). Social support as a moderator of life stress. *Psychosomatic Medicine, 38*(5), 300–314.

Diagnostic and Statistical Manual of Mental Disorder. (2013). Fifth Edition. American Psychiatric Association.

Durst, R., & Rosca-Rebaundengo, P. (1991). The disorder named koro. *Behavioural Neurology, 4*(1), 1–13.

Edwards, J. W. (1983). Semen anxiety in South Asian cultures: Cultural and transcultural significance. *Medical Anthropology, 7*, 51–67.

Eysenck, H. J. (1970). Personality and attitude to sex: A factorial study. *Personality, 1*, 355–376.

Eysenck, H. J. (1972). Personality and sexual behaviour. *Journal of Psychometric Research, 16*, 141–152.

Eysenck, H. J., & Claridge, G. (1962). The position of hysterics and dysthymics in a two-dimensional frame-work of personality description. *Journal of Abnormal Social Psychology, 69*, 46–53.
Eysenck, H. J., & Eysenck, S. B. J. (1975). *Manual of the Eysenck Personality Questionnaire*. Hodder and Stoughton.
Fisher, S. (1959). Extensions of theory concerning body image and body reactivity. *Psychosomatic Medicine, 21*, 142–149.
Fisher, S., & Cleveland, S. E. (1958). Body-Image boundary and sexual behaviour. *Journal of Psychology, 45*, 207–211.
Guazzo, F. M. (1608). *Compendium Maleficarum* (English Translation by E. A. Ashwin, 1929).
Gwee, A. L. (1963). Koro—A cultural disease. *Singapore Medical J, 4*, 119–122.
Gwee, A. L. (1968). Koro - Its origin and nature as a disease entity. *Singapore Medical Jorunal, 9*, 3–6.
Hall, W., Degenhardt, L., & Lynskey, M. (1994). *The health and psychological consequences of Cannabis use. Commonwealth of Australia* (Monograph Series No. 44, 2nd ed.).
Harington, J. A. (1982). Epidemic psychosis. *The British Journal of Psychiatry, 141*, 98–99.
Illechukwu, S. T. C. (1992). Magical penis loss in Nigeria: Report of a recent epidemic. *Transcultural Psychiatric Research Review, 29*, 91–108.
Kirmayer, L. J. (1992). From the Witche's hammer to the Oedipus complex: Castration anxiety in Western society. *Transcultural Psychiatric Research Review, 29*, 133–138.
Lappierre, Y. D. (1972). Koro in a French Canadian. *Canadian Psychiatric Association Journal of, 17*, 333–334.
Mechanic, D. (1972). Social psychologic factors affecting the presentation of bodily complaints. *New England Journal of Medicine, 286*, 1132–1139.
Mechanic, D. (1975). Socio-cultural and social psychological factors affecting personal response to psychological disorders. *Journal of Health & Social Behaviour, 16*, 394–404.
Mechanic, D. (1977). Illness behaviour, social adaptation and management of illness. *Journal of Nervous & Mental Disease, 165*, 79–87.
Menzel, H. (1960). Innovation, integration, and marginality: A survey of physicians. *American Sociological Review, 25*, 707–708.
Mookerjee, A., & Khanna, M. (1989). *The tantric way: Art, science, ritual* (pp. 59–65). Thames and Hudson Ltd.
Mookerjee, A. (1965). *Tantric Art: Times of India Annual*. New Delhi.

Mosher, D. L. (1966). The development of multitrait multimethod matrix analysis of three measures of three aspects of guilt. *Journal of Consulting Psychology, 30*, 35–41.
Mosher, D. L., & Cross, H. J. (1971). Sex-guilt and premarital sexual experience of college students. *Journal of Consulting Psychology, 36*, 27–31.
Murphy, H. B. M. (1982). *Comparative psychiatry: The international and intercultural distribution of mental illness* (pp. 269–277). Springer-Verlag.
Murthy, H. N. (1965). *Development of the paranoid, depressive, manic and anxiety scale* (AIIMH Transaction, No. 5, Bangalore, pp. 50–54).
Murthy, H. N., & Lakshminarayan, C. S. (1968). *A note on the development of hysteria scale* (AIIMH Transaction, No. 8, Bangalore, pp. 42–45).
Ngui, P. W. (1969). The Koro epidemic in Singapore. *Australian & New Zealand Journal of Psychiatry, 3*, 263–266.
O'Neill, M., & Kempler, B. (1969). Approach and avoidance response of the hysterical personality to sexual stimuli. *Journal of Abnormal Psychology, 74*, 300–305.
Prince, R. H. (1992). A symposium on the vulnerable male: Cultural variations on the castration theme. *Transcultural Psychiatric Research Review, 29*, 87–90.
Raman, A. C., & Murphy, H. B. M. (1972). Failure of traditional prognostic indicators in Afro-Asian psychotics: Results of a longterm followup survey. *Journal of Nervous & Mental Disease, 154*, 238–247.
Rin, H. (1965). A study of the aetiology of Koro in respect to the Chinese concept of illness. *International Journal of Social Psychiatry, 11*, 7–13.
Spielberger, C. D., Gorsuch, R. L., & Lushene, R. E. (1970). *Manual of the state-trait anxiety inventory (Self-evaluation questionnaire)*. Consulting Psychologists Press.
Sprenger, J., & Kramer, H. (1489). *Malleus Maleficarum*. English Translation by Montague Summer, 1928.
Swensen, C. H. (1963). Sexual behaviour and psychopathology: A study of college men. *Journal of Clinical Psychology, 19*, 403–408.
Wells, B. W. P. (1969). Personality characteristics of V. D. patients. *British Journal of Social & Clinical Psychology, 8*, 246–249.
Westermeyer, J. (1989). A case of koro in a refugee family: Association with depression and folie a deux. *Journal of Clinical Psychiatry, 50*, 181–183.
Wilkinson, R. L. (1932). *A Malay-English Dictionary*. Maytilene.
WittKower, E. D., & Rin, H. (1965). Transcultural psychiatry. *Archives of General Psychiatry, 13*, 387–394.

Yap, P. M. (1965). Koro—A culture-bound depersonalization syndrome. *British Jouranl of Psychiatry, 111*, 43–50.
Zysk, K. G. (1991). *Asceticism and healing in ancient India.* Oxford University Press.

10

Risk Assessment and Forensic Aspect of Koro

Introduction

Risk assessment in Koro is a severe clinical issue, but unfortunately, this aspect is never received an appropriate focus in any of the Koro repotting to date. At least six large epidemics are reported from Singapore, Thailand, Indonesia, China, and India. Still, except for three reports, no mention of any health hazards of social treatment, including death or penile injury, was reported. Some Koro case reports, mainly associated with secondary psychiatric diagnoses (psychosis) mentioned self-inflicted penile wounds. This brief review will highlight the importance of risk assessment in Koro from an individual and community response perspective.

Methods

A thorough Koro literature search was done in English language journals between 1895 and 2020. A total of 394 publications are critically reviewed and searched for risk and forensic issues related to Koro. Only

A. N. Chowdhury, *Koro*,
https://doi.org/10.1007/978-3-030-87962-4_10

five epidemic reports and seven case reports mentioned Koro's risk aspect, which is discussed below with a case study done at the background of a Koro epidemic in India.

Results and Discussion

Social Paranoia Induced Koro

The relationship between paranoid social cognition or social anxiety and psychiatric epidemic or Mass Psychogenic Illness (MPI) is well documented in the literature (Boss, 1997; Gallay et al., 2002). Social paranoia about the epidemic cause (and effect) may trigger risky behavior in the individual or threaten the community to risky or threatening collective behavior. News media may further amplify this iatrogenic propensity of social cognition (Vasterman et al., 2005). Unfortunately, this aspect was never studied sufficiently in any of the available large-scale Koro epidemic reports, but some examples of risk issues may be worth considering.

Singapore Koro epidemic: It is a glaring example where paranoid social cognition triggered Koro attacks among the population's vulnerable section. In the spring of 1967, a swine-fever epidemic took place in Malaysia and then spread to Singapore. In July 1967, the Singapore Government took a massive program to inoculate all swine with an anti-swine-fever vaccine. On October 29, 1967, a rumor emerged that inoculated pork consumption would cause the penis to retract. This rumor mainly affected the Chinese population as the pork was their staple food, and the epidemic was triggered. From October 29 to November 30, a total of 496 cases attended the hospital. On 7 November 1967, the news daily "Straits Times" published a piece of sensational news, "A strange Malady Hits Singapore Men." The government's conjoint efforts, press media, and Singapore Medical Association were able to check the spread of the epidemic by active advocacy. Though some author believes that "The *Koro* hysteria reflected potentially explosive racial aggravations and religious sensitivities at a politically difficult moment, both domestically and internationally" (Everest-Philips, 2018), but fortunately there was no report of ethnic or racial clash or violence centering around the Koro epidemic. Though the inherent racial tension and religious divide remain suppressed, it flared up after 18 months. In Malaysia, a race riot against ethnic Chinese triggered violence against Malays in Singapore—4 people were killed and 80 injured (Everest-Philips, 2018).

Ngui (1969) mentioned out of 159 male cases, 72.3% manually grasped their penis either by themselves or by relatives, only 3 cases used the chopsticks, and 2 cases tied a string around the penis. He provided the picture of the Jeweler's instrument "lit eng hok," but no injury was reported. Koro Study Team (1969) also mentioned this instrument by Koro patients, but no numbers were mentioned, and no significant injury was reported except some "superficial issue." Among 227 males, manual restraint was applied in 72% of the cases.

Thailand Koro Epidemic: A similar social conspiracy rumor triggered the epidemic in the Thailand Koro epidemic (1976). The epidemic took place between November and December 1976 in five provinces in Northeast Thailand, where at least 350 cases were reported (Suwanlert, 1978a, 1978b). The role of news media was significant in the generation and propagation of social paranoia. It was said that people would develop Koro (in male—shrinking of penis and in female—increased appetite for sex) after either consuming foods, water, or tobacco that are poisoned by chemicals by migrant Vietnamese. It was believed that the rumor originated from political refugees from Laos (Jilek & Jilek-Aall, 1977a, 1977b). As an aftermath of this social, racial tension, a harmful impact was observed on the fruit industry and other commercial enterprises, affecting the local Vietnamese and Thai farmers later. The social after-effect of the epidemic, which resulted in the Vietnamese' ostracism and fear of social stability, was also reported (Suwanlert & Coates, 1979).

Social or Folk Treatment-Induced Health Risk in Koro

Indian Koro epidemic: Chowdhury (1991) reported several health hazards from Koro patients' social treatments from the 1982 Koro epidemic. He provided very shocking data, including deaths from the social therapies. He reported four deaths (all male) from West Bengal and 32 cases with severe medical complications resulted from the social therapy of water pouring/immersion or forced feeding of standard salt solution.

Penile injury due to traction: Chowdhury (1991) reported several penile injuries ranging from mild to severe soft tissue injury and manual and mechanical traction infection among 65 male Koro cases. Manual traction usually was induced by the patient himself (16 cases), but others always imposed mechanical traction (49). It was reported that at least six types of mechanical penile traction were applied with a resultant penile injury, of which at least 17 needed surgical attention and intervention at hospital A & E or from local general practitioners.

Penile injury due to use of irritants: Four self-inflicted severe injuries like a burning or scalding of prepuce or glans were reported. The patients locally applied different irritant materials like potassium permanganate, raw Dettol, washing soda, or common salt (NaCl) solutions.

Chakraborty and Sanyal (2011) studied a mini Koro epidemic among 19 Jute mill workers (all males) in West Bengal. They found 5.26% of cases attempted mechanical penile traction, resulting in abrasive injury on the glans penis.

China Koro epidemic: Report from 1984 to 1985 Koro epidemic in Haikang County of Guandong, China: Mo et al. (1987), in their study of 195 Suo-yang (Koro) victims, reported nine fatalities from folk intervention. A child died of asphyxia, a young woman was beaten to death, another woman was drowned at sea, and numerous men suffered penile injuries due to mechanical handling to pull the penis. Some women sustained injury and infection after an iron pin was inserted through their nipples.

Koro Induced Social Paranoia

Case study: There was a mini Koro epidemic in the South 24 Parganas district of West Bengal, India, in 1993. The present case study was from a village called Taldi. Four male cases of Koro (A, B, C, D) from different families were reported from this hamlet of 31 families. The mother of

Case C (19-year-old single) and brother of Case D (24-year-old newly married male) raised a concern that the Koro illness (they designated it as "Disco fever") was due to some malevolent tricks ("Tuk-tak") perpetuated by a widower in their neighborhood. This man, Mr. Gp, lost his wife long back and had no issues. He maintains a sedentary life with religious pursuits with minimal social interactions. The complainants raised the reason for Mr. Gp's allegedly suspicious behavior because he visited the homes of those affected families within 1–3 days before the Koro attack. As a matter of more substantial proof, they alleged that when the brother of Case D informed him of the illness's occurrence, he is a very "calmly way with a suspicious smile", answered, "I knew that." This assessment concluded that he is the perpetrator of sorcery to inflict *Disco* illness on their family members. A section of villagers supported this allegation. A group of few villagers, including the family members of Case C and D went to Mr. Gp's house and challenged him directly, which he vehemently denied. They verbally and quite severely physically assaulted him (with a fracture of the right ulna bone) and threatened that if any further *Disco fever* incident takes place in the village, they will either kill or throw him out from the village. Mr. Gp was too terrified to report the incident of abuse and physical assault to the police. With the timely interference from some good-minded village-elders, the matter stopped there. It is reported that after this incident, Mr. Gp was absconded from the village (possibly out of fear).

Report from Kerala (India) epidemic (2010): It is reported (Promodu et al., 2012) that a Koro epidemic took place among the migrant workers in Kochi, a town in Kerala, South India. About 100 construction laborers were affected. Most of them fled to their native North Indian states, but some remained in their temporary labor camps. They were socially boycotted by the local community and violently prevented from visiting local shops and restaurants in fear of Koro contamination.

Risk to Self or from Others

It is quite evident from many of the Koro reports that the individual, out of their acute anxiety and fear tried traction of the penis to prevent its retraction toward the abdomen. Usually, this method is by manual traction but often with mechanical traction. The penis is a soft tissue organ, and applying strong or inappropriate force to drag it outside may cause serious injury to the penis. When mechanical methods are used for the traction, other people usually do it, often a very self-inspired voluntary community people. They apply different mechanical traction methods like tying the penis with ropes, wire, iron pincer, or special devices. A historical report by Palthe (1935) from Dutch-Indies mentioned a long-held custom of inserting a "penis rod" into the penis; it is a 4 cm long slender rod with rounded tips. These rods are inserted inside the penis by perforation to prevent the shooting of the penis.

Koro delusion: There are quite a few published reports in the literature where Koro symptom is associated with another psychiatric diagnosis, especially psychosis. Historically, the first report of Koro with forensic and legal importance was reported by Palthe (1937), where Koro attack precipitated Amok's onset, leading to the murder of his wife in a 40-year-old Badjavanese fisherman. The second report was from New Zealand by Chowdhury and Faulkner (1997), where a 25-year Pacific islander was arrested for "wilful damage" and "threaten to injure" his wife and family members with a risk of self-harming behavior. After a gap of almost 50 years, two Koro reports appeared in the literature—one from the USA by Lewis and Ednie (1997)—where a 25-year black American was admitted to a forensic hospital after murdering a stranger under command hallucination and with a 6-year diagnosis of chronic paranoid schizophrenia. He had chronic Koro symptoms, and the voices directed him to kill himself or others to get rid of his penile symptom. The nucleus of his paranoid ideation was his belief in a gradual retraction of the penis.

Besides this, Koro's other five specific reports with forensic relevance also deserved mention where Koro perception triggered self-inflicting injury with risky and threatening behavior, often with psychotic illness. These are:

Fernando (1988) reported a case of monosymptomatic hypochondriacal psychosis with a Koro-like symptom (delusional conviction of genital deformity), who, because of his dysmorphic distress, attempted suicide by therapeutic drug overdose.

Chen (1991) reported a delusion of genital shrinkage in a 69-year-old married Englishman, referred from a surgical ward with urethral trauma. "He had inserted a knitting needle into his urethra in the belief that his penis was shrinking into his abdomen, thus obstructing urine flow." The patient was on L-dopa therapy for his idiopathic Parkinsonism. He was diagnosed as a Koro symptom complex with an organic psychosis caused by L-dopa therapy.

Chowdhury (1992) reported a Koro case with schizophrenia, who believed that some black magic ("tuk-tak") was cast on him to make him impotent. He accused few fellow workers and attacked them physically, and police were involved.

Chiniwala et al. (1996) reported a case with Koro-like symptoms in a 41-year-old single Muslim West-African man at the background of paranoid schizophrenia, from New York, USA. After an attempt to kidnap a nursing home inmate, who he believed was his father.

Kim et al. (2000) reported a 65-year-old Korean man presented with penile pain, who believed that his penis would shrink and retract into the abdomen and prevent this malady put an "anti-retraction device" around the glans penis seven months ago. This was a steel bottle cap with a hole in the center. The steel cap had penetrated to penile tissue and caused severe infection with inflammatory granulation. Surgical intervention was needed to take out the steel cap.

Penis-Theft Epidemic in Africa—A Koro Variant with High Forensic Risk

Since mid-1990s some epidemics concerning "penis vanishing or genital theft" (breast/vagina vanishing also) are reported from several West-African nations. It is variously described in the literature as Koro-like or magical penis loss (Ilechukwu, 1992), or "Vanishing Sexual/genital Organ Syndrome" (VSOS) (Sackey, 1997) or as "Genital Shrinking Panic" (GSP) or Mass Psychogenic Illness (Adams & Dzokoto, 2007) or "penis snatching phenomena" (Mather, 2005). The victim suddenly discovers genital loss after encountering a stranger, and he accused him of stealing. The public then tortures the accused, and they demand a high amount of money as ransom. In the strict nosological sense, they are not Koro but may be designated as a Koro variant. The forensic aspect of these epidemics was alarming as the violent mob attacked accused individuals and lynched them ("instant or street justice"). There were reports of more than a hundred dead. Dzokoto and Adams (2005) analyzed media reports of 36 such deaths from different African nations. In some countries, security alarms and the military were used to stop mass violence, and in some cases, criminal charges were booked for stealing, and legal claims were framed in court against the alleged accused.

Conclusion

Koro involves penile pull or traction either by self or by others is potential for penile injury and vasoconstriction with its associated complication. Social or folk treatments are also potential for different types of health hazards, including death. As a part of delusion in psychosis, Secondary Koro poses a definite forensic risk to self or others. Social anxiety or paranoia relating to Koro's alleged cause in epidemic form is highly potential for violence and ethnic or familial clash toward the accused person or alleged racial group. Unfortunately, there is minimal mention of risk issues in female Koro cases in the literature. It is a significant gap in our understanding of the nature and degree of injuries or health hazards of female Koro cases (Chowdhury & Chawla, 2019). So, be it a sporadic or epidemic case, risk assessment and mitigation of risk factors should constitute management.

Koro epidemic poses a public health threat and emergency. When the Koro epidemic involves school or community, a mass-psychogenic response threatens public health and administration severely. Four issues need immediate attention. These are: (1) The risk to self (injury or self-harming behavior); (2) The risk imposed by others (mechanical penile traction, social/folk therapy, etc.), (3) Presence of social paranoia or accusation with potential risk behavior in the community, and (4) The rapid spread of the illness in the community. It creates fear and chaos and imposes a burden on the health care system. The risk prevention strategy should include an intersectoral approach involving a proactive effort by public health administration, local healthcare providers, security administration, and news media. This conjoint strategy will also help mitigate the epidemic of fear (Slovic, 1987) because the whole community and the individual victims are terrified by the Koro superstition, potent cultural myth, and belief (Cheng, 1979).

References

Adams, G., & Dzokoto, V. A. (2007). Genital-shrinking in Ghana: A cultural-psychological analysis. *Culture & Psychology, 13*, 83–104.

Boss, L. P. (1997). Epidemic hysteria: A review of the published literature. *Epidemiologic Reviews, 19*(2), 233–243.

Chakraborty, S., & Sanyal, D. (2011). An outbreak of Koro among 19 workers in a jute mill in South Bengal. *Industrial Psychiatry J, 20*(1), 58–60.

Chen, E. (1991). Drug induced Koro in a non-Chinese man. *British Journal of Psychiatry, 158*, 721.

Cheng, S. T. (1979). Epidemic genital retraction syndrome: Environmental and personal risk factors in Southern China. *Journal of Psychology & Human Sexuality., 9*(1), 57–70.

Chiniwala, M., Alfonso, C. A., Torres, J. R., & Lefer, J. (1996). Koro in an immigrant from Guinea with brief psychotic disorder. *American Journal of Psychiatry, 153*(5), 736.

Chowdhury, A. N. (1991). Medico-cultural cognition of Koro epidemic: An ethnographic study. *Journal of Indian Anthropological Society, 26*, 155–170.

Chowdhury, A. N. (1992). Koro in schizophrenia with a case report from industrial set up. *Industrial Psychiatry Journal, 5*(1), 47–59.

Chowdhury, A. N., & Chawla, M. (2019). Koro in female. A case report and a mini review. *European Jounal of Psychiatry, 33*(4), 182–185.

Chowdhury, A. N., & Faulkner, R. (1997). Koro and offending behaviour: A report from New Zealand. *Transcultural Psychiatry, 34*, 545–546.

Dzokoto, V. A., & Adams, G. (2005). Understanding genital-shrinking epidemics in West Africa: Koro, juju, or mass psychogenic illness? *Culture, Medicine & Psychiatry, 29*(1), 53–78.

Everest-Phillips, M. (2018). Anxiety politics in Singapore: The "Koro Crisis" of 1967. *Asian J Public Affairs, 10*(2), 53–66.

Fernando, N. (1988). Monosymptomatic hypochondriasis treated with a tricyclic antidepressant. *British Journal of Psychiatry, 152*, 851–852.

Gallay, A., Van Loock, F., Demarest, S., van der Heyden, J., Jans, B., & Oyen, H. V. (2002). Belgian coca-cola- related outbreak: Intoxication, mass sociogenic illness, or both? *American Journal of Epidemiology, 155*(2), 140–147.

Illechukwu, S. T. C. (1992). Magical penis loss in Nigeria: Report of a recent epidemic. *Transcultural Psychiatric Research Review, 29*, 91–108.

Jilek, W., & Jilek-Aall, L. (1977). A Koro epidemic in Thailand. *Transcultural Psychiatric Research Review, 14*, 57–59.

Jilek, W., & Jilek-Aall, L. (1977). Mass hysteria with koro symptom in Thailand. *Schweizer Archieve Neurologic Neurochirurgie Und Psychiatrie, 120*, 257–259.

Kim, J., Kim, M., Lee, N., & Park, Y. (2000). A case of urethrocutaneous fistula with koro syndrome. *Journal of Urology, 164*(1), 123.

Koro Study Team (Chairman: AL Gwee). (1969). The Koro epidemic in Singapore. *Singapore Medical Journal, 10*, 234–242.

Lewis, C. F., & Ednie, K. (1997). Koro and homicidal behavior. *American Journal of Psychiatry, 154*(8), 1169.

Mather, C. (2005). Accusations of genital theft: A case from northern Ghana. *Culture, Medicine & Psychiatry, 29*(1), 33–52.

Mo, K. M., Li, L. S., & Ou, L. W. (1987). Report of koro epidemic in Leizhou Peninsula, Hainan Island. *Chinese Journal of Neuropsychiatry, 20*, 232–234.

Ngui, P. W. (1969). The Koro epidemic in Singapore. *Australian & New Zealand Journal of Psychiatry, 3*, 263–266.

Palthe, P. M. van W. (1935). Koro-Eine Merkwurdige Angsthysterie. *Internationale Zeitschrift Fur Psychoanalyse, 21*, 249–257.

Palthe, P. M. van W. (1937). It significanto forense del 'Koro'. *Archivio Di Anthropological Criminale, Psychiatry Medicina Legale, 57*, 173–182.

Promodu, K., Nair, K. R., & Pushparajan, S. (2012). Koro syndrome: Mass epidemic in Kerala, India. *Indian Journal of Clinical Psychology, 39*, 152–156.

Sackey, B. M. (1997). The vanishing organ phenomenon in the context of Ghanaian religious beliefs. *African Anthropology, 4*(2), 110–125.

Suwanlert, S. (1978). Koro epidemic in northeast Thailand. *Journal of Psychiatric Association of Thailand, 23*(1), 1–38.

Suwanlert, S. (1978). Thai cultural concepts related to Koro syndrome. *Journal of Psychiatric Association of Thailand, 23*(3), 261–275.

Suwanlert, S., & Coates, D. (1979). Epidemic Koro in Thailand: Clinical and social aspects. *Transcultural Psychiatric Research Review, 16*, 64–66.
Slovic, P. (1987). Perception of risk. *Science, 236*(4799), 280–285.
Vasterman, P., Yzermans, C. J., & Dirkzwager, A. J. E. (2005). The role of the media and media hypes in the aftermath of disasters. *Epidemiological Review, 27*(1), 107–114.

11

Koro Research Methodology

Introduction

Over the years, Koro publication numbers are increasing globally. Koro is now reported from diverse ethnicities, various medical, psychiatric, neurological, and urological diseases, and many countries. It is hoped that many more publications on Koro will emerge in the years to come and enrich our understanding of Koro's phenomenology and psychodynamics. The epidemic form is still confined to Southeast Asian countries, including India. Simultaneously, a Koro-variant epidemic of "penis theft" or "penis (or breast) vanishing" is reported from some African nations. Any careful analysis of Koro's concept and clinical construct's historical evolution will focus on many discrepancies and confusion in its assessment and diagnostic labeling—both in sporadic and in epidemic forms. By DSM-5 (2013) pruning, Koro has lost its legendary tag of "culture-bound syndrome," but still, I believe that careful analysis of cases shows some cultural association, background, or psychodynamic vulnerability. Construct of sexuality, at any rate, is always heavily culture-dependent. Koro being a genitally focused psychological abnormality, socio-cultural concept, and construct of sexuality and sexual abnormality in some way

A. N. Chowdhury, *Koro*,
https://doi.org/10.1007/978-3-030-87962-4_11

or other (pathogenic or pathoplastic) would play a role in this illness phenomena. One of the aims of this discourse is to share some of our Koro research methodology understanding with all the new researchers so that they can contribute more precisely and scientifically coherent documentation of the Koro phenomena in their research work. It is noted that much of the reporting lacks crucial clinical findings and draws a very superficial conclusion about the Koro phenomenon. Following is a brief suggestion about some of the methodological clinical standards that the researchers should address in their work.

Research Issues

Koro—clinical diagnostic issues: The three following symptoms must be present to diagnose it a Koro: (1) sudden perception of acute inward retraction of the penis (or breast or vulva in female); (2) acute panic-like reaction (with both psychological and bodily manifestations); and (3) acute fear of impending danger, most commonly death (or sexual disability) from this disorder. The whole episode lasts from a few minutes to an hour. This episode is accompanied by a preventive maneuver (by self or by others) either by manual or mechanical means of pulling the penis (or breast in female) outwardly to prevent retraction. Commonly, there is a myth or community folk belief about this Koro illness prevailing in the background in an epidemic situation. The suddenness of the episode and the clinical picture described above constitute the culture-bound classical Koro (Chowdhury, 1996). If the retraction is chronic over days or weeks or months with intense sexual or somatic concern but without the fear of impending death and acute anxiety—it is not usually the classical Koro but either Koro-like symptom (KLS) or chronic Koro (Chowdhury, 2008a; Kar, 2005). This clinical differentiation is necessary to put the clinical narrative in the proper perspective. Historically the ideational component of Koro fear is "death anxiety," but recently, some other issues have been reported, such as fear of sex change, loss of fecundity, or impotence. In recent years, few reports from urogenital services noted the complaints of gradual "shortening of penis" secondary to some urogenital pathology, and these were designated as Koro (Caballero et al., 2000; Kim et al., 2000). Slow and gradual "shortening of the penis" is different from retraction of the penis (with accompanied acute anxiety and fear of death) in Koro. However, a retracting penis is obviously shortened in length! The dynamics of inward pull are important in Koro (Bernstain & Gaw, 1990). In adolescent sexual clinics, more and more cases are reporting for "false penis shortness" (Fontana et al., 1998), or feelings of "penile deficiency" due to the small penis (Rosso et al., 1998) makes the contextual understanding of penile symptoms in Koro more confounding and challenging.

Moreover, in the psychotic background, the delusion of penile dissolution by malevolent force or envious person(s) (Bayer, 2000; Ungvari & Mullen, 1994) also needs a careful differentiation from Koro symptom. In Koro, the penile pull is a dynamic phenomenon with marked suddenness and rapidity. Still, delusional complaints (or in hypochondriacs) are usually a long-standing or slow process with a different conceptual component (psychotic or health-related anxiety). They generally present with other features of the primary disorder. So appropriate delineation of clinical symptoms is beneficial for correct Koro diagnosis, and that, in turn, will yield more precision without any other clinical contamination.

***Clinical data recording*:** It would be a good clinical practice to record the clinical presentation or symptom spectrum in different clinical categories like:

A. *Demographic features*
B. *History of illness/operation*
C. *Habits and addiction history*
D. *Clinical features:*

   i. Onset type
   ii. Onset time
   iii. Place and situation of attack
   iv. Duration of attack

E. *Clinical Symptoms:*

   i. Precipitating or Triggering factor or condition, if any

ii. Premonitory symptoms (symptoms before the attack)
iii. Physical symptoms
iv. Mental symptoms
v. Genital symptoms

F. *Clinical aftermath:*

i. Risk to self or from others
ii. Frequency of attack
iii. Relapse or recurrence

G. .*Associated morbidity (physical or mental).*

Let us discuss some of the issues in greater detail.

Demography of cases: Ethnicity, age, sex, marital status, and education data are essential to understand the global comparative distribution of Koro cases—be it in an epidemic setting or a sporadic occurrence. World Koro research data shows that adolescents or young adults with fewer academic years are more prone (Cheng, 1979), but no such trend is noted in sporadic cases. Sporadic case reports show age variation between 16 and 80 years with average education (not very high). Koro in the same family (kinship) is an exciting area. It should be looked for as it sheds focus on the role of shared psychopathology in a psychiatric epidemic or even in sporadic cases in the same family or community (Chowdhury, 1989a).

History of illness or operation: This is an essential component that may have some potential for Koro vulnerability, especially any illness or operation relating to genital organ morphology (e.g., phimosis, scrotal filarial, hydrocele, atrophied testis, venereal diseases) or functions (e.g., urinary hesitancy, impotence, delayed ejaculation, Dhat syndrome, coital difficulties, prostate operation). These abnormalities may heighten hypochondriacal or obsessive genital concern (Chowdhury, 1992a; Yap, 1965).

Habits and addiction: This area is gaining more attention in Koro research recently. Two important reasons are: diagnostic placement of Koro under ORCD by DSM-5, and several substance cases of abuse are reported with Koro. OCD personality traits may manifest in pre-Koro issues like gambling habits or sexual obsessive rumination in checking and rechecking genital organs or excessive somatic concern about genito-urinary function. Some substances are associated with the experience of depersonalization with Koro perception like cannabis (Chowdhury & Bera, 1994; Kalaitzi & Lalantzis, 2006), heroin (Chowdhury & Bagchi, 1993), and buprenorphine (Chowdhury & Banerjee, 1996). Amphetamine causes perceptible penile vasoconstriction (Bloor, 2004).

Place and situation of attack: This history is vital to assess Koro psychopathology's environmental risk factors, especially in epidemic form. In recent years, Koro's incidence immediately after viewing Koro news on television or receiving mobile telephone messages is reported.

Duration of attack: Koro is a short-lived acute attack similar to a panic attack. A careful analysis of Koro attack duration (chronic, slow and lengthy hours or days) may indicate the elements of hypochondriacal/obsessive or delusional component of Koro perception.

Triggering or precipitating factor or situation: There are quite a few reports where Koro was precipitated immediately after some sexual behavior (after masturbation, intercourse, failed intercourse, intercourse with a prostitute) or due to some environmental situation (insect bite on the penis, penile exposure to cold) or after micturation or defecation. This triggering factor or situation may indicate some personality or an environmental issue that increases the individual's Koro vulnerability (Chowdhuty et al., 1988).

Clinical symptoms: Though genital retraction (or breast or labial retraction in females) is the main clinical complaint, a host of premonitory symptoms, physical and mental, usually accompany genital symptoms. In addition to genital retraction, more and more different types of genital symptoms are reported. These are loss of penile sensation or muscular tone, insensitive penis (Cai, 1982); alteration of penis morphology like reduced glans size, reduced penis-shaft girth (Chowdhury, 1991a, 1993a) and thus making the Koro presentation as a multi-symptom complex.

Comorbidity—With other mental and physical illnesses: This is an essential issue in differentiating Secondary Koro from Primary Koro. In recent literature, schizophrenia, affective disorders, medical disorders, neurological and urological disorders with Koro have been reported. So this information will help to clarify the role of primary morbidity in the dysmorphophobic penile perception of the victim. A good example here is Koro's report with the affective disorder, which is mood-congruent, i.e., the perception of the small penis in the depressive phase and the big penis in a manic state is quite typical (Damodaran & Nizamie, 1993; Weller & Ameen, 1982). A delusion of penile retraction/shortening in psychosis (made or enacted by envious others or by magic or witchcraft) is an example of secondary Koro (Afonso et al., 2013). The detailed sexual history is vital to examine the role of psychosexual dysfunction or guilt (Aneja et al., 2015) in the genesis of patho-perception of penile morphology (Chowdhury, 1989b, 1993b). Comorbidity in Koro is an exciting and expanding research area, and thus every researcher should be alert not to miss the opportunity.

DSM-5 (2013) placed Koro under "Other specified Obsessive-Compulsive and Related Disorders" (300.3), and some research has already been published pointing Koro as an OCD manifestation (Silva et al., 2016). So it would be wise to inquire about the OCD spectrum in Koro cases, which will enrich our insight into the Koro phenomenology. It is worth remembering that Koro lost its culture-bound tag after the publication of DSM-5 in 2013, and it is now the researchers' task to examine the Koro symptoms in the clinical frame of OCD spectrum.

A detailed medical and psychiatric history, including psychosexual history and physical examination of the genitalia, is mandatory. This is to exclude body dysmorphic disorder and any morphological abnormality of the external genitalia. Some physical abnormality of the penis deserves mention. These are: Hypospadias (congenital defect where the opening of the urethra is on the underside of the penis instead of at the tip), or epispadias (where urethra does not form properly), or Peyronie's disease (causes reduction of penis size because of scar tissue development in the tunica albuginea that prevents full expansion of an erection and causes flaccid penis retraction) and buried penis state (normally developed penis but partially covered by suprapubic fat).

Epidemic Specificity: If it is a report of Koro epidemic, then the nature of the spread of the epidemic (geographical epicenter, the radius of epidemicity/epidemic type) should be outlined, the index case, number of cases, and their timeline and demographic features, mode of transmission of news (mobile phone, radio, newspaper, TV news) (Ghosh et al., 2013; Roy et al., 2011), previous acquaintance, individual and community/professional response (Chowdhury, 1992b); and timeline, etc., should be sufficiently reported. The aftermath of mitigation measures, administrative and public health approaches, and the media's role is an essential part of the documentation. These will enrich our understanding of the psycho-social dynamics and social pathology-networking of the psychiatric epidemic. In recent years, the role of mobile phones or other social media is a novel research agenda in the spread of Koro or other mass-psychogenic illnesses (Adams & Dzokoto, 2007). Many extraordinary or unusual incidents of clinical importance happen in the community during an epidemic. It would be a rich research contribution to report all these in the context of an ongoing epidemic (Ghosh et al., 2013). Social cognition and communication are important research areas in any psychiatric epidemic (Chowdhury, 1991b, 1991c, 1992b, 2008c).

Cognitive mapping and Explanatory Model Analysis: Cognitive mapping is an important research tool to visually represent a person's illness model or concept. The patient's perception of the illness is a precious component in the understanding of Koro phenomena. It needs a very detailed qualitative research approach to probe the patient's perception about the specific cause (causes) of his/her disorder in their verbatim and may be asked to engage in participatory mapping of pathology, which may unfold a folk cultural focus (Chowdhury, 2008a, 2008b). Most of the Koro reporting in the literature lacks this vital aspect. It needs a skill of good rapport with active listening, empathic persuasion, and sufficient time. The patient should have some familiarity with using a pen or pencil and some minimal drawing ability.

Risk assessment and prevention: Different maneuvers are reported either enacted by the individual (usually in sporadic cases) or by others (generally in epidemic cases) to prevent the retraction of penis or breast, causing soft tissue injury, often of a severe nature (Chowdhury,

1991d, 1991e; Tseng et al., 1988). Social or folk healing rituals in the epidemic form are reported with many health hazards, including death. In epidemic forms where psycho-social ethnic or racial tension is present, racial clashes or community violence is also reported. These are issues of public health concern. These are Koro's risks to the person or the community and should be adequately studied and documented. This is still a neglected area in Koro research.

Boundness with Culture: This is a vital and debated aspect of Koro's cultural boundness. The researcher should elicit any particular cultural myth or belief present behind the presentation, or the sufferer has any such beliefs or any such cultural construct in circulation in the community during the Koro episodes. Even in sporadic cases, there are different cultural-social cognition plays a role. This is a very dearth area, and more elaborative research is needed. Narratives from the victims (or family members/folk healers) would be a valuable contribution (Mitchell, 2010). Culture-boundness is visible in epidemic settings (Koro Study Team, 1969; Suwanlert, 1978) and sometimes in sporadic or secondary cases (Ilechukwu, 1988; Lucier, 1984–1985; Menezes, 1992; Ogunlesi, 1986) also.

The concept "Culture-bound" has undergone a sea-change in recent years. A few new constructs emerged in place of "culture-bound," like idiom for distress (Nichter, 1981), culture-specific disorder, cultural concept of distress (Kaiser & Weaver, 2019) or culturally interpreted symptom (Low, 1985), or folk illness or ethno-behavioral model (Carr, 1978). Current prevalent consensus supports the construct that every illness is culture-bound. Because of the illness experience and communication of distress (Mechanic, 1972; Nichaikovit et al., 1993), help seeking, family role, social support (Garro, 2000), care delivery, and treatment compliance (Kleinman et al., 1978)—all are culture-dependent. All components and stages are, in the true sense, influenced by cultural disposition. So the specific focus of culture on a particular illness is misleading or not correct. DSM-5 (APA, 2013) used the term "cultural concept of distress". Indian culture-bound illnesses (Chabra et al., 2008) are a vast research area to explore (Chowdhury & Brahma, 2004).

Treatment—Traditional or Modern: Detailed treatment and its outcome should be recorded along with the specifics and healing time. If any psychotropic medications were helpful, that should be noted in detail. It is applied to folk treatment as well—the details of such treatment should be recorded with its reason for application and/or complication (health hazard), if any. Analysis of help-seeking behavior sheds light on the cultural and or personality dynamics of Koro patients.

Recurrent Koro: This is a very important aspect of the course of Koro morbidity. Be it in the epidemic setting or solitary case, recording this information is valuable. There will be a definite time gap between two or more Koro episodes, ranging from a few hours to days or even months and years. At least two reports in the literature noted recurrent Koro over a reasonable length of time (Barett, 1978; Chowdhury et al., 1994). An unusually long time gap usually indicates the probability of some secondary psychiatric diagnosis.

Conceptual Model of Koro: Given the recent DSM-5 classification of Koro under ORCD, the following flow chart may be helpful as a guide to diagnostic precession of Koro (Table 11.1).

Suppose these issues are carefully addressed in any research on Koro. In that case, we may expect more robust scientific clinical material that would help us substantiate Koro's elaborate psychosomatic presentation either in their socio-cultural context or as a part of underlying secondary psychiatric pathology (Chowdhury, 2015).

Table 11.1 Diagnostic steps in Koro

Step 1: Diagnostic screening	Koro with predominant OCD symptoms	Koro without predominant OCD symptoms
Step 2: Diagnostic label	Primary (only genital symptom)	Secondary (with associated other disorder—Dual diagnosis or KLS) a. With Psychiatric disorder b. With Medical disorder c. With Neurological disorder d. With urogenital disorder e. With substance abuse disorder f. With other disorders (e.g., another culture-bound disorder like Dhat syndrome, etc.)
Step 3: Type	Sporadic	Epidemic
Step 4: Nature	Single episode	Recurrent or multiple episodes
Step 5: Health seeking behavior	Details of treatments received or attempted, including traditional or folk treatment	
Step 6: Risk Assessment	Risk of injury to self or from others concerning manual penile traction; in epidemic situation public health threat assessment and mitigation	
Step 7: Explanatory Model of Illness	Details to be elicited from the patient or significant others, including cause(s), illness experiences, local name, and treatment expectations	
Step 8: Role of Culture	Definite cultural issues present	No cultural issues present

References

Adams, G., & Dzokoto, V. A. (2007). Genital-shrinking in Ghana: A cultural-psychological analysis. *Culture & Psychology, 13*, 83–104.

Afonso, P., Sarauva, S., & Gameiro, Z. (2013). Schizophrenia presenting with koro-like symptoms. *Journal of Neuropsychiatry & Clinical Neuroscience, 25*, E32.

Aneja, J., Grover, S., Avasthi, A., Mahajan, S., Pokhrel, P., & Triveni, D. (2015). Can masturbatory guilt lead to severe psychopathology: A case series. *Indian Journal of Psychological Medicine, 37*(1), 81–86.

Barret, K. (1978). Koro in a Londoner. *Lancet, ii, 1319.*

Bayer, R. S. (2000). Koro-like symptoms and transient post-ictal psychosis. *Qatar Medical Journal, 9*(2), 68–69.

Berntein, R. L., & Gaw, A. C. (1990). Koro: Proposed classification for DSM-IV. *American Journal of Psychiatry, 147*, 1670–1674.

Bloor, R. N. (2004). Whizz-dick: Side effect, urban myth or amphetamine-related koro-like syndrome? *International Journal of Clinical Practice, 58*(7), 717–719.

Caballero, J. M., Avila, A., Cardona, X., Sastre, F., & Bello, M. P. (2000). Genital pain without urogenital pathology: The koro-like syndrome. *The Journal of Urology, 163*(1), 243.

Cai, J. B. (1982). Five case reports of suo-yang zen. *Chinese Journal of Neuropsychiatry, 4*, 206–288.

Carr, J. E. (1978). Ethno-behaviorism and the culture-bound syndromes: The case of *amok*. *Culture, Medicine & Psychiatry, 2*, 269–293.

Cheng, S. T. (1979). Epidemic genital retraction syndrome: Environmental and personal risk factors in Southern China. *Journal of Psychology & Human Sexuality, 9*(1), 57–70.

Chhabra, V., Bhatia, M. S., & Gupta, R. (2008). Culture Bound syndromes in India. *Delhi Psychiatry Journal, 11*(1), 15–18.

Chowdhury, A. N. (1989a). Koro among kinships. *Indian Journal of Social Psychiatry, 5*, 24–26.

Chowdhury, A. N. (1989b). Neuroticism, extraversion and sex-guilt cognition in the genesis of Koro. *Journal of Indian Psychoanalytical Society, 4*, 57–64.

Chowdhury, A. N. (1991a). Penis-shaft perception of Koro patients. *Journal of Indian Academy of Applied Psychology, 17*, 41–44.

Chowdhury, A. N. (1991b). Medico-cultural cognition of Koro epidemic: An ethnographic study. *Journal of Indian Anthropological Society, 26*, 155–170.

Chowdhury, A. N. (1991c). Role of medical cognition in psychiatric outbreaks: Study from North Bengal Koro epidemic. *Indian Journal of Behavioural Sciences, 1*, 64–67.

Chowdhury, A. N. (1991d). Medico-cultural cognition of Koro epidemic: An ethnographic study. *Journla of Indian Anthropological Society, 26*, 155–170.

Chowdhury, A. N. (1991e). Role of medical cognition in psychiatric outbreaks: Study from North Bengal Koro epidemic. *Indian Journal Behavioural Sciences, 1*, 64–67.

Chowdhury, A. N. (1992a). Clinical analysis of 101 Koro cases. *Indian Journal of Social Psychiatry, 7*, 67–70.

Chowdhury, A. N. (1992b). Koro social response (*urban*): A longitudinal study of North Bengal Koro epidemic. *Indian Journal of Psychiatry, 34*, 46–52.

Chowdhury, A. N. (1993a). Glans penis perception of Koro patients. *Acta Psychiatrica Scandinavica, 87*, 355–357.

Chowdhury, A. N. (1993b). Variations in the perception of penis. *Journal of Sexual Health, 3*, 156–160.

Chowdhury, A. N. (1996). Definition and classification of Koro. *Culture, Medicine & Psychiatry, 20*, 41–65.

Chowdhury, A. N. (2008a). Cultural Koro and Koro-like symptom (KLS). *German Journal of Psychiatry, 11*, 81–82.

Chowdhury, A. N. (2008b). Ethnomedical concept of heat and cold in Koro: Study from Indian patients. *World Cultural Psychiatry Research Review, 3*, 146–158.

Chowdhury, A. N. (2008c). Koro social response during an epidemic: Study from India. *Scientific-Practical Reviewed Journal (Moscow), 3*, 41–42.

Chowdhury, A. N. (2015). Koro. In R. L. Cautin & S. O. Lilienfeld (Eds.), *The encyclopedia of clinical psychology* (1st ed., 1626–1629). Wiley.

Chowdhury, A. N., & Bagchi, D. (1993). Koro in heroin withdrawal. *Journal of Psychoactive Drugs, 25*, 257–258.

Chowdhury, A. N., & Banerjee, G. (1996). Recurrent Koro in repeated IV buprenorphine withdrawal. *Addiction, 91*, 145–146.

Chowdhury, A. N., Banerjee, G., Sen, K. D., Bera, N. K., & Sharma, N. K. (1994). Koro in West Bengal again: Report of nine cases. *Indian Journal Social Psychiatry, 10*, 27–30.

Chowdhury, A. N., & Bera, N. K. (1994). Koro following cannabis smoking. *Addiction, 89*, 1017–1020.

Chowdhury, A. N., & Brahma, A. (2004). A case of dhat syndrome with borderline personality disorder. *Indian Journal Psychiatry, 46*, 373–374.

Chowdhury, A. N., Pal, P., Chatterjee, A., Roy, M., & Das Chowdhury, B. B. (1988). Analysis of North Bengal Koro epidemic with three years follow-up. *Indian Journal of Psychiatry, 30*, 60–72.

Damodaran, S. S., & Nizamie, S. H. (1993). "Incomplete Koro"—A fore-runner for mood disorders: Two case reports. *Indian Journal of Psychiatry, 35*, 60–62.

Diagnostic and Statistical Manual of Mental Disorder. (2013). *Fifth edition.* American Psychiatric Association.

Fontana, I., Rolle, C., Ceruti, G., Datta, F., Ragni, A., & Tamagnone, A. (1998). False penile shortness. *Archivo Italiano Urologia, Andrologia, 70*(5), 241–245.

Garro, L. C. (2000). Cultural meaning, explanations of illness, and the development of comparative frameworks. *Ethnology, 39*(4), 305–334.

Ghosh, S., Nath, S., Brahma, A., & Chowdhury, A. N. (2013). Fifth Koro epidemic in India: A review report. *World Cultural Psychiatry Research Review, 8*(1), 8–20.

Illechukwu, S. T. C. (1988). Koro-like syndrome in Nigeria. *Transcultural Psychiatry Research Review, 25*, 310–314.

Kaiser, B. N., & Weaver, L. J. (2019). Culture-bound syndromes, idioms of distress, and cultural concept of distress: New directions for an old concept in psychological anthropology. *Transcultural Psychiatry, 56*(4), 589–598.

Kalaitzi, C. K., & Kalantzis, A. (2006). Cannabis-induced koro-like syndrome. A case report and mini review. *Urologia Internationalis, 76*(3), 278–280.

Kar, N. (2005). Chronic koro-like symptoms—Two case reports. *BMC Psychiatry, 5*(1), 1–3.

Kim, J., Kim, M., Lee, N., & Park, Y. (2000). A case of urethrocutaneous fistula with koro syndrome. *Journal of Urology, 164*(1), 123.

Kleinman, A., Eisenberg, L., & Good, B. (1978). Culture, illness, and care. Clinical lessons from anthropologic and cross-cultural research. *Annals Internal Medicine, 88*, 251–258.

Koro Study Team (Chairman: AL Gwee). (1969). The Koro epidemic in Singapore. *Singapore Medical Journal, 10*, 234–242.

Low, S. M. (1985). Culturally interpreted symptoms or culture-bound syndromes: A cross-cultural review of nerves. *Social Science & Medicine, 21*(2), 187–196.

Lucieer, W. M. (1984–1985). The bitter taste of liberty. *Psychopathologic Africaine, 20*, 17–40.

Mechanic, D. (1972). Social psychologic factors affecting the presentation of bodily complaints. *New England Journal Medicine, 286*, 1132–1139.
Menezes, S. B. (1992). A case of Koro and folie a deux in a Shona family. *South African Medical Journal, 82*(6), 483.
Mitchell, D. (2010). Koro in Eastern Indonesia 1999 to 2010. *Asia-Pacific Psychiatry, 2*(3), A7.
Nichter, M. (1981). Idioms of distress: Alternatives in the expression of psychosocial distress: A case study from South India. *Culture, Medicine & Psychiatry, 5*, 379–408.
Nilchaikovit, T., James, D., Jimmie, D., & Holland, C. (1993). The effects of culture on illness behavior and medical care: Asian and American differences. *General Hospital Psychiatry, 15*(1),:41–50.
Ogunlesi, A. O. (1986). Koro symptomatology associated with paranoid psychosis in a Nigerian patient: A case report. *West African Journal Medicine, 5*(4), 305–307.
Rosso, C., Ostacoli, L., Garbolino, S., & Furlan, M. (1998). The "small penis": Considerations about subjective penile deficiency. *Achivio Italiano Urologica Andrologia, 70*(5), 227–233.
Roy, D., Hazarika, S., Bhattacharya, A., Das, S., Nath, K., & Saddichha, S. (2011). Koro: Culture bound or mass hysteria? *Australian & New Zealand Journal Psychiatry, 45*(8), 683.
Silva, L., Rapso-Lima, C., Soares, C., Cerqueira, J. J., & Morgado, P. (2016). Koro syndrome in an obsessive compulsive disorder. *European Psychiatry, 33*, S618.
Suwanlert, S. (1978). Thai cultural concepts related to koro syndrome. *Journal Psychiatric Association of Thailand, 23*(3), 261–275.
Tseng, W. S., Mo, M. K., Hsu, J., Li, L. S., Ou, L. W., Chen, G. Q., & Jiang, D. W. (1988). A socio-cultural study of Koro epidemic in Guangdong, China. *American Journal of Psychiatry, 145*, 1538–1543.
Ungvari, G. S., & Mullen, R. S. (1994). Koro: The delusion of penile retraction. *Urology, 43*(6), 883–885.
Weller, M. P. I., & Ameen, N. (1982). Elvis Presley, reactive hypomania and Koro. *American Journal of Psychiatry, 13*(7), 970.
Yap, P. M. (1965). Koro—A culture-bound depersonalization syndrome. *British Journal of Psychiatry, 111*, 43–50.

Index

A. N. Chowdhury, *Koro*,
https://doi.org/10.1007/978-3-030-87962-4

I

N

Q

R